Artificial Intelligence in Urology

Editor

ANDREW J. HUNG

UROLOGIC CLINICS
OF NORTH AMERICA

www.urologic.theclinics.com

Editor-in-Chief
KEVIN R. LOUGHLIN

February 2024 • Volume 51 • Number 1

ELSEVIER

1600 John F. Kennedy Boulevard ● Suite 1800 ● Philadelphia, Pennsylvania, 19103-2899

http://www.theclinics.com

UROLOGIC CLINICS OF NORTH AMERICA Volume 51, Number 1
February 2024 ISSN 0094-0143, ISBN-13: 978-0-443-13035-9

Editor: Kerry Holland
Developmental Editor: Nitesh Barthwal

Urologic Clinics of North America (ISSN 0094-0143) is published quarterly by Elsevier Inc., 360 Park Avenue South, New York, NY 10010-1710. Months of issue are February, May, August, and November. Business and Editorial Offices: 1600 John F. Kennedy Blvd., Suite 1800, Philadelphia, PA 19103-2899. Periodicals postage paid at New York, NY and additional mailing offices. Subscription prices are $427.00 per year (US individuals), $100.00 per year (US students and residents), $483.00 per year (Canadian individuals), $100.00 per year (Canadian students/residents), $557.00 per year (foreign individuals), and $240.00 per year (foreign students/residents). For institutional access pricing please contact Customer Service via the contact information below. Foreign air speed delivery is included in all *Clinics* subscription prices. All prices are subject to change without notice. **POSTMASTER:** Send address changes to *Urologic Clinics of North America*, Elsevier Health Sciences Division, Subscription Customer Service, 3251 Riverport Lane, Maryland Heights, MO 63043. **Customer Service: 1-800-654-2452 (US). From outside the United States, call 1-314-447-8871. Fax: 1-314-447-8029. E-mail: JournalsCustomerServiceusa@elsevier.com (for print support)** and **JournalsOnlineSupport-usa@elsevier.com (for online support)**.

Reprints. For copies of 100 or more, of articles in this publication, please contact the Commercial Reprints Department, Elsevier Inc., 360 Park Avenue South, New York, New York 10010-1710. Tel.: 212-633-3874; Fax: 212-633-3820; E-mail: reprints@elsevier.com.

Urologic Clinics of North America is covered in MEDLINE/PubMed (*Index Medicus*), *Excerpta Medica, Current Contents/Clinical Medicine, Science Citation Index,* and *ISI/BIOMED.*

Contributors

EDITOR-IN-CHIEF

KEVIN R. LOUGHLIN, MD, MBA
Emeritus Professor of Surgery (Urology),
Harvard Medical School, Visiting Scientist,
Vascular Biology Research Program at Boston
Children's Hospital, Boston, Massachusetts,
USA

EDITOR

ANDREW J. HUNG, MD
Vice Chair for Academic Development, Acting
Associate Professor, Department of Urology,
Cedars-Sinai Medical Center, Los Angeles,
California, USA

AUTHORS

RAYYAN ABID
Undergraduate Student, Case Western
Reserve University, Cleveland, Ohio,
USA

ANDRE LUIS ABREU, MD
Assistant Professor, USC Institute of Urology,
Catherine and Joseph Aresty Department of
Urology, Keck School of Medicine of USC,
Artificial Intelligence Center at USC Urology,
Center for Image-Guided Surgery, Focal Therapy
and Artificial Intelligence for Prostate Cancer,
Department of Radiology, University of Southern
California, Los Angeles, California,
USA

**JAIME ALTAMIRANO-VILLARROEL, MD,
FRCS**
Department of Urology, University of California,
Irvine, Orange, California, USA

PURIA AZADI MOGHADAM, MSc
Department of Electrical and Computer
Engineering, School of Biomedical
Engineering, University of British Columbia,
Vancouver, British Columbia, Canada

ALI BASHASHATI, PhD
Assistant Professor, School of Biomedical
Engineering, Department of Pathology and
Laboratory Medicine, University of British
Columbia, Vancouver, British Columbia,
Canada

GIOVANNI E. CACCIAMANI, MSc, MD, FEBU
Assistant Professor of Research Urology,
Assistant Professor of Research Radiology,
USC Institute of Urology, Catherine and
Joseph Aresty Department of Urology, Keck
School of Medicine of USC, Director, Artificial
Intelligence Center at USC Urology, Center for
Image-Guided and Focal Therapy for Prostate
Cancer, Department of Radiology, University of
Southern California, Los Angeles, California,
USA

ANDREW CHEN, MD
USC Institute of Urology, Catherine and Joseph
Aresty Department of Urology, Keck School of
Medicine of USC, Center for Image-Guided
Surgery, Focal Therapy and Artificial Intelligence
for Prostate Cancer, University of Southern
California, Los Angeles, California, USA

TIMOTHY N. CHU, BS
USC Institute of Urology, Catherine and Joseph Aresty Department of Urology, Keck School of Medicine of USC, Center for Image-Guided Surgery, Focal Therapy and Artificial Intelligence for Prostate Cancer, University of Southern California, Los Angeles, California, USA

ANDREI D. CUMPANAS, MD
LIFT Research Fellow, Department of Urology, University of California, Irvine, Orange, California, USA

VINAY A. DUDDALWAR, MD, FRCR
Professor, Department of Radiology, Viterbi School of Engineering, University of Southern California, Los Angeles, California, USA

MICHAEL EPPLER, BA
USC Institute of Urology, Catherine and Joseph Aresty Department of Urology, Keck School of Medicine of USC, Artificial Intelligence Center at USC Urology, Center for Image-Guided and Focal Therapy for Prostate Cancer, University of Southern California, Los Angeles, California, USA

DAVID FISHER, BS
Department of Radiology, University of Southern California, Los Angeles, California, USA

INDERBIR GILL, MD
Chairman and Professor, USC Institute of Urology, Catherine and Joseph Aresty Department of Urology, Keck School of Medicine of USC, Artificial Intelligence Center at USC Urology, Center for Image-Guided and Focal Therapy for Prostate Cancer, University of Southern California, Los Angeles, California, USA

KARANVIR GILL, BA
USC Institute of Urology, Catherine and Joseph Aresty Department of Urology, Keck School of Medicine of USC, Artificial Intelligence Center at USC Urology, Center for Image-Guided and Focal Therapy for Prostate Cancer, University of Southern California, Los Angeles, California, USA

MITCHELL G. GOLDENBERG, MBBS, PhD, FRCSC
Assistant Professor, Catherine and Joseph Aresty Department of Urology, USC Institute of Urology, University of Southern California, Los Angeles, California, USA

S. LARRY GOLDENBERG, OC, CM, MD, FRCSC, FACS, FCAHS
Professor, Department of Urologic Sciences, University of British Columbia, Vancouver, British Columbia, Canada

ANTONIO R.H. GORGEN, MD
Research Associate, Department of Urology, University of California, Irvine, Orange, California, USA

KHURSHID A. GURU, MD
Professor of Urologic Oncology, Department of Urology, Roswell Park Comprehensive Cancer Center, Buffalo, Erie County, New York, USA

JACOB S. HERSHENHOUSE, BS
USC Institute of Urology, Catherine and Joseph Aresty Department of Urology, Keck School of Medicine of USC, Artificial Intelligence Center at USC Urology, Center for Image-Guided and Focal Therapy for Prostate Cancer, University of Southern California, Los Angeles, California, USA

AHMED A. HUSSEIN, MD
Assistant Professor, Department of Urology, Roswell Park Comprehensive Cancer Center, Buffalo, Erie County, New York, USA

MD TAUHIDUL ISLAM, PhD
Postdoctoral Scholar, Department of Radiation Oncology, Stanford University School of Medicine, Stanford, California, USA

DONYA S. JADVAR
Dornsife School of Letters and Science, University of Southern California, Los Angeles, California, USA

C.-C. JAY KUO, MS, PhD
Professor, Ming Hsieh Department of Electrical and Computer Engineering, University of Southern California, Los Angeles, California, USA

MASATOMO KANEKO, MD, PhD
Assistant Professor, USC Institute of Urology, Catherine and Joseph Aresty Department of Urology, Keck School of Medicine of USC, Center for Image-Guided Surgery, Focal

Therapy and Artificial Intelligence for Prostate Cancer, University of Southern California, Los Angeles, California, USA; Department of Urology, Graduate School of Medical Science, Kyoto Prefectural University of Medicine, Kyoto, Japan

J. EVERETT KNUDSEN, BSE
Catherine and Joseph Aresty Department of Urology, USC Institute of Urology, Center for Robotic Simulation and Education, University of Southern California, Los Angeles, California, USA

SEYEDEH-SANAM LADI-SEYEDIAN, MD
Catherine and Joseph Aresty Department of Urology, Center for Robotic Simulation and Education, Norris Comprehensive Cancer Center, University of Southern California, Los Angeles, California, USA

JAIME LANDMAN, MD
Chair, Department of Urology, University of California, Irvine, Orange, California, USA

MARK A. LAURIE, MS
Departments of Urology and Radiation Oncology, Stanford University School of Medicine, Institute for Computational and Mathematical Engineering, Stanford University School of Engineering, Stanford, California, USA; Veterans Affairs Palo Alto Health Care System, Palo Alto, California, USA

JOSEPH C. LIAO, MD
Professor and Vice Chair for Academic Affairs, Department of Urology, Stanford University School of Medicine, Stanford, California, USA; Veterans Affairs Palo Alto Health Care System, Palo Alto, California, USA

JINYUAN LIU, MS
PhD Student, Ming Hsieh Department of Electrical and Computer Engineering, University of Southern California, Los Angeles, California, USA

RUNZHUO MA, MD
Catherine and Joseph Aresty Department of Urology, USC Institute of Urology, Center for Robotic Simulation and Education, University of Southern California, Los Angeles, California, USA

VASILEIOS MAGOULIANITIS, MS
PhD Student, Ming Hsieh Department of Electrical and Computer Engineering, University of Southern California, Los Angeles, California, USA

DANIEL MOKTAR, BS
USC Institute of Urology, Catherine and Joseph Aresty Department of Urology, Keck School of Medicine of USC, Artificial Intelligence Center at USC Urology, Center for Image-Guided and Focal Therapy for Prostate Cancer, University of Southern California, Los Angeles, California, USA

CALEB P. NELSON, MD, MPH
Associate Professor of Surgery, Harvard Medical School, Director, Clinical and Health Services Research, Department of Urology, Boston Children's Hospital, Boston, Massachusetts, USA

CHRYSOSTOMOS L. NIKIAS, MS, PhD
Ming Hsieh Department of Electrical and Computer Engineering, University of Southern California, Los Angeles, California, USA

ASSAD OBERAI, PhD
Professor, Viterbi School of Engineering, University of Southern California, Los Angeles, California, USA

DIVYANGI PARALKAR, MD
USC Institute of Urology, Catherine and Joseph Aresty Department of Urology, Keck School of Medicine of USC, Artificial Intelligence Center at USC Urology, Center for Image-Guided Surgery, Focal Therapy and Artificial Intelligence for Prostate Cancer, University of Southern California, Los Angeles, California, USA

LORENZO STORINO RAMACCIOTTI, MD
USC Institute of Urology, Catherine and Joseph Aresty Department of Urology, Keck School of Medicine of USC, Center for Image-Guided Surgery, Focal Therapy and Artificial Intelligence for Prostate Cancer, University of Southern California, Los Angeles, California, USA

ALEX G. RAMAN, MS
Department of Radiology, University of Southern California, Los Angeles, California,

USA; Western University of Health Sciences, Pomona, California, USA

JOSEPH M. RICH, BS
Catherine and Joseph Aresty Department of Urology, USC Institute of Urology, Center for Robotic Simulation and Education, University of Southern California, Los Angeles, California, USA

ALLEN ROJHANI, MD
Research Fellow, Department of Urology, University of California, Irvine, Orange, California, USA

HSIN-HSIAO SCOTT WANG, MD, MPH, MBAN
Assistant Professor of Surgery, Harvard Medical School, Director, Computational Healthcare Analytics Program, Department of Urology, Boston Children's Hospital, Boston, Massachusetts, USA

EUGENE SHKOLYAR, MD
Urologic Oncologist, Department of Urology, Stanford University School of Medicine, Stanford, California, USA; Veterans Affairs Palo Alto Health Care System, Palo Alto, California, USA

ZACHARY E. TANO, MD
Urology specialist, Department of Urology, University of California, Irvine, Orange, California, USA

RANVEER VASDEV, MD, MS
Urology Resident, Department of Urology, Mayo Clinic, Rochester, Minnesota, USA

ELYSSA Y. WONG, BS
Catherine and Joseph Aresty Department of Urology, Center for Robotic Simulation and Education, Norris Comprehensive Cancer Center, University of Southern California, Los Angeles, California, USA

LEI XING, PhD
Professor, Department of Radiation Oncology, Stanford University School of Medicine, Stanford, California, USA

JINTANG XUE, MS
PhD student, Ming Hsieh Department of Electrical and Computer Engineering, University of Southern California, Los Angeles, California, USA

JIAXIN YANG, MS
PhD student, Ming Hsieh Department of Electrical and Computer Engineering, University of Southern California, Los Angeles, California, USA

YIJING YANG, MS, PhD
Ming Hsieh Department of Electrical and Computer Engineering, University of Southern California, Los Angeles, California, USA

FELIX YAP, MD
Radiology Associates, San Luis Obispo, California, USA

STEVE R. ZHOU, MD
Department of Urology, Stanford University School of Medicine, Stanford, California, USA

Contents

The application of artificial intelligence (AI) on prostate magnetic resonance imaging (MRI) has shown promising results. Several AI systems have been developed to automatically analyze prostate MRI for segmentation, cancer detection, and region of interest characterization, thereby assisting clinicians in their decision-making process. Deep learning, the current trend in imaging AI, has limitations including the lack of transparency "black box", large data processing, and excessive energy consumption. In this narrative review, the authors provide an overview of the recent advances in AI for prostate cancer diagnosis and introduce their next-generation AI model, Green Learning, as a promising solution.

Artificial intelligence (AI) has the potential to transform pathologic diagnosis and cancer patient management as a predictive and prognostic biomarker. AI-based systems can be used to examine digitally scanned histopathology slides and differentiate benign from malignant cells and low from high grade. Deep learning models can analyze patient data from individual or multimodal combinations and identify patterns to be used to predict the response to different therapeutic options, the risk of recurrence or progression, and the prognosis of the newly diagnosed patient. AI-based models will improve treatment planning for patients with prostate cancer and improve the efficiency and cost-effectiveness of the pathology laboratory.

Artificial intelligence (AI) is revolutionizing prostate cancer genomics research. By leveraging machine learning and deep learning algorithms, researchers can rapidly analyze vast genomic datasets to identify patterns and correlations that may be missed by traditional methods. These AI-driven insights can lead to the discovery of novel biomarkers, enhance the accuracy of diagnosis, and predict disease progression and treatment response. As such, AI is becoming an indispensable tool in the pursuit of personalized medicine for prostate cancer.

show great promise for better understanding of disease and patient care, we should be realistic about the challenges arising from the nature of pediatric urologic conditions and practice, in order to continue to produce high-impact research.

Surgical Artificial Intelligence in Urology: Educational Applications 105

Mitchell G. Goldenberg

Surgical education has seen immense change recently. Increased demand for iterative evaluation of trainees from medical school to independent practice has led to the generation of an overwhelming amount of data related to an individual's competency. Artificial intelligence has been proposed as a solution to automate and standardize the ability of stakeholders to assess the technical and nontechnical abilities of a surgical trainee. In both the simulation and clinical environments, evidence supports the use of machine learning algorithms to both evaluate trainee skill and provide real-time and automated feedback, enabling a shortened learning curve for many key procedural skills and ensuring patient safety.

Artificial Intelligence in Urology: Current Status and Future Perspectives 117

Rayyan Abid, Ahmed A. Hussein, and Khurshid A. Guru

Surgical fields, especially urology, have shifted increasingly toward the use of artificial intelligence (AI). Advancements in AI have created massive improvements in diagnostics, outcome predictions, and robotic surgery. For robotic surgery to progress from assisting surgeons to eventually reaching autonomous procedures, there must be advancements in machine learning, natural language processing, and computer vision. Moreover, barriers such as data availability, interpretability of autonomous decision-making, Internet connection and security, and ethical concerns must be overcome.

Comprehensive Assessment of MRI-based Artificial Intelligence Frameworks Performance in the Detection, Segmentation, and Classification of Prostate Lesions Using Open-Source Databases 131

Lorenzo Storino Ramacciotti, Jacob S. Hershenhouse, Daniel Mokhtar, Divyangi Paralkar, Masatomo Kaneko, Michael Eppler, Karanvir Gill, Vasileios Mogoulianitis, Vinay Duddalwar, Andre L. Abreu, Inderbir Gill, and Giovanni E. Cacciamani

Numerous MRI-based artificial intelligence (AI) frameworks have been designed for prostate cancer lesion detection, segmentation, and classification via MRI as a result of intrareader and interreader variability that is inherent to traditional interpretation. Open-source data sets have been released with the intention of providing freely available MRIs for the testing of diverse AI frameworks in automated or semiautomated tasks. Here, an in-depth assessment of the performance of MRI-based AI frameworks for detecting, segmenting, and classifying prostate lesions using open-source databases was performed. Among 17 data sets, 12 were specific to prostate cancer detection/classification, with 52 studies meeting the inclusion criteria.

UROLOGIC CLINICS OF NORTH AMERICA

SERIES OF RELATED INTEREST
Surgical Clinics of North America
https://www.surgical.theclinics.com/

Foreword

Artificial Intelligence in Urology: The Final Frontier?

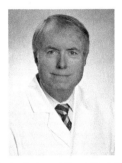

Kevin R. Loughlin, MD, MBA
Consulting Editor

Most urologists remember the opening lines of the iconic television show, *Star Trek*, "Space, the final frontier. These are the voyages of the Starship Enterprise. Its five-year mission. To explore new worlds." In this issue of *Urologic Clinics*, Dr Andrew Hung has assembled recognized experts to provide insight into the emerging applications of artificial intelligence (AI) to urologic practice. The question to be posed is whether AI is our "final frontier"? As the reader glances at the table of contents, he or she will get a glimpse of how AI is changing and will continue to change urology. AI will touch all areas of urology, including oncology, imaging, pathology, and pediatric urology, just to name some of its applications. This issue of *Urologic Clinics* provides the reader with the opportunity to pull back the curtain and peek at the future of urology.

We are on the cusp of the development of AI in medical practice. AI has already been applied to

oncology utilizing the Deep Learning diagnostics for bladder tumor identification. LYNA (Lymph Node Assistant algorithm) has been applied to detect cancer in lymph node biopsies, and the Decipher biopsy test can analyze the metastatic potential of tumors. Exciting applications of AI have been utilized to enhance urologic imaging, including MRI/TRUS Fusion for prostate biopsies. AI applications also represent the potential for enhanced drug discovery for a variety of urologic disorders.

However, AI will not replace physicians; it will simply provide us with the tools to enable us to make better decisions. Urologists are comfortable with change, and the history of our specialty illustrates that. Our first biomarker, acid phosphatase, was discovered in the 1930s and decades later was replaced by prostate-specific antigen (PSA). PSA testing evolved into a variety of PSA permutations,

Urol Clin N Am 51 (2024) xi–xii
https://doi.org/10.1016/j.ucl.2023.08.004
0094-0143/24/© 2023 Published by Elsevier Inc.

and we are now entering an era where genetic testing is used to assess prostate cancer risk and prognosis.

Two generations ago, the intravenous pyelogram was the sine qua non of urologic imaging, and it evolved into an era of CT and MRI scans, which have evolved further into molecular imaging. In the 1980s, the open radical prostatectomy was introduced only to be replaced within two to three decades with robotic radical prostatectomy. Indeed, the urologic tradition is to relentlessly make ourselves obsolete.[1]

With this background, it should be clear to most urologists that AI is not the final frontier, but rather, the next frontier. Urologists will take the lead as to what are both the applications and the limitations of AI in urologic practice. We would be wise to remember the words of Mr Spock, "Change is the essential process of existence."

Kevin R. Loughlin, MD, MBA
Vascular Biology Research Laboratory
Boston Children's Hospital
300 Longwood Avenue
Boston, MA 02115, USA

E-mail address:
kloughlin@partners.org

REFERENCE

1. Loughlin KR. Relentlessly make yourself obsolete: Robot assisted radical cystectomy, the emerging standard of care. Urol Oncol 2021;39(1):13–4.

Preface

A Glance at the Present and Future of Artificial Intelligence in Urology

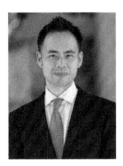

Andrew J. Hung, MD
Editor

While there has been tremendous interest in artificial intelligence (AI) and its potential impact on health care, substantive work has already been done in applying AI to the field of Urology. This comes through significant partnerships between clinicians and data scientists.

In this issue of *Urologic Clinics*, we share the most contemporary work, presented by the leading authorities in the respective areas. We cover the hot topics of AI, radiomics, pathomics, and genomics for prostate cancer; AI, pathomics, genomics, and radiomics for renal cell carcinoma; and AI applications for bladder cancer. We further present AI applications in pediatric urology, endourology, surgical education, and autonomous surgery. A final article covers the large publicly available data sets, and their importance for the continued successful development of AI models.

While exploring the current state-of-the-art advances, authors also spell out where the important next steps will be. Outstanding issues of reproducibility, ethics, and transparency transcend any one application of AI. The only sustainable path forward is if the clinician and patient trust the technology. As the innovations continue to occur in machine learning, so will the applications and advances in Urology.

Andrew J. Hung, MD
Department of Urology
Cedars-Sinai Medical Center
8635 West 3rd Street, Suite 1070W
Los Angeles, CA 90048, USA

E-mail address:
Andrew.hung@cshs.org

Urol Clin N Am 51 (2024) xiii
https://doi.org/10.1016/j.ucl.2023.06.017
0094-0143/24/

The Novel Green Learning Artificial Intelligence for Prostate Cancer Imaging
A Balanced Alternative to Deep Learning and Radiomics

Masatomo Kaneko, MD, PhD[a,b,c], Vasileios Magoulianitis, MS[d],
Lorenzo Storino Ramacciotti, MD[a,b], Alex Raman, MS[e],
Divyangi Paralkar, MD[a,b], Andrew Chen, MD[a,b], Timothy N. Chu, BS[a,b],
Yijing Yang, MS, PhD[d], Jintang Xue, MS[d], Jiaxin Yang, MS[d], Jinyuan Liu, MS[d],
Donya S. Jadvar[f], Karanvir Gill, MS, BA[a,b], Giovanni E. Cacciamani, MD[a,b,g],
Chrysostomos L. Nikias, MS, PhD[d], Vinay Duddalwar, MD, FRCR[g],
C.-C. Jay Kuo, MS, PhD[d], Inderbir S. Gill, MD[a], Andre Luis Abreu, MD[a,b,g,*]

KEYWORDS

- Prostate cancer • Prostate biopsy • Magnetic resonance imaging • Artificial intelligence
- Machine learning • Radiomics • Deep learning • Computer vision

KEY POINTS

- Artificial intelligence (AI) models achieve accurate prostate segmentation, prostate cancer (PCa) detection, and lesion characterization on magnetic resonance imaging (MRI).
- Combination models of MRI AI and clinical information further improve PCa detection performance.
- Most of the evidence is based on retrospective single-center studies, and further robust studies including multicenter randomized control trials are warranted.
- Deep learning models have some limitations including "black box" lack of transparency, large data processing, and excessive energy consumption.
- Green Learning models that can achieve high accuracy while still being explainable and sustainable are ongoing in the medical field.

INTRODUCTION

Multiparametric MRI (mpMRI) is recommended by several guidelines for all men with suspicions of prostate cancer (PCa) before undergoing a prostate biopsy (PBx). However, approximately 25% of clinically significant PCa (CSPCa) can be missed by mpMRI.[1]

The application of artificial intelligence (AI) on prostate MRI has shown encouraging results. Several AI systems have been developed to automatically analyze MRI for prostate segmentation,

[a] USC Institute of Urology and Catherine & Joseph Aresty Department of Urology, Keck School of Medicine, University of Southern California, Los Angeles, CA, USA; [b] USC Institute of Urology, Center for Image-Guided Surgery, Focal Therapy and Artificial Intelligence for Prostate Cancer; [c] Department of Urology, Graduate School of Medical Science, Kyoto Prefectural University of Medicine, Kyoto, Japan; [d] Ming Hsieh Department of Electrical and Computer Engineering, University of Southern California, Los Angeles, CA, USA; [e] Western University of Health Sciences. Pomona, CA, USA; [f] Dornsife School of Letters and Science, University of Southern California, Los Angeles, CA, USA; [g] Department of Radiology, Keck School of Medicine, University of Southern California, Los Angeles, CA, USA
* Corresponding author. 1441 Eastlake Avenue, Suite 7416, Los Angeles, CA 90089.
E-mail address: andre.abreu@med.usc.edu

Urol Clin N Am 51 (2024) 1–13
https://doi.org/10.1016/j.ucl.2023.08.001

cancer detection, and region of interest characterization, thereby assisting clinicians in their decision-making process.[2–16] The utilization of AI-assisted imaging holds potential for improved, objective, and reproducible diagnostic performance, enhanced decision-making, efficiency, and reduced workload.[17]

AI approaches for PCa imaging can be classified into radiomics combined with the machine learning (ML) method and deep learning (DL) approach depending on the difference of the imaging feature extraction methods used. However, these methods have limitations such as modest performance and "black box" decisions.

In this narrative review, the authors provide an overview of the recent advances in AI for PCa diagnosis and introduce their next-generation AI model, Green Learning (GL), as a promising solution.[18]

RATIONALE FOR ARTIFICIAL INTELLIGENCE IN PROSTATE CANCER IMAGING
Radiomics

Radiomics is one of the widely and powerfully used libraries for extracting features from medical images.[19] Different statistical, shape-based, or texture-based features aim at capturing the different characteristics of MRI signal depicted on the voxels. As there are certain mathematical formulas for calculating those features, the process is very transparent and explainable. Yet, those features are not data-dependent and do not take into account the overall training data distribution into the feature extraction process. After feature extraction, in a separate step, a classifier needs to be trained to find the decision boundaries between classes.

Random forest (RF) is a popular ML algorithm that uses multiple decision trees, each trained on a random subset of features from the dataset.[20] Another variant that offers improvements over RF is the Extreme Gradient Boosting Tree (XGBoost),[21] in which each decision tree is trained over improving the loss function based on past decision tree errors.

Another popular ML algorithm, support vector machine, finds a higher-dimensional hyperplane that best separates the classes.[22] For classification tasks, data-driven feature extraction usually leads to better results because it optimizes the features to be more accurate in classifying the data.

The advantages of radiomics include the transparent, explainable, light-weight, and efficient feature extraction process. However, regions of interest (ROI) and features need to be predefined by

humans, and the performance is limited compared with data-driven approaches.

Deep Learning

With the advent of DL in the past decade, data-driven end-to-end methods such as Convolutional Neural Networks (CNN) provide a holistic way for feature extraction and classification, without separating the 2 processes as in radiomics pipeline. Data-driven methods adapt their feature learning process targeting a specific dataset. Those features are calculated during an optimization process, by maximizing an objective function such as classification/segmentation accuracy.

Although these features are very powerful, they have received a lot of criticism especially in the medical analysis field because there is no mathematically transparent process behind their extraction process ("black box" decision module). Furthermore, DL models are usually very complex, requiring a large number of samples for training and storage of a massive number of parameters, and this entails a considerably higher power consumption both for training and testing of those models. In addition, to successfully train those models, a sufficiently large number of data is required, which may limit its use for medical applications.

Pre-DL methods including radiomics pipeline use a very small number of parameters for solving the problem, and also do not require large datasets, whereas DL methods' complexity is an order of higher magnitude, entailing a greater demand for larger training datasets. If a massive amount of training data can be provided, and power consumption and interpretability are not major concerns, DL methods are the best option to achieve the highest performance using AI. However, in high-stakes decision-making tasks, such as predicting cancer presence in a patient, transparent pipelines are of high preference.

Green Learning, the Next-Generation Approach

Recently, GL, a novel feature extraction method, arose in computer vision field, aiming at reconciling aspects of the DL paradigm and pre-DL methods by using lightweight models with faster training/testing time, explainability, and less power consumption (**Fig. 1**).[18] Although mathematical knowledge is necessary to understand how GL makes decisions, it uses a transparent feature extraction process. In this process, each feature holds a physical meaning. It decomposes the input image into different spatial-spectral representations. In comparison with DL, the GL requires

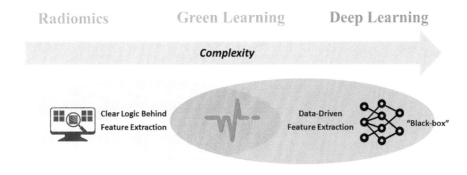

Radiomics　　Green Learning　　Deep Learning

Complexity

Clear Logic Behind Feature Extraction　　Data-Driven Feature Extraction　　"Black-box"

Explainability

	Radiomics	Green Learning	Deep Learning
Power consumption	Very low	Low	Very High
Model size	Very low	Low	Very High
Performance	Moderate	High	Very High
Number of training data needed	Small	Moderate	Very High
Interpretability	Very High	High	Low

Fig. 1. A comparison of different types of pipelines for medical image analysis. GL stands among DL and radiomics, because GL has data-driven and explainable logic behind feature extraction, providing a competitive and responsible alternative for medical image analysis tasks. Radar chart shows the performance of each method. Computing speed is determined by model size, training efficiency means how much training data are needed, and power efficiency indicates how much electricity is consumed. Impressively, the model complexity is several thousand times more in DL compared with GL. AI, artificial intelligence; GL, Green Learning; DL, deep learning.

less training data, as it has a more stable and formulated way of calculating the features. This advantage is extremely relevant for certain medical applications where the data are sparse. Furthermore, the model size, including the number of parameters, is several times less than the DL models. In terms of performance, GL falls between radiomics and DL.

Thus, the GL approach may be optimal to develop an automated PCa detection system that offers a very lightweight model package with a transparent feature extraction process that contributes to understanding the nature of those features, making the AI system's decisions more trustworthy from physicians.

ARTIFICIAL INTELLIGENCE FOR MRI PROSTATE SEGMENTATION
Technical Aspects

Because prostate organ segmentation is useful for generating an input for radiomics-based classification and grading, there is active interest in segmenting the prostate organ on mpMRI.

The research for a fully automated prostate gland segmentation increased tremendously with the advent of DL. Different CNN architectures have been proposed to be trained from human annotations and learn the prostate shape and textures. The most popular architecture is the U-Net.[3,4] It is named after its shape of the letter "U." The U-Net has 2 main branches, the downstream (contracting path) and the upstream (expansive path). The input volume is fed in the downstream branch, where multiple convolutional layers learn the shape and texture features at different spatial scales of the prostate gland, as well as its zonal segments. Overall, there are architectures that can operate on 2-dimensional (2D) images (ie, slice by slice processing) or on 3-dimensional (3D) images, thus exploiting the interslice correlations of prostate structures. All those DL models can learn a rich feature representation at multiple scales, at the expense of conveying a very high number of parameters.

On the other hand, the GL has been designed to address the segmentation problem using a significantly smaller number of parameters and avoiding an unnecessary high volume of computations. The first stage segments the prostate gland and the second stage zooms into the predicted prostate area to further delineate the transition zone (TZ) and peripheral zone (PZ). Both stages share a lightweight feed-forward GL system (**Fig. 2**), inspired from the U-Net architecture of DL, but having far fewer parameters. Different from the

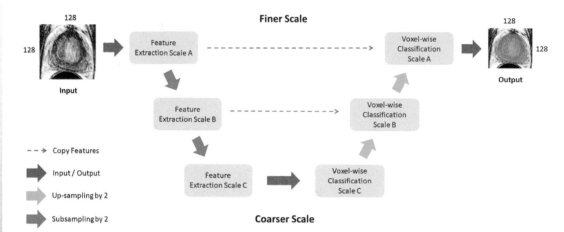

Fig. 2. Automated prostate gland segmentation technical pipeline is illustrated. Features are extracted at different scales by subsampling the input by two at each layer. In the coarsest scale, a rough segmentation of the prostate segmentation is initially derived. It is refined in the finer scale layers, up to the original resolution that matches with the input size of the MRI.

DL, the GL feature extraction consists of local Principal Component Analysis[23] units, instead of neurons, named the Hop layer. Having learned multiscale features, the right decoding branch trains different classifiers such as RF or XGBoost at each scale to get predictions on whether the voxel is on the prostate gland or the background; this is a supervised local refinement strategy, obtaining the predictions from coarser scales and progressively integrating them into finer scales using interpolation and concatenation. After that, the heat map, which shows the probability of prostate region, is obtained from the last classifier in the finer scale. Our group developed GL model from 119 prebiopsy T2-W images and validated it with 5-fold cross-validation.[24] The GL model with web-based software interface achieved a Dice similarity coefficient (DSC) of 0.85, 0.81, and 0.62 and the Pearson correlation coefficient for volumes of 0.92, 0.93, and 0.63 (all $P < .01$) for whole prostate, TZ, and PZ segmentation, respectively.

Recent Findings

Because a manual segmentation of the prostate on MRI is a time-consuming task with significant interreader variability, the use of AI algorithms, particularly those of ML and DL, resulted in ever-improving outcomes.[25] Vincent and colleagues used an active appearance model built from 50 transverse T2-weighted images (T2WI) and achieved a DSC of 0.88.[26] Although initial segmentation by automated algorithms were effective, the development and advancement of ML algorithms resulted in greater improvements in segmentation.[27]

Other methods of segmentation include uniquely designed DL networks. Tian and colleagues fine-tuned an already developed fully convolutional network (FCN) of natural image segmentation for the prostate.[6,28] The FCN of Long and colleagues was itself a modification of an existing classification CNN. Previous CNNs had been applied to handle 2D medical image segmentation. Wang and colleagues was one of the first groups to apply a 3D FCN with deep supervision to capture more volumetric features of anatomic structures of the prostate and achieved a DSC of 0.88 tested on a public dataset of 50 T2WI.[29] More recently, Ushinsky and colleagues, using a hybrid 3D-2D modified CNN technique based on U-Net, was able to achieve a DSC score of 0.898 on a large cohort of clinically acquired images.[30] A comparison of various DL models demonstrated the success of the nnUNet algorithm for prostate gland segmentation.[31,32] The model achieved a DSC score of 0.93, which was about 2% higher than all other models tested.

In addition to the whole prostate gland segmentation, separation of the PZ and the TZ is also under investigation. Bardis and colleagues used 2 U-Nets in parallel to segment the PZ and TZ.[33] They demonstrated a DSC score of 0.940 for the whole prostate, 0.910 for the TZ, and 0.774 for the PZ.

Although the initial results are promising, this still leaves room for improvement of delineation within the prostate gland. Progress in the field of prostate segmentation has clearly accelerated within the last 5 years. Further applications of this work can improve automated PCa detection, MRI fusion techniques, as well as improved mapping for radiation therapy.

ARTIFICIAL INTELLIGENCE FOR PROSTATE CANCER DETECTION AND CHARACTERIZATION
Technical Aspects

Prostate cancer detection

After segmenting the prostate gland, the subsequent region detection module is applied. Several DL-based methods have been proposed for automatically detecting lesion areas in the prostate MRI.

FocalNet was proposed earlier to predict the grade group (GG) histology from biparametric MRI (bpMRI) input. It uses a novel attention mechanism and loss function for training that aims to discover the most discriminant visual features, shared between T2WI and apparent diffusion coefficient (ADC).[7] In addition, although the dataset consisted of the imbalanced data (abundant negative regions vs very few positive ones), FocalNet properly learned the features of high-grade lesions with large focal weight and accurately predicted the underrepresented class.

Other researchers used 3D-CNNs that comprise convolutional operations on 3 planes (XYZ).[10] As

such, AI can learn the cancer appearance over benign regions by looking at different slices of MRI. In general, 3D-based systems entail more parameters and heavier model sizes; however, a good performance can be obtained if trained with a large dataset.

The GL paradigm can be also used for prostate cancer detection. In particular, for feature extraction in the detection pipeline, IPHOP-II (**Fig. 3**) method is used to decompose the input signal into a spatial-spectral representation, where the discriminant dimensions are kept through feature selection and eventually fed to the classifier. IPHOP-II takes T2WI, ADC, and diffusion-weighted imaging high b-value images independently as input. After resampling onto the T2WI reference system, it generates per voxel features for classification. The classifier is trained to discern between malignant and benign areas. In the testing phase, per-voxel feature extraction and malignant probability prediction (heatmap) are performed. The authors' preliminary experiment showed GL trained by 1200 prostate biparametric

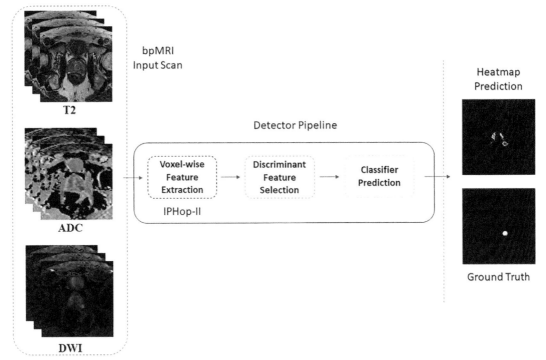

Fig. 3. Prostate lesion detection pipeline in Green Learning. Green Learning model receives bpMRI input to capture all different modalities of MRI and lesion appearance. After confining the search space into the prostate gland area using the prostate segmentation module predictions, all 3 sequences are used for feature extraction. To search for lesion areas, the prostate is divided into patches. Then, the IPHop-II method transforms each patch into a spatial-spectral representation that constitutes the features. Subsequently, feature selection cuts down the feature space to a much smaller discriminant subset before getting to the classifier for predicting the probability of a voxel being suspicious. After all, a heat map with predicted probabilities per voxel is outputted. bpMRI, biparametric MRI.

MRI images with Prostate Imaging-Reporting and Data System (PI-RADS) 3 to 5 legion accurately detected ROIs with a per-patient area under the curve (AUC) of 0.81 and a sensitivity of 0.92 at a 0.43 false-positive rate.[34]

Prostate Cancer Characterization on MRI

For the ROI characterization task, radiomics prevail in literature, as they offer a more explainable approach, crucial for physicians. Also, having detected first the suspicious ROIs, it is easier to extract radiomic features. Radiomics can provide extensive analysis to the ROI and further use popular feature selection modules such as analysis of variance and classifiers for characterizing the ROI into benign or malignant.[14–16] A more recent study used a CNN (XmasNet) to classify the detected ROIs into CSPCa versus non-CSPCa, and the model achieved the second highest AUC of 0.84 in the PROSTATEx challenge.[13] However, the feature extraction process is unclear and makes it hard to interpret decisions from such a model.

ROIs on PZ and TZ have different features for predicting prostate cancer. Therefore, the GL paradigm aims to extract the best spectral components of each region. For this, independent modules are used for classifying ROIs from each region. For feature extraction and ROI classification, the IPHOP-II feature extraction process is adopted (**Fig. 4**). This process offers certain advantages over DL due to a small model size, an explainable and transparent feature extraction process. Moreover, the feature extraction process decomposes the signal into different spectral components and can also lead to understanding what the differences are between suspicious and nonsuspicious ROIs. The authors' preliminary experiment demonstrated GL trained by 205 prostate biparametric MRI with PI-RADS score 3 to 5 precisely discriminated ROIs with CSPCa (defined as GG $\geq$ 2) confirmed on targeted biopsy versus those without CSPCa with an AUC of 0.82 for PZ and 0.79 for TZ. Interestingly, if combined with prostate specific antigen (PSA) density greater than or equal to 0.15 ng/mL and abnormal digital rectal examination findings, the AUC for PZ and TZ increased to 0.85.[35]

Recent Findings

Several recent publications have explored AI and radiomics for PCa detection and characterization. Certain studies have taken a non-DL approach, by carefully selecting radiomics features that correlate with PCa. One study demonstrated the success of radiomics features extracted from the gray-level co-occurrence matrix of mpMRI in predicting CSPCa.[36] In their cohort, the radiomics features were more than 30% a better predictor of CSPCa than both PI-RADS and PSA density. In addition, work by Varghese and colleagues proposed a systematic way of training and evaluating multiple ML classifiers that use radiomics metrics for PCa prediction.[37] Classifier evaluation was performed using the Friedman-Nemenyı test, and their optimal classifier achieved a higher precision and recall in predicting high-risk PCa than PI-RADS.[38]

Hosseinzadeh and colleagues assessed DL algorithm based on PI-RADS for detecting PCa with bpMRI.[39] The algorithm was trained with 1586 cases and validated with 366 cases. PI-RADS 4 to

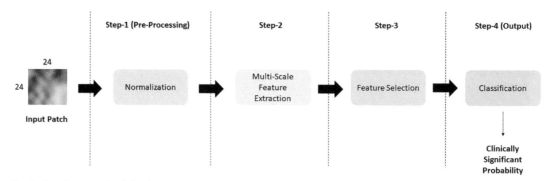

Fig. 4. IP-HOP-II method for feature extraction in Green Learning framework. For ROI characterization, a 16x16 patch is cropped around the center of an identified ROI and then IPHOP-II is followed to extract features for the classifier. Feature extraction is derived in 2 scales, using Hop-1 and -2, cascaded to each other. IPHOP-II consists of 2 features: the spatial and spectral ones. Spatial features correspond to the feature representation at specific areas of the ROI. On the other hand, spectral features do not have any spatial meaning but rather encode more the global pattern of the ROI. At the output of the feature extraction, both spatial and spectral features are concatenated together. After feature selection, a binary classifier is trained on predicting clinically significant cancer. ROI, region of interest.

5 was used to train the DL model. The study found that the performance of the AI to detect PI-RADS 4 to 5 ROI was significantly affected by the number of cases trained, with the AUC varying from 0.80 (50 cases) to 0.87 (1586 cases), even at 1952 cases. Adding zonal segmentation as prior knowledge to the AI model improved performance significantly. Despite achieving high diagnostic performance (AUC = 0.85) for predicting biopsy-proven CSPCa, a consensus panel of expert radiologists still performed significantly better. Based on these results, the investigators suggest that DL AI for prostate bpMRI should be trained with more than 2000 cases to achieve expert-level detection of PCa.

The use of mpMRI to evaluate the aggressiveness of PCa has also been investigated.[7] Specifically, a DL model called FocalNet was used to predict GS based on the mpMRI characteristics. A prostate mpMRI dataset from 417 patients was extracted to validate and train the model. At one false positive per patient, FocalNet achieved 89.7% and 87.9% sensitivity for histopathology-proven index and CSPCa (GS $\geq$ 7) lesion detection, respectively. For GS group classification, FocalNet received an AUC of 0.81 for GS greater than or equal to 3 + 4 and 0.79 for GS greater than or equal to 4 + 3. Compared with highly experienced radiologists, FocalNet's detection sensitivity for index and clinically significant lesions was only 3.4% and 1.5% lower, respectively, with no statistical significance.

A study demonstrates the effectiveness of a fully automatic pipeline for GG prediction of PCa from mpMRI.[40] In this study, the Retina UNet was trained by mpMRI with targeted PBx and achieved a lesion level sensitivity and specificity of 1.0 and 0.80, respectively, for predicting the presence of GG greater than or equal to 2 lesions. The model similarly received a sensitivity and specificity of 1.0 and 0.79 on a test set from the publicly available dataset.

A retrospective study was conducted on 644 patients to evaluate the performance of radiomics and DL models in detecting CSPCa on mpMRI.[41] Both models were trained by MRI-target biopsy yields. Although the DL model was designed to automatically segment CSPCa legions, radiomics models differentiate the ROIs defined by a radiologist into CSPCa or non-CSPCa. Although DL model demonstrated higher AUC than radiomics model (0.89 vs 0.83) with internal cross-validation, the radiomics model outperformed the DL model on 3 unseen test cohorts including external cohorts, achieving AUCs of 0.88, 0.91, and 0.65, compared with 0.70, 0.73, and 0.44, respectively. The DL model's higher performance on internal dataset but lower performance on external dataset indicates the issue of overfitting. Identifying predisposed patients can have significant implications for optimizing treatment decisions and planning regarding neoadjuvant or adjuvant systemic therapies. Bourbonne and colleagues developed a radiomics model for predicting biochemical recurrence (BCR), based on a single predictive feature—"size zone emphasis"—and validated the model on an independent dataset from outside of their institution.[42] The model had an accuracy of 78% on the initial dataset and an accuracy of 76% on the outside dataset, demonstrating its robustness.

In another retrospective multicenter study involving 485 patients, a newly developed DL-trained AI model was tested to predict the risk of BCR in patients who underwent radical prostatectomy (RP).[43] The model incorporated quantitative features of prostate MRI from T2 delineated tumors. The AI model outperformed existing methods, with a C-index of 0.802 in both primary and validating cohorts.

Evaluation of extraprostatic extension (EPE) of cancer is important for determining treatment decisions. A study used radiomics features derived from segmented prostate lesions, along with an RF model to predict EPE. Their model received an AUC of 0.74, noted to be comparable with the radiologist interpretation, which received an AUC of 0.75.[44]

FUTURE DIRECTIONS

Current standard of MRI for PCa detection, PI-RADS, has several limitations including the risk of false negatives, nonlinear correlation between PI-RADS score and the risk of CSPCa, not fully quantitative evaluation, moderate interreader agreement, and dependence on radiologists' factors (need of expertise, workload, exhaustion, risk of burnout, and search satisfaction).[1,45,46]

The authors would propose Prostate *Artificial Intelligence* Imaging-Reporting and Data System (PAIRADS) as a taxonomy for AI-aid PI-RADS.

AI-aid prostate MRI has shown considerable potential in precise prostate annotation, ROI detection, cancer identification, and prediction of PSA recurrence and EPE. Combination models of AI and clinical information have been shown to further increase the AUC in PCa detection compared with AI-only models (**Table 1**).[47–53] Fully quantitative prostate MRI evaluation by AI, a concept the authors name PAIRADS, may improve CSPCa detection even in the case of PI-RADS 1 to 2, consistent/reproducible performance, and more accurate and quantitative prognosis contributing more personalized decision-making and reduce

Table 1
Recent studies comparing MRI AI–only model versus AI + clinical/radiologic parameter model for prostate cancer diagnosis

Author, Year	Study Design	No. of Patients	Imaging Modality Analyzed by AI	AI Algorithm[a]	Reference Standard	Performance[b] of AI-Only vs Combination (AI + Clinical/ Radiologic Parameters) Model AUC/Sensitivity/Specificity
Qi Y et al,[47] 2020	Single-center, retrospective study	Total: 199 Training: 133 Test: 66	T2WI, ADC, and DCE	RF	12-core SB + at least 1-core TB	PCa characterization AI only: 0.90/0.78/0.81 AI + age + PSAD + DRE + PIRADS: 0.93/0.82/0.92
Li M et al,[48] 2020	Single-center, retrospective study	Total: 381 Training: 229 Test: 152	T2WI and ADC	LASSO	10-core SB + 2–4	CSPCa characterization AI only: 0.98/0.95/0.87 AI + age + tPSA + PSAD: 0.98/0.82/0.97
Hiremath A et al,[49] 2021	Multicenter, retrospective study	Total: 592 Training: 368 Test: 224	T2WI and ADC	AlexNet	12-core SB and MRI-guided and US fusion–guided biopsies or RP	CSPCa detection/ characterization AI only: 0.76/69%/67% AI + PIRADS + PSA + prostate volume + lesion volume: 0.81/83%/59%
Roest C et al,[50] 2021	Multicenter, retrospective study	Total: 1434 Training: 1291 Test: 143	T2W, ADC, and sequential MRI	U-Net + SVM	MRI-targeted or systematic biopsy	CSPCa detection/ characterization AI only: 0.81/0.76/0.79 AI + age + PSA + PSAD: 0.86/0.9/0.75
Li T et al,[51] 2022	Multi center, retrospective study	Total: 371 Training: 199 Test: 107 External validation: 65	T2WI, ADC, and DCE	LASSO with SMOTE	12-core SB + at least 2-core TB or RP with PIRAD 3 lesion	CSPCa characterization Test group AI only: 0.84/0.85/0.73 AI + PSAD: 0.88/0.79/0.82 External validation group AI only: 0.83/0.75/0.85 AI + PSAD: 0.90/0.75/0.95

Gui S et al,[52] 2022	Single-center, retrospective study	Total: 146 Training: 103 Test: 43	T2W	LASSO algorithm	Histopathologic confirmation TRUS Bx or RP	PCa characterization AI only: 0.74/0.73/0.75 AI + PSA: 0.86/0.93/0.82
Lu Y et al,[53] 2022	Single-center, retrospective study	Total: 136 Training: 95 Test: 41	T2WI and ADC	Fusion radscore (RF, SVM, LR, LASSO, LDA, NB, and KNN)	Histologic confirmation of SB	PCa characterization AI only: 0.84/80.0%/84.6% AI + transitional zone volume: 0.87/73.3%/84.6%

Abbreviations: ADC, apparent diffusion coefficient; AUC, area under the curve; CSPCa, clinically significant prostate cancer; DCE, dynamic contrast-enhanced; DRE, digital rectal examination; KNN, K-nearest neighbor; LASSO, least absolute shrinkage and selection operator; LDA, linear discriminant analysis; LR, logistic regression; MRI, magnetic resonance imaging; NB, naive Bayes; PCa, prostate cancer; PIRADS, prostate imaging reporting and data system; PSA, prostate-specific antigen; PSAD, prostate-specific antigen density; RF, random forest; RP, radical prostatectomy; SB, systematic biopsy; SMOTE, synthetic minority oversampling technique; SVM, support vector machine; T2WI, T2-weighted imaging; TB, targeted biopsy.

[a] AI algorithm that achieved the best AUC in the paper.
[b] Performance is from the model that achieved the best AUC in the test dataset.

workload of radiologists who should focus on more complicated tasks.

To implement PAIRADS in society there are many issues that need to be addressed. So far, most of the studies were retrospective and single centric; therefore, their generalizability has not been well demonstrated yet. Because the performance of data-driven AI highly relies on the training dataset, the performance may be biased in the case that biased training dataset is used. Several AI support systems for PCa imaging are already available.[54] However, details of training data used to develop these AI systems are not readily available. Diverse, generalizable, and high-quality data sets ideally collected from multi-center and variable imaging scanners should be used throughout the AI development process to cover all patients. In addition, to prove generalizability, further robust studies, such as multicenter RCTs, are needed.

Current prostate MRI AI models have shown promising performance for specific single tasks mainly for PCa diagnosis. However, prostate MRI is not used only for detecting PCa but also for evaluating other prostatic diseases and anatomic features including surrounding organs. Therefore, current single-task prostate MRI AI cannot completely undertake radiologists' task. Because radiologists eventually need to review the images following AI, workload is not reduced much. To enhance the value and effectiveness of AI, a multi-task AI system that comprehensively evaluates prostate MRI as radiologists do is desired.

The current trend in PCa imaging AI is DL, but this approach suffers from the black box decision-making, which makes it difficult to explain the basis of the diagnostic decisions. To ensure that AI is used for medical professionals' and patients' responsible shared decision-making, an explainable AI system is necessary. Developing an explainable AI system would also contribute to a deeper clinical understanding of PCa.

DL models also require significantly more computing power energy consumption and carbon emissions for training and posttraining inference than non-DL ML models, which are not assumed as sustainable.[54,55] Therefore, there is a need for novel AI models such as GL that can achieve high accuracy while still being explainable and sustainable.

AI models can be vulnerable to cyberattacks. Adversarial attacks on medical AI systems may lead to unauthorized access to sensitive patients' privacy data and could affect patient safety. To ensure robust security measures, light model AI is preferable, because it can run in a secured local (offline) environment.

The development of guidelines, regulations, and legal frameworks has not kept pace with the explosive advancement of AI technology.[56] Establishing and spreading clear guidelines and policies that address concerns of liability, accountability, and the ethical use of AI is needed in the health care field.

To spread AI-aid prostate imaging, reimbursement is also important. To get better reimbursement from regulatory authorities, prostate imaging AI should clearly show the added value of AI-aid imaging over standard radiologist evaluation.

If advances in AI technology continue, it may be possible to diagnose and plan the treatment of PCa using AI prediction "virtual biopsy," bypassing invasive prostate needle biopsy. To prepare for the coming AI era, physicians must be familiar with imaging AI for PCa diagnosis.

SUMMARY

Prostate MRI is an area where the application of AI has shown promising results in recent years. Several AI systems have been developed to automatically analyze prostate MRI images for prostate segmentation, cancer detection, and region characterization, thereby assisting clinicians in their decision-making process. The current trend in PCa imaging AI is DL, but this approach suffers from the black box issue and excessive energy consumption. Therefore, next-generation non-DL AI models such as GL that can achieve high accuracy while still being explainable and sustainable are desired. To prepare for the coming AI era, physicians must be familiar with imaging AI for PCa diagnosis.

CLINICS CARE POINTS

- AI models achieve DSC for the whole prostate segmentation on MRI as high as 0.9.
- AI models show comparable CSPCa detection performance on MRI with radiologists.
- AI models precisely predict BCR and EPE following RP from presurgery MRI.
- Combination models of MRI AI and clinical information further improve CSPCa detection performance.
- Most of the evidence is retrospective single center study, and further robust studies including multicenter randomized controlled trials are warranted.

- DL models have some limitations including "black box" issues and excessive energy consumption.
- Non-DL AI models that can achieve high accuracy while still being explainable and sustainable are reasonable in the medical field.
- Fully quantitative prostate MRI evaluation by AI "PAIRADS" may realize improved CSPCa detection, consistent/reproducible performance, and more accurate and quantitative prognosis and reduce workload of radiologists.

DISCLOSURE

I.S. Gill is an unpaid advisor for Steba (Unpaid Advisor) and has equity interest in OneLine Health. Andre Luis Abreu is consultant for Koelis and Quibim and speaker for EDAP.

FUNDING

None.

ACKNOWLEDGMENTS

None.

REFERENCES

1. Ahmed HU, El-Shater Bosaily A, Brown LC, et al. Diagnostic accuracy of multi-parametric MRI and TRUS biopsy in prostate cancer (PROMIS): a paired validating confirmatory study. Lancet 2017;389: 815–22.
2. Rundo L, Han C, Nagano Y, et al. USE-Net: Incorporating Squeeze-and-Excitation blocks into U-Net for prostate zonal segmentation of multi-institutional MRI datasets. Neurocomputing 2019;365:31–43.
3. Zhou Z, Rahman Siddiquee MM, Tajbakhsh N, et al. A nested u-net architecture for medical image segmentation. Lect Notes Comput Sci 2018;3–11, 11045 LNCS.
4. Ronneberger O, Fischer P, Brox T. U-Net: Convolutional Networks for Biomedical Image Segmentation. IEEE Access 2015;9:16591–603.
5. Milletari F, Navab N, Ahmadi SA. V-Net: Fully convolutional neural networks for volumetric medical image segmentation. Proc - 2016 4th Int Conf 3D Vision, 3DV 2016. 2016:565-571.
6. Tian Z, Liu L, Zhang Z, et al. PSNet: prostate segmentation on MRI based on a convolutional neural network. J Med Imaging 2018;5:1.
7. Cao R, Mohammadian Bajgiran A, Afshari Mirak S, et al. Joint Prostate Cancer Detection and Gleason Score Prediction in mp-MRI via FocalNet. IEEE Trans Med Imag 2019;38:2496–506.
8. Cao R, Zhong X, Scalzo F, et al. Prostate cancer inference via weakly-supervised learning using a large collection of negative MRI. Proc - 2019 Int Conf Comput Vis Work ICCVW 2019;434–9.
9. Saha A, Hosseinzadeh M, Huisman H. End-to-end prostate cancer detection in bpMRI via 3D CNNs: Effects of attention mechanisms, clinical priori and decoupled false positive reduction. Med Image Anal 2021;73:102155.
10. Yu X, Lou B, Shi B, et al. False Positive Reduction Using Multiscale Contextual Features for Prostate Cancer Detection in Multi-Parametric MRI Scans. Proc - Int Symp Biomed Imaging 2020;1355–9.
11. Mehralivand S, Yang D, Harmon SA, et al. Deep learning-based artificial intelligence for prostate cancer detection at biparametric MRI. Abdom Radiol 2022;47:1425–34.
12. Liu Z, Jiang W, Lee KH, et al. A two-stage approach for automated prostate lesion detection and classification with mask R-CNN and weakly supervised deep neural network. Vol 11850 LNCS. Cham, Switzerland: Springer International Publishing; 2019.
13. Liu S, Zheng H, Feng Y, et al. Prostate Cancer Diagnosis using Deep Learning with 3D Multiparametric MRI. SPIE Med Imaging 2017;10134:1–4.
14. Fehr D, Veeraraghavan H, Wibmer A, et al. Automatic classification of prostate cancer Gleason scores from multiparametric magnetic resonance images. Proc Natl Acad Sci U S A 2015;112: E6265–73.
15. Ginsburg SB, Algohary A, Pahwa S, et al. Radiomic features for prostate cancer detection on MRI differ between the transition and peripheral zones: Preliminary findings from a multi-institutional study. J Magn Reson Imag 2017;46:184–93.
16. Algohary A, Viswanath S, Shiradkar R, et al. Radiomic features on MRI enable risk categorization of prostate cancer patients on active surveillance: Preliminary findings. J Magn Reson Imag 2018;48:818–28.
17. Cacciamani GE, Sanford DI, Chu TN, et al. Is Artificial Intelligence Replacing Our Radiology Stars? Not Yet. Eur Urol Open Sci 2023;48:14–6.
18. Kuo CCJ, Madni AM. Green learning: Introduction, examples and outlook. J Vis Commun Image Represent 2023;90:103685.
19. Sugano D, Sanford D, Abreu A, et al. Impact of radiomics on prostate cancer detection: a systematic review of clinical applications. Curr Opin Urol 2020;30:754–81.
20. Qi Y. Random forest for bioinformatics. Ensemble Mach Learn Methods Appl 2012;307–23.
21. Chiu PKF, Shen X, Wang G, et al. Enhancement of prostate cancer diagnosis by machine learning techniques: an algorithm development and validation study. Prostate Cancer Prostatic Dis 2022;25:672–6.

22. Wang J, Wu CJ, Bao ML, et al. Machine learning-based analysis of MR radiomics can help to improve the diagnostic performance of PI-RADS v2 in clinically relevant prostate cancer. Eur Radiol 2017;27:4082–90.

23. Roweis S. EM algorithms for PCA and SPCA. Adv Neural Inf Process Syst. Published online 1998;626–32.

24. Kaneko M, GiE Cacciamani, Yang Y, et al. MP09-05 Automated prostate gland and prostate zones segmentation using a novel mri-based machine learning framework and creation of software interface for users annotation. J Urol 2023;209:105–6.

25. Becker AS, Chaitanya K, Schawkat K, et al. Variability of manual segmentation of the prostate in axial T2-weighted MRI: A multi-reader study. Eur J Radiol 2019;121:108716.

26. Salimi A, Pourmina MA, Moin MS. Fully automatic prostate segmentation in MR images using a new hybrid active contour-based approach. Signal, Image Video Process. 2018;12:1629–37.

27. Litjens G, Toth R, van de Ven W, et al. Evaluation of prostate segmentation algorithms for MRI: The PROMISE12 challenge. Med Image Anal 2014;18:359–73.

28. Shelhamer E, Long J, Darrell T. Fully Convolutional Networks for Semantic Segmentation. IEEE Trans Pattern Anal Mach Intell 2017;39:640–51.

29. Wang B, Lei Y, Tian S, et al. Deeply supervised 3D fully convolutional networks with group dilated convolution for automatic MRI prostate segmentation. Med Phys 2019;46:1707–18.

30. Ushinsky A, Bardis M, Glavis-Bloom J, et al. A 3D-2D Hybrid U-Net Convolutional Neural Network Approach to Prostate Organ Segmentation of Multiparametric MRI. AJR Am J Roentgenol 2021;216(1):111–6.

31. Isensee F, Jaeger PF, Kohl SAA, et al. nnU-Net: a self-configuring method for deep learning-based biomedical image segmentation. Nat Methods 2021;18:203–11.

32. Rodrigues NM, Silva S, Vanneschi L, et al. A Comparative Study of Automated Deep Learning Segmentation Models for Prostate MRI. Cancers 2023;15:1–21.

33. Bardis M, Houshyar R, Chantaduly C, et al. Segmentation of the prostate transition zone and peripheral zone on mr images with deep learning. Radiol Imaging Cancer 2021;3.

34. Abreu AL, Cacciamani G, Kaneko M, et al. MP09-06 Assessment of a novel bpmri-based machine learning framework to automate the detection of clinically significant prostate cancer using the pi-cai (prostate imaging: cancer ai) challenge dataset. J Urol 2023;209:2023.

35. Kaneko M, Cacciamani GE, Magoulianitis V, et al. MP55-20 a novel machine learning framework for automated detection of prostate cancer lesions confirmed on mri-informed target biopsy. J Urol 2023;209:771–2.

36. Ogbonnaya CN, Zhang X, Alsaedi BSO, et al. Prediction of clinically significant cancer using radiomics features of pre-biopsy of multiparametric MRi in men suspected of prostate cancer. Cancers 2021;13.

37. Varghese B, Chen F, Hwang D, et al. Objective risk stratification of prostate cancer using machine learning and radiomics applied to multiparametric magnetic resonance images. Sci Rep 2019;9:1–10.

38. Demšar J. Statistical comparisons of classifiers over multiple data sets. J Mach Learn Res 2006;7:1–30.

39. Hosseinzadeh M, Saha A, Brand P, et al. Deep learning–assisted prostate cancer detection on biparametric MRI: minimum training data size requirements and effect of prior knowledge. Eur Radiol 2022;32:2224–34.

40. Pellicer-Valero OJ, Marenco Jiménez JL, Gonzalez-Perez V, et al. Deep learning for fully automatic detection, segmentation, and Gleason grade estimation of prostate cancer in multiparametric magnetic resonance images. Sci Rep 2022;12:1–13.

41. Castillo Tovar JM, Arif M, Starmans MPA, et al. Classification of clinically significant prostate cancer on learning and radiomics. Cancers 2022;14:12.

42. Bourbonne V, Fournier G, Vallières M, et al. External validation of an MRI-derived radiomics model to predict biochemical recurrence after surgery for high-risk prostate cancer. Cancers 2020;12.

43. Yan Y, Shao L, Liu Z, et al. Deep learning with quantitative features of magnetic resonance images to predict biochemical recurrence of radical prostatectomy: A multi-center study. Cancers 2021;13.

44. Losnegård A, Reisæter LAR, Halvorsen OJ, et al. Magnetic resonance radiomics for prediction of extraprostatic extension in non-favorable intermediate- and high-risk prostate cancer patients. Acta Radiol 2020;61:1570–9.

45. Turkbey B, Rosenkrantz AB, Haider MA, et al. Prostate Imaging Reporting and Data System Version 2.1: 2019 Update of Prostate Imaging Reporting and Data System Version 2. Eur Urol 2019;76:340–51.

46. Smith CP, Harmon SA, Barrett T, et al. Intra- and interreader reproducibility of PI-RADSv2: A multi-reader study. J Magn Reson Imag 2019;49:1694–703.

47. Qi Y, Zhang S, Wei J, et al. Multiparametric MRI-Based Radiomics for Prostate Cancer Screening With PSA in 4–10 ng/mL to Reduce Unnecessary Biopsies. J Magn Reson Imag 2020;51:1890–9.

48. Li M, Chen T, Zhao W, et al. Radiomics prediction model for the improved diagnosis of clinically significant prostate cancer on biparametric MRI. Quant Imag Med Surg 2020;10:368–79.

49. Hiremath A, Shiradkar R, Fu P, et al. An integrated nomogram combining deep learning, Prostate Imaging–Reporting and Data System (PI-RADS) scoring, and clinical variables for identification of clinically significant prostate cancer on biparametric MRI: a retrospective multicentre study. Lancet Digit Heal 2021;3:e445–54.

50. Roest C, Kwee TC, Saha A, et al. AI-assisted biparametric MRI surveillance of prostate cancer: feasibility study. Eur Radiol 2023;33:89–96.

51. Li T, Sun L, Li Q, et al. Development and Validation of a Radiomics Nomogram for Predicting Clinically Significant Prostate Cancer in PI-RADS 3 Lesions. Front Oncol 2022;11:1–9.

52. Gui S, Lan M, Wang C, et al. Application Value of Radiomic Nomogram in the Differential Diagnosis of Prostate Cancer and Hyperplasia. Front Oncol 2022;12:1–8.

53. Lu Y, Li B, Huang H, et al. Biparametric MRI-based radiomics classifiers for the detection of prostate cancer in patients with PSA serum levels of $4\sim10$ ng/mL. Front Oncol 2022;12:1–12.

54. Sunoqrot MRS, Saha A, Hosseinzadeh M, et al. Artificial intelligence for prostate MRI : open datasets , available applications , and grand challenges. Eur Radiol Exp 2022. https://doi.org/10.1186/s41747-022-00288-8.

55. Strubell E, Ganesh A, McCallum A. Energy and Policy Considerations for Deep Learning in NLP. 2019. Available at: http://arxiv.org/abs/1906.02243.

56. Crossnohere NL, Elsaid M, Paskett J, et al. Guidelines for Artificial Intelligence in Medicine: Literature Review and Content Analysis of Frameworks. J Med Internet Res 2022;24.

Artificial Intelligence and Pathomics: Prostate Cancer

Puria Azadi Moghadam, MSc[a,1], Ali Bashashati, PhD[b,c,1],
S. Larry Goldenberg, OC, CM, MD, FRCSC, FCAHS[d,2,*]

KEYWORDS

- Digital pathology • Artificial intelligence • Machine learning • Deep learning • Pathomics

KEY POINTS

- The ability of computers to perform cognitive tasks is reshaping our world and our health care system, with exponentially growing interest in pathomic applications.
- Machine learning applied to digitally scanned histology slides enables the rapid and accurate diagnosis of cancerous lesions, resulting in improved workflow, efficiency, reproducibility, decreased costs, and training opportunities.
- Fusing clinical and molecular data with manually engineered and convolutional neural network–extracted features from hematoxylin and eosin and alternatively stained tissue yields markedly better risk models for predicting tumor behavior, individual response to treatment options as well as overall survival.
- Medicine is rapidly adapting to the application of AI to pathomics; however, challenges remain in applying algorithms to populations from diverse sites and with yet unexplored ethical and regulatory challenges of data privacy, data security, transparency, accountability and the potential for algorithm bias and discrimination.

INTRODUCTION

Since the introduction of the hematoxylin and eosin (H&E)-stained slide in 1876 as the primary tool in the pathologist's toolbox up until the last decade, few tools, other than the invention of immunohistochemistry in 1974 and the introduction of DNA sequencing in the 1970s have been created to enhance diagnostics and prognostics in cancer care. Today, we are in an exciting, paradigm-shifting era with high-resolution digitized histology slides and artificial intelligence (AI) applications offering the capacity to not only diagnose various grades of cancer in a histopathologic slide but to identify features that may not be appreciated by the human occipital lobes, such as targetable mutations, which may alter treatment decisions and provide the opportunity for personalized care and prognosis; this will be doable without the need to interrogate actual tissue with costly and often unavailable molecular assays. Today, AI offers the reality of more accurate and efficient differentiation of benign from malignant cells, of decreasing inter- and intraobserver variability in the grading of cancer lesions, of correlating to molecular features of a heterogeneous tumor, and ultimately aiding the patient and the bedside physician in making more informed treatment decisions.

[a] Department of Electrical and Computer Engineering, University of British Columbia, 2332 Main Mall, Vancouver, British Columbia V6T 1Z4, Canada; [b] School of Biomedical Engineering, University of British Columbia, 2222 Health Sciences Mall, Vancouver, British Columbia V6T 1Z3, Canada; [c] Department of Pathology and Laboratory Medicine, University of British Columbia, 2211 Wesbrook Mall, Vancouver, BC V6T 1Z7, Canada; [d] Department of Urologic Sciences, University of British Columbia, 2775 Laurel Street, Vancouver British Columbia V5Z 1M9, Canada
[1] Co-first authors.
[2] Senior author.
* Corresponding author.
E-mail address: l.gold@ubc.ca

Urol Clin N Am 51 (2024) 15–26
https://doi.org/10.1016/j.ucl.2023.06.001
0094-0143/24/Crown Copyright © 2023 Published by Elsevier Inc. All rights reserved.

Digitization and Workflow of a Pathology Laboratory

Fig. 1 depicts the workflow of tissue processing and analysis in a modern pathology laboratory. When a specimen is received, it is first assigned a block accession number, and its visual characteristics, including tissue type, size, and description are documented; this is a tedious and time-intensive process.

The next steps are tissue processing, embedding, sectioning, and staining. Tissue processing and staining are largely automated; however, the 2 middle steps, embedding and sectioning, are highly technical and crucially important tasks; automation of these processes is in its early days. Once the stained tissue slides are dry, they are manually sorted and distributed among the laboratory's pathologists.

High-throughput pathology slide scanners are now capable of digitizing routine histopathology slides in an unprecedented scale. For example, a next-generation scanner is capable of scanning a slide at 40x magnification in just 32 seconds, delivering 450 high-quality, high-resolution slide images in less than 6 hours. These scanners are essentially robotic microscopes that move a slide underneath a microscope's objective lens, record the images, and stitch them together to create a digital copy.

These advances open up the opportunities for the implementation of digital pathology workflows for clinical sign-out as well as new exciting opportunities for the use of diagnostic support tools powered by machine learning and AI.

Artificial Intelligence Applied to Pathology

The microscopic study of diseased tissue by pathologists has been a cornerstone in cancer diagnosis and prognostication for more than a century. But histologic diagnoses face many challenges, including cellular variations in heterogeneous tumors that are a mosaic of cells containing different genetic and molecular alterations. Questions remain about how well histologic similarity reflects tumor biological similarity, given that tumors with the same histology can progress in different ways, and tumors that have contrasting histology can progress in the same way.

In recent years, there has been a surge of interest in applying computational tools (computer vision algorithms; deep learning [DL] methods such as deep convolutional neural networks [CNN] and their extensions) that allow machine-learning (ML) processes to analyze and classify digitized histology slides into several classes such as benign, low-grade cancer, and high-grade cancer. In this approach, a computer is "trained" using a data set of sample images of tumors that have been annotated and classified by pathologists. Because of their extremely large size, in the order of 0.1 to 10 gigapixels, classification of digitized whole slide images presents a challenge in processing. This challenge can be overcome by dividing each slide into many smaller image "patches," which are typically square and only a few thousand pixels in size (**Fig. 2**). ML techniques then extract a set of prespecified hand-crafted features from each patch or region of interest, and the computer uses the classification information to develop its own pattern-recognition criteria with which to differentiate benign prostate from cancerous lesions. Common examples of explicit features in a region of interest include number of glands, individual cells, or the nuclei per unit area. The computed features are then fed into a standard classifier such as support vector machines, random forests, or Bayesian classifiers to perform the classification.

Another class of methods that have become popular in recent years are based on DL, which are not limited to the hand-crafted features that can be biased by the existing domain knowledge (see **Fig. 2**). DL avoids the feature engineering step by performing the feature learning and classification in a single framework.[1] Given sufficient training data and proper training, these should be able to discover better discriminative visual patterns and lead to superior results, but in the medical domain these are challenged by a scarcity of labeled training data.

ARTIFICIAL INTELLIGENCE PATHOMICS IN PROSTATE CANCER
Cancer Diagnosis and Gleason Grading

The AI-based identification of prostate cancer on a histology slide and its grading remains challenging. It is a highly relevant and prevalent

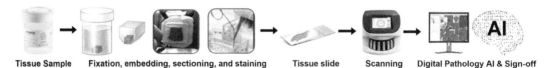

Tissue Sample   Fixation, embedding, sectioning, and staining   Tissue slide   Scanning   Digital Pathology AI & Sign-off

Fig. 1. Modern pathology laboratory workflow.

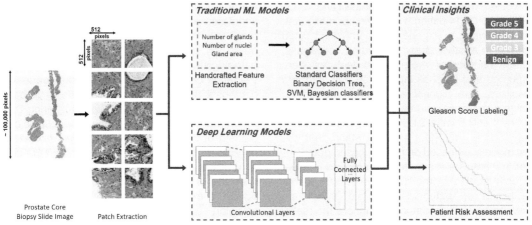

Fig. 2. Artificial intelligence–based pathology image analysis of a prostate core biopsy. Histopathology slide images are first divided into small patches (eg, 512 × 512 pixels). Next, they are fed into traditional ML (eg, SVM, RF) or DL models (eg, convolutional neural networks) for training to identify specific patterns in the images. The trained model provides the labels for each patch as well as the overall predictions (eg, Gleason score, risk of disease recurrence) for a given patient. RF, random forest; SVM, support vector machine.

disease and is also very heterogeneous, both within and between individuals. The Gleason scoring system dates back to 1966, and its application by the pathologist[2] has been at the core of predicting tumor behavior, leading to the stratification of tumors into low-, intermediate-, and high-risk categories. Despite its indisputable role in prognostication and patient management, Gleason scoring by pathologists is a subjective exercise and suffers from suboptimal interobserver and intraobserver variability, with reported Gleason score discordance ranging from 30% to 53%[3–6] (**Fig. 3**).

With the increase of AI in computer vision, various models have been developed for prostate cancer diagnosis and grading.[7] Initial ones were based on ML of handcrafted features for "cancer versus benign" or "low- versus high-grade" classification on small cohorts of patients.[8,9] Doyle and colleagues,[8] for instance, achieved a positive

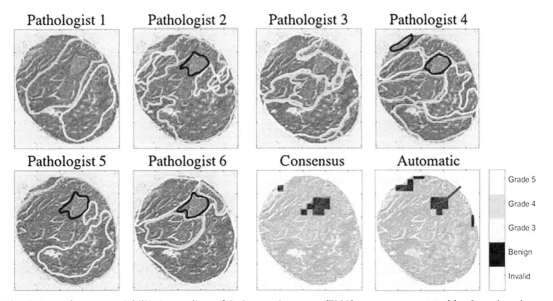

Fig. 3. Interobserver variability in grading of 2 tissue microarray (TMA) cores as annotated by 6 genitourinary (GU) pathologists and an example of an automatic classifier in good overall agreement with the consensus of the multiple pathologist annotations. Upgraded and downgraded areas are still in agreement with some pathologists. Arrow indicates a benign focus (Unpublished; from the authors' laboratory).

predictive value of 86% in classifying 2000 patches from 214 patients as benign or malignant, similar to what an experienced pathologist could achieve. In another study by Nir and colleagues, a large number of morphologic features were computed and used as input to several standard classifiers. The highest accuracy in classifying benign versus cancerous and grade 3 versus grades 4 and 5 were 91.6% and 79.1%, respectively.[10] It is important to understand that the best models are based on patient-based patch images that have been annotated for ground truth (ie, correctly labeled) by multiple experts. Studies that are based on patch-wise images and/or are reviewed by a single pathologist ignore the reality of interobserver variability and lead to less reliable classification and overfitting (see **Fig. 3**).[7]

Next, DL CNN-based models were developed, which automatically "learned" to extract the correlated morphologic patterns from individually scanned patches. In 2018, Arvanity and colleagues[11] introduced an AI algorithm for Gleason grading of tissue microarray cores using detailed pathologists' annotations of a discovery cohort of 641 patients. They evaluated their model on a test cohort of 245 patients and achieved a 0.71 inter-annotator agreement with pathologists (Cohen's quadratic kappa statistical) and achieved pathology expert-level stratification of patients into prognostically distinct groups (based on cohort survival data). Also in 2018, Nir and colleagues published[10] a grading CNN model based on 333 cores from 231 patients and approximately 16,000 patches. Their patient-based cross-validation accuracy, sensitivity, and specificity for cancer detection (benign vs malignant) and cancer grading (3 vs 4 and 5) were 85.8, 86.3, 85.5 and 81.2, 82.4, 82.0, respectively. They proved the importance of multiple expert annotations to the development of an accurate ML model.

Karimi and colleagues described a method of combining the predictions of 3 separate CNNs that work with different patch sizes to augment the available training data and improve the accuracy of classification. Their method achieved an accuracy of 92% in classifying cancerous patches versus benign patches and an accuracy of 90% in classifying low-grade (ie, Gleason grade 3) from high-grade (ie, Gleason grades 4 and 5) patches. These experiments indicated that data augmentation with DL-based methods can achieve expert-level performance.[12]

Subsequent breakthroughs in the applicability of DL models toward reproducible prostate cancer AI diagnostic tools started in 2019 with the introduction of models trained and tested on *very large* cohorts. A team at Google health used 112 million annotated patches from 1226 slides of prostatectomy patients to train a DL model and then validated on a set of 331 slides.[13] Although 29 pathologists had a mean accuracy of 0.61 on the validation cohort, the DL framework produced a diagnostic accuracy of 0.70. In another large database, a team from Memorial Sloan Kettering Cancer Center evaluated a DL framework at scale on a dataset of 24,859 whole slide images from 7159 patients without any form of detailed image-level annotations. Although achieving an area under the curve of 0.991, their model could allow pathologists to exclude 65% to 75% of slides while retaining 100% sensitivity.[14]

In 2020, Bulten and colleagues[15] collected 5759 biopsies from 1243 patients at the Radboud University Medical Center to develop a DL system for biopsy-level grading. Their model achieved high agreement with the reference (kappa 0·918) with high scores at several important clinical decision thresholds (benign vs malignant, the International Society of Urological Pathology [ISUP] grade of 2 or more, and ISUP of 3 or more). Also, in a subsequent observer experiment on 100 biopsy specimens, their system scored kappa of 0·854, outperforming 10 of 15 pathologist observers (median kappa 0·819). In a similar study, an AI model was trained with a total of 6953 slides, and its performance was assessed on a test set and external validation set with 1631 and 330 biopsies, respectively.[16] Although this method could get 0.96 kappa score on the test set, it also performed well on the external dataset (kappa 0.87).

These encouraging results of several DL systems led to the largest histopathology competition (up to now) called PANDA,[17] which was joined by 1290 developers who proposed weakly supervised and automated AI methods for prostate Gleason grading. A total of 10,616 digitized multicenter prostate biopsies were used in this challenge. The algorithms were evaluated, fully blinded to developers, on external sets from different continents and showed agreements of 0.862 (quadratically weighted kappa) and 0.868 with expert genitourinary (GU) pathologists. This competition proved that multiple AI models could generalize well on diverse populations of patients from different centers for Gleason grading.

Finally, in 2021, the US Food and Drug Administration (FDA) authorized the marketing of software, called Paige Prostate,[18] as the first-to-market AI-based software designed to identify an area of interest on a scanned prostate biopsy image for it to be further reviewed and signed off by a pathologist. This software is a cloud-based service accessed through a Web browser that compares the tissue patterns using a model that was trained on a large database collected at the Memorial Sloan Kettering Cancer Center and assists in the differentiation of benign from malignant glands.

Prediction and Prognostication

Although most of the research efforts, so far, have focused on the deployment of AI models for diagnostics and grade classification, the holy grail of biomarker research lies in the potential for ML to provide, in a prospective manner, both predictive and prognostic information that an individual and his physician would use to make an informed decision on the type of, timing of, and duration of individualized treatment. The National Comprehensive Cancer Network (NCCN) risk categories are predictive to a degree, but a spectrum of outcomes still exists within each of the current 6 categories (very low risk, low risk, favorable intermediate, unfavorable intermediate, high and very high risk[19]). Molecular assays based on RNA expression markers have been developed to enhance the predictive power of these clinical variables.[20–23] But these genomic markers require access to and consumption of prostate tissue, and since nearly all of these tests lack validation in prospective randomized clinical trials in the intended use population, have significant costs, laboratory requirements, and processing time,[24] there has been little to no adoption outside of the United States. Liquid biopsy[25] (circulating tumor DNA) has the potential to avoid tissue acquisition; however it has low sensitivity in early stage cancers. Modern imaging with multiparametric MRI is useful for diagnostics, less so for prognostics. And all of these approaches are also limited by the need for human labor, availability, and cost.

Thus, an ML histology–based predictive biomarker would be reliable, lower cost, massively scalable, and rapidly and readily available in a digital world through the distribution of scanned slides over the cloud to centers of expertise; no need for tissue sacrifice, shipping across borders, or processing as is required for molecular genomic markers via RNA extraction from tissue! And with high specificity, it could potentially diminish overtreatment and diminish toxicity while maximizing effectiveness of a personalized therapy.

Until recently, the correlation between digital pathologic algorithms and ultimate disease outcome has been relatively underexplored, mainly due to the extensive difficulty of tracking patients through a long multiyear follow-up period. In 2021, Wulczyn and colleagues[26] from Google Health introduced a cohort of prostatectomy cases with 2807 patients (Gleason grades are reported in the original path report for 1517 cases), who were tracked for 5 to 25 years. They developed a DL risk assessment model for prostate cancer–specific mortality. Following the patients' stratification into subgroups, based on the model's risk scores, this tool achieved a concordance index (c-index) of 0.82, confirming the AI tools' potential for substantial performance in prognostic applications compared with traditional hazard models.

Clinical, biochemical, pathologic, imaging, and other biological features have all been included in the creation of ever-larger "fused" databases to enable better predictive and prognostic stratification of patients with newly diagnosed prostate cancer.[27–29] So could AI-derived histopathologic interrogations similarly be improved by combining with other markers in a multimodal approach, such as integrating histopathology features and genomic data through deep neural networks? This was explored in 2 studies by Ren and colleagues for predicting recurrence among patients with prostate cancer diagnosed with Gleason score 7 cancer.[30,31] They used CNN features plus genomic data injected into long short-term memory networks (a popular version of recurrent neural networks) and could identify a set of biomarkers for risk of recurrence prediction with a c-index of 0.74 and a hazard ratio of 5.73. In comparison with conventional markers, histogenomic patterns showed a stronger link with outcome, and the authors demonstrated with their model that higher risks are associated with 4 + 3 Gleason score compared with 3 + 4.[30]

Another example of a DL multimodal approach is work being conducted by the investigators in the highly relevant clinical situation involving the issue of overtreatment, as it relates to choosing invasive therapy versus active surveillance at the time of prostate cancer diagnosis. Our team has built an automatic ML pipeline for risk assessment that combines clinicopathologic data with manually engineered and CNN-extracted features from H&E and Ki67-stained histology slides.[32] This pipeline yielded better risk models in predicting biochemical recurrence as well as overall survival compared with the state-of-the-art CAPRA-S model. We validated the utility of the proposed pipeline on a dataset of 502 patients. In a striking finding we reclassified 10 CAPRA-S high-risk patients as low-risk and another 10 low-risk patients as high-risk. These findings emphasize the potential of a multimodal DL-based biomarker to guide patients through choosing between active surveillance and definitive treatment and could potentially introduce significant changes in prostate cancer management.

ArteraAI is a multimodal digital pathology–based platform recently approved for the purpose of identifying patients who will benefit from therapy intensification with androgen deprivation therapy (ADT) and thus help guide treatment decisions for men with localized intermediate-risk prostate cancer undergoing radiation therapy. A self-supervised[33] multimodal DL architecture was developed to learn from both clinicopathologic and digital imaging histopathology data and identify differential outcomes by treatment type. The model was trained on clinical and digitized pathology data from 5 radiation therapy randomized controlled trials that included 5654 patients with more than 1000 high-risk individuals. The training cohort included 3935 patients with a median follow-up of 13.6 years, and the ADT classifier was validated on a cohort of 1719 men with a median follow-up of 17.6 years.[34] Esteva and colleagues[35] showed that the Artera model could outperform the standard NCCN risk models by 9.2% to 14.6% on a validation set.

In the diagnosis of colorectal cancer (CRC), Tsai and colleagues[36] have recently reported the exciting development of a Multi-omics Multicohort Assessment (MOMA) ML framework for connecting whole-slide digital histopathology images with multiomics biomarkers and survival outcomes. Their model was trained using patients' age, sex, cancer stage, and outcomes, as well as genomic, epigenetic, protein, and metabolic profiles of the tumors of approximately 2000 patients with CRC. They were able to predict the response to specific therapies, overall survival, disease-free survival, and copy-number alterations and identify interpretable pathology patterns predictive of gene expression profiles, microsatellite instability status, and clinically actionable genetic alterations. MOMA outperformed human pathologists and other current AI models.

For patients with prostate cancer it is highly probable that in the near future, multimodal (MOMA) approaches will combine digital histopathology with radiomics, genomics, and clinical variables to further optimize predictive and prognostic models and inform treatments.

IMPLEMENTATION IN THE CLINIC: CHALLENGES AND NEXT STEPS

Although significant progress has been made in improving the utility of digital pathology ML models within the context of prostate cancer, we believe that several advancements are still required before massive scaling and adoption of these models should occur in the clinical realm.

Digital Pathology Infrastructure and Model Reliability

The implementation of AI digital pathology tools in the clinic requires significant investments in whole slide image scanners and information technology infrastructure. Several studies have analyzed the costs and benefits associated with transitioning from traditional to digital pathology frameworks,[37,38] and although these upfront costs are significant, gains in efficiency and productivity in the long run do justify their implementation. For the wider applicability of AI systems in low-resourced countries or in parts of the world that lack access to prostate pathology expertise, other strategies such as the AI-driven augmented reality microscope built by Google Health could be beneficial.[39] This system projects the classification results from a trained DL network onto a display that is in line with the ocular lens of a microscope providing real-time feedback while a pathologist views the slides.

AI models will also be required to have robust performance on data derived from different hospitals and health settings. As an example, the performance of AI diagnostic models can be negatively affected by color variations in whole slide images due to variations in staining protocols, tissue thickness, stain concentration, reagent manufacturer, scanner models, digitization protocols,[40] or even room conditions.[41,42] In an ideal scenario, AI software should be able to handle this variability in the quality of slides. As such, several strategies to handle or harmonize color variations have been proposed such as through various statistical matching,[43,44] color-deconvolution,[45,46] or generative adversarial networks (GAN).[47] These technologies still require further improvements to increase the robustness of the AI models in multiple settings.

Artificial Intelligence as the Pathologist's Diagnostic Adjunct: Prospective Evaluation

The need to explore the utility and impact of AI on a pathologist's case-to-case decision-making is important for understanding the possible limitations and biases of digital pathomics. Automation and overreliance biases are among the significant potential challenges that need to be evaluated in real scenario trials. The former is defined as a tendency to accept AI decisions instead of a diagnosis based on the physician's scientific knowledge and expertise.[48] The latter refers to overreliance on AI that causes gradual erosion of the skills needed to perform the automated tasks independently.[49] A randomized, controlled study by Harada and colleagues[50] examined the effect of an AI support system that was based on patients' clinical information on a physician's differential diagnosis. The investigators report that the differential diagnosis provided by the AI tool had a significant influence on 15% of physician's working diagnosis. Cabitza and colleagues[51] performed a study on the impact of 2 DL models supporting 12 certified radiologists' double reading of knee lesions on MRI. They showed that an appropriate interaction between AI tools and radiologists can outperform the performance of either alone. Such studies need to be done in digital pathology to assess the utility of AI systems and how they could affect the final clinical decision-making process.

Role of Artificial Intelligence in Pathology Training

Generative adversarial networks are among the most seminal recent ideas in the field of AI.[47] Although discriminative methods intend to map data (eg, images, genomics, texts) to a limited domain such as a subtype or grade, generative methods are able to learn the underlying distribution of a dataset and can synthesize random samples similar to the training dataset (**Fig. 4**). One such generative model is DALL-E,[52] which is an AI tool to synthesize high-quality images from text inquiries. ChatGPT is another generative tool that is able to produce sequences of text based on the user prompt.

Similarly, generative models have multiple applications in histopathology such as creating indefinite numbers of synthetic histology images for educational purposes or proficiency testing,[53,54]

especially when there is a lack of labeled data for uncommon malignancies. GANs could also overcome privacy protection regulations,[54] as synthetic pathology images generated within a specific center can easily be shared with collaborators anywhere on the globe. In addition, time, labor, and economic costs associated with gathering and labeling histology slides increase the chance of AI tools overfitting.[55] Synthetic generated pathology images can be used to augment training datasets as a potential solution for such overfitting.

The most common generative models are GAN-based[47] networks. Levine and colleagues[53] used a progressive GAN (ie, a GAN model that gradually increases the size of images) to produce high-quality diagnostic images of multiple cancer types. However, GAN models suffer from extensive instability during their training process. Recently, a newer set of generative models called diffusion models[56] were introduced with a stable training advantage, and these are the backbone of some of the current famous tools such as DALL-E.[52] Inspired by similar approaches, it is interesting to synthesize histopathology patches from gene expressions or mutation information to have numerous novel paired samples for rare cases. Azadi and colleagues,[54] have introduced a diffusion probabilistic model to generate synthetic images of low-grade glioma from genotypes including various isocitrate dehydrogenase (*IDH*) mutations. Prostate pathology AI, similar to other cancer types, can benefit from synthesized images in educational, privacy, and performance aspects.

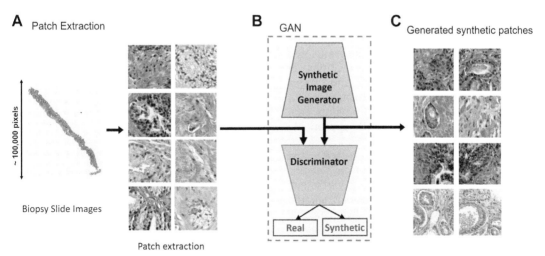

A Patch Extraction   **B** GAN   **C** Generated synthetic patches

~ 100,000 pixels

Biopsy Slide Images

Patch extraction

Synthetic Image Generator

Discriminator

Real | Synthetic

Fig. 4. Generative Adversarial Network's framework for synthesizing histopathology images. (*A*) A set of original patches are extracted from whole slide images. (*B*) Generator produces synthetic images, and the discriminator intends to distinguish between the real and synthetic samples. The discriminator provides feedback to the generator to improve the quality of the synthetic images. (*C*) Samples of synthesized images.

Regulatory Considerations

AI has the potential to change pathology practice; however, it is not likely that such algorithms will replace pathologists[57] and much is being written about the introduction and updating of regulations on the applications of AI models in pathology.[58,59]

When a new solution for a health need is proposed based on medical research, regulatory science is responsible for review and evaluation of the existing legislation and submission/approval policies and the related risks and benefits.[60] It is important that the implemented regulations balance the risks and profits coming from using AI systems and should not cause overregulation, underregulation, or misregulation. The former may prevent the introduction of innovative products, whereas the latter may increase the risk of harm for the patients.[58,59]

The data used in developing the contemporary AI algorithms should contain the adequate number of datapoints with the highest quality and integrity (ie, without crucial errors), while preserving the privacy of the participating patients.[48,61] Therefore, updated data-sharing protocols are needed to balance the quality of data and patients' privacy without causing a significant limitation on developing generalized AI models, which need to be trained and validated on diverse and large datasets.

POTENTIAL NEW DIRECTIONS AND TECHNOLOGIES

Although the morphologic assessment of H&E-stained slides has not changed in the past 100 years as the basis of the surgical pathology practice, researchers are exploring other tissue imaging modalities to derive more biological insights from tissue sections. These underexplored optical modalities as a single source of data or their combination with each other and normal H&E images may result in better biomarkers for precise and quick classification of prostate cancer into clinically relevant and appropriate subgroups.

Hyperspectral imaging is able to record scene information through a high number of wavelengths (normally more than 200 bands) in the visible and invisible range of the spectrum, including infrared or ultraviolet domain. As a result, hyperspectral cameras provide a wealth of information about the scene, allowing for greater knowledge even when they are invisible to the human eye or RGB-based camera systems. There are a variety of uses for them in the military, remote sensing, pollution monitoring, and so on.[62,63] They are also valuable in the medical field such as for early skin cancer detection[64] or vein visualization.[65] Recently, individual application of hyperspectral imaging or its combination with histopathology slides in solid tumor detection,[66] breast cancer cell segmentation,[67] or prostate cancer identification[68] has been explored as a rich source of information for improving AI multimodal strategies.

High-throughput 3-dimensional (3D) light-sheet microscopic imaging has enabled the 3D study of biospecimens.[69] Compared with 2D histology sections, the interpretation of prostate needle biopsies from a nondestructive 3D-glandular structure is more accurate.[70] In addition to providing bigger specimens, volumetric imaging, and measurement of microstructures that are important for diagnosis, 3D pathology also preserves the specimen structure for further investigation.[71] In a recent study published in 2022, Xie and colleagues[70] scanned 300 biopsies (118 with tumor), and by using them in an end-to-end AI framework, they showed the superior performance of 3D pathology structures for stratification of patients with prostate cancer.

Raman spectroscopy is another optical tool that can have a high utility in tissue and/or biofluid analysis.[72] This modality examines the molecular signature of endogenous cellular biomolecules under biocompatible settings with great spatial resolution and can offer prostate cancer biopsy examination (fast-acquisition approaches function in near real-time), surgical margin evaluation, and treatment efficacy monitoring.[72] Grosset and colleagues[73] released their case-control study with multicohort validation on identification of intraductal carcinoma in prostate, high-grade prostatic intraepithelial neoplasia, prostate cancer, and benign tissue using the combination of an AI tool and Raman microspectroscopy. Their results indicate that Raman microspectroscopy may improve high-risk patients with prostate cancer classification and provide higher reliability on intraductal carcinoma detection.

SUMMARY

We are in a very exciting time in the practice of surgical pathology that has remained largely unaltered for almost 150 years. The staggering rate of expansion of DL applications over the past decade and our ability to digitize slides have opened novel and exciting avenues for rapid, efficient, and accurate prostate cancer diagnosis, prediction, and prognostication. Workflow systems and high-throughput slide scanners are allowing for more efficient, faster, and cheaper systems and opens the door to improved slide management, access and preservation, telepathology, image manipulation, collaborative research, teaching, and training. With the increasing number of biopsy specimens, decreasing number of general pathologists and especially the scarcity of subspecialty-trained GU pathologists, fewer medical trainees entering pathology training programs, and the increasing quantity and complexity of pathology cases, taking advantage of AI will be crucial to preserve and increase efficiency and diagnostic accuracy in pathology laboratories, whether in a high-throughput academic setting or in a small hospital in a remote geography. In fact, prostate cancer is already the first area in pathology to adopt AI-based solutions to decrease pathology workload by triaging benign biopsy samples and directing pathologists to review the biopsy samples that potentially contain tumor deposits without expelling any slides containing cancer; this approach has led to the first FDA-approved AI-based pathology product for in vitro diagnostics.

Obtaining a comprehensive molecular profile of a tumor specimen is certainly useful, especially when combined with microscopic examination, and might be the way forward, as medical treatments become ever-more personalized to the characteristics of an individual's tumor. However, for now, histology remains indispensable for disease classification because the standard approaches for specimen preservation and examination by microscopy offer the most accessible and universal entry point in the routine diagnostic workflow used in clinical laboratories worldwide. A disease can manifest itself in both molecular and cellular changes; therefore, an approach that integrates both molecular analysis and visual inspection might strengthen diagnostic capabilities.

Despite the potential benefits of AI in prostate pathology, there are also several limitations and challenges that need to be addressed. One of the main challenges is the availability and quality of data. In order to train and validate AI systems large and diverse data sets are required. There is currently a lack of standardization in the field that can make it difficult to compare the performance of different systems and limit the generalizability of software trained on specific data sets that may not perform as well when applied to different populations or settings. False-negative and false-positive results may be mitigated by AI's use as an adjunct and by the professional evaluation by the pathologist who can take into account the patient's clinical information and who may perform additional laboratory studies on the samples before rendering a final diagnosis. There are important ethical and legal considerations that need to be taken into account when developing and applying AI systems in pathology. These considerations include issues related to data privacy, data security, transparency, accountability, and the potential for algorithm bias and discrimination.

The PANDA challenge has cemented the position of AI-based analysis of digitized slides as beyond hype and as today's reality. In the future, AI will not replace pathologists—it will only replace those who do not use AI in their daily practice.

DISCLOSURE

None of the authors have any commercial or financial conflicts of interest to disclose. This work was supported by a Canadian Institutes of Health Research (CIHR) grant to AB and LG and Michael Smith Health Research BC Scholar grant to AB.

REFERENCES

1. Goldenberg SL, Nir G, Salcudean SE. A new era: artificial intelligence and machine learning in prostate cancer. Nat Rev Urol 2019;16(7):391–403.
2. Epstein JI, Zelefsky MJ, Sjoberg DD, et al. A Contemporary Prostate Cancer Grading System: A Validated Alternative to the Gleason Score. Eur Urol 2016;69(3):428–35.
3. Persson J, Wilderäng U, Jiborn T, et al. Interobserver variability in the pathological assessment of radical prostatectomy specimens: Findings of the Laparoscopic Prostatectomy Robot Open (LAPPRO) study. Scand J Urol 2014;48(2):160–7.
4. Egevad L, Ahmad AS, Algaba F, et al. Standardization of Gleason grading among 337 European pathologists. Histopathology 2013;62(2):247–56.
5. Netto GJ, Eisenberger M, Epstein JI. Interobserver Variability in Histologic Evaluation of Radical Prostatectomy Between Central and Local Pathologists: Findings of TAX 3501 Multinational Clinical Trial. Urology 2011;77(5):1155–60.
6. Allsbrook WC, Mangold KA, Johnson MH, et al. Interobserver reproducibility of Gleason grading of prostatic carcinoma: General pathologist. Hum Pathol 2001;32(1):81–8.
7. Nir G, Karimi D, Goldenberg SL, et al. Comparison of Artificial Intelligence Techniques to Evaluate Performance of a Classifier for Automatic Grading of Prostate Cancer From Digitized Histopathologic Images. JAMA Netw Open 2019;2(3):e190442.
8. Doyle S, Feldman M, Tomaszewski J, et al. A boosted Bayesian multiresolution classifier for prostate cancer detection from digitized needle biopsies. IEEE Trans Biomed Eng 2012;59(5):1205–18.
9. Gorelick L, Veksler O, Gaed M, et al. Prostate histopathology: learning tissue component histograms

for cancer detection and classification. IEEE Trans Med Imag 2013;32(10):1804–18.

10. Nir G, Hor S, Karimi D, et al. Automatic grading of prostate cancer in digitized histopathology images: Learning from multiple experts. Med Image Anal 2018;50:167–80.

11. Arvaniti E, Fricker KS, Moret M, et al. Automated Gleason grading of prostate cancer tissue microarrays via deep learning. Sci Rep 2018;8(1): 12054.

12. Karimi D, Nir G, Fazli L, et al. Deep Learning-Based Gleason Grading of Prostate Cancer From Histopathology Images—Role of Multiscale Decision Aggregation and Data Augmentation. IEEE J Biomed Health Inform 2020;24(5):1413–26.

13. Nagpal K, Foote D, Liu Y, et al. Development and validation of a deep learning algorithm for improving Gleason scoring of prostate cancer. Npj Digit Med 2019;2(1):1–10.

14. Campanella G, Hanna MG, Geneslaw L, et al. Clinical-grade computational pathology using weakly supervised deep learning on whole slide images. Nat Med 2019;25(8):1301–9.

15. Bulten W, Pinckaers H, Boven H van, et al. Automated deep-learning system for Gleason grading of prostate cancer using biopsies: a diagnostic study. Lancet Oncol 2020;21(2):233–41.

16. Ström P, Kartasalo K, Olsson H, et al. Artificial intelligence for diagnosis and grading of prostate cancer in biopsies: a population-based, diagnostic study. Lancet Oncol 2020;21(2):222–32.

17. Bulten W, Kartasalo K, Chen PHC, et al. Artificial intelligence for diagnosis and Gleason grading of prostate cancer: the PANDA challenge. Nat Med 2022;28(1):154–63.

18. Commissioner O of the. FDA Authorizes Software that Can Help Identify Prostate Cancer. FDA. Published October 1, 2021. Accessed April 24, 2023. https://www.fda.gov/news-events/press-announcements/fda-authorizes-software-can-help-identify-prostate-cancer.

19. Moses KA, Sprenkle PC, Bahler C, et al. NCCN Guidelines® Insights: Prostate Cancer Early Detection, Version 1.2023: Featured Updates to the NCCN Guidelines. J Natl Compr Cancer Netw 2023;21(3):236–46.

20. Capitanio U, Briganti A, Gallina A, et al. Predictive models before and after radical prostatectomy. Prostate 2010;70(12):1371–8.

21. Kattan MW, Cuzick J, Fisher G, et al. Nomogram incorporating PSA level to predict cancer-specific survival for men with clinically localized prostate cancer managed without curative intent. Cancer 2008;112(1):69–74.

22. Tewari A, Johnson CC, Divine G, et al. Long-term survival probability in men with clinically localized prostate cancer: a case-control, propensity modeling study stratified by race, age, treatment and comorbidities. J Urol 2004;171(4):1513–9.

23. Kornberg Z, Cooperberg MR, Spratt DE, et al. Genomic biomarkers in prostate cancer. Transl Androl Urol 2018;7(3). 45971-45471.

24. Gaudreau PO, Stagg J, Soulières D, et al. The Present and Future of Biomarkers in Prostate Cancer: Proteomics, Genomics, and Immunology Advancements: Supplementary Issue: Biomarkers and their Essential Role in the Development of Personalised Therapies (A). Biomarkers Cancer 2016. 8s2: BIC.S31802.

25. Herberts C, Annala M, Sipola J, et al. Deep whole-genome ctDNA chronology of treatment-resistant prostate cancer. Nature 2022;608(7921):199–208.

26. Wulczyn E, Nagpal K, Symonds M, et al. Predicting prostate cancer specific-mortality with artificial intelligence-based Gleason grading. Commun Med 2021;1(1):1–8.

27. Thurtle DR, Greenberg DC, Lee LS, et al. Individual prognosis at diagnosis in nonmetastatic prostate cancer: Development and external validation of the PREDICT Prostate multivariable model. PLoS Med 2019;16(3):e1002758.

28. Stephenson AJ, Scardino PT, Eastham JA, et al. Postoperative nomogram predicting the 10-year probability of prostate cancer recurrence after radical prostatectomy. J Clin Oncol Off J Am Soc Clin Oncol 2005;23(28):7005–12.

29. Kattan MW, Eastham J. Algorithms for prostate specific antigen recurrence after treatment of localized prostate cancer. Clin Prostate Cancer 2003; 1(4):221–6.

30. Ren J, Karagoz K, Gatza M, et al. Differentiation among prostate cancer patients with Gleason score of 7 using histopathology whole-slide image and genomic data. Proc SPIE-Int Soc Opt Eng 2018; 10579:1057904.

31. Ren J, Karagoz K, Gatza ML, et al. Recurrence analysis on prostate cancer patients with Gleason score 7 using integrated histopathology whole-slide images and genomic data through deep neural networks. J Med Imaging Bellingham Wash 2018;5(4): 047501.

32. Shao Y, Bazargani R, Karimi D, et al. Improved Prostate Cancer Risk Stratification by Digital Histopathology and Deep Learning. In: Medical Image Computing and Computer Assisted Interventions (MICCAI) Conference. ; 2023.

33. Jing L, Tian Y. Self-Supervised Visual Feature Learning With Deep Neural Networks: A Survey. IEEE Trans Pattern Anal Mach Intell 2021;43(11):4037–58.

34. Spratt DE, Sun Y, Van der Wal D, et al. An AI-derived digital pathology-based biomarker to predict the benefit of androgen deprivation therapy in localized prostate cancer with validation in NRG/RTOG 9408. J Clin Oncol 2022;40(6_suppl):223.

35. Esteva A, Feng J, van der Wal D, et al. Prostate cancer therapy personalization via multi-modal deep learning on randomized phase III clinical trials. NPJ Digit Med 2022;5(1):71.

36. Tsai PC, Lee TH, Kuo KC, et al. Histopathology images predict multi-omics aberrations and prognoses in colorectal cancer patients. Nat Commun 2023; 14(1):2102.

37. Ho J, Ahlers SM, Stratman C, et al. Can Digital Pathology Result In Cost Savings? A Financial Projection For Digital Pathology Implementation At A Large Integrated Health Care Organization. J Pathol Inf 2014;5:33.

38. Hanna MG, Reuter VE, Samboy J, et al. Implementation of Digital Pathology Offers Clinical and Operational Increase in Efficiency and Cost Savings. Arch Pathol Lab Med 2019;143(12):1545–55.

39. Chen PHC, Gadepalli K, MacDonald R, et al. An augmented reality microscope with real-time artificial intelligence integration for cancer diagnosis. Nat Med 2019;25(9):1453–7.

40. Yagi Y. Color standardization and optimization in Whole Slide Imaging. Diagn Pathol 2011;6(Suppl 1):S15.

41. Lyon HO, De Leenheer AP, Horobin RW, et al. Standardization of reagents and methods used in cytological and histological practice with emphasis on dyes, stains and chromogenic reagents. Histochem J 1994;26(7):533–44.

42. Bancroft JD. Theory and Practice of Histological Techniques. Elsevier Health Sciences; 2008.

43. Jain AK. Fundamentals of Digital Image Processing. Prentice-Hall, Inc.; 1989.

44. Reinhard E, Adhikhmin M, Gooch B, et al. Color transfer between images. IEEE Comput Graph Appl 2001;21(5):34–41.

45. Khan AM, Rajpoot N, Treanor D, et al. A Nonlinear Mapping Approach to Stain Normalization in Digital Histopathology Images Using Image-Specific Color Deconvolution. IEEE Trans Biomed Eng 2014;61(6):1729–38.

46. Vahadane A, Peng T, Sethi A, et al. Structure-Preserving Color Normalization and Sparse Stain Separation for Histological Images. IEEE Trans Med Imag 2016;35(8):1962–71.

47. Goodfellow IJ, Pouget-Abadie J, Mirza M, et al. Generative adversarial nets. In: Proceedings of the 27th International Conference on Neural Information Processing Systems - Volume 2. NIPS'14. MIT Press 2014;2672–80.

48. Coppola F, Faggioni L, Gabelloni M, et al. Human, All Too Human? An All-Around Appraisal of the "Artificial Intelligence Revolution" in Medical Imaging. Front Psychol 2021;12.

49. Cabitza F, Rasoini R, Gensini GF. Unintended Consequences of Machine Learning in Medicine. JAMA 2017;318(6):517–8.

50. Harada Y, Katsukura S, Kawamura R, et al. Effects of a Differential Diagnosis List of Artificial Intelligence on Differential Diagnoses by Physicians: An Exploratory Analysis of Data from a Randomized Controlled Study. Int J Environ Res Publ Health 2021;18(11):5562.

51. Cabitza F, Campagner A, Sconfienza LM. Studying human-AI collaboration protocols: the case of the Kasparov's law in radiological double reading. Health Inf Sci Syst 2021;9(1):8.

52. Ramesh A, Pavlov M, Goh G, et al. Zero-Shot Text-to-Image Generation. Published online February 26, 2021. doi:10.48550/arXiv.2102.12092.

53. Levine AB, Peng J, Farnell D, et al. Synthesis of diagnostic quality cancer pathology images by generative adversarial networks. J Pathol 2020; 252(2):178–88.

54. Moghadam P.A., Van Dalen S., Martin K.C., et al., A Morphology Focused Diffusion Probabilistic Model for Synthesis of Histopathology Images. In: Proceedings of the IEEE/CVF Winter Conference on Applications of Computer Vision (WACV); 2023, 2000-2009.

55. Lan L, You L, Zhang Z, et al. Generative Adversarial Networks and Its Applications in Biomedical Informatics. Front Public Health 2020;8:164.

56. Ho J, Jain A, Abbeel P. Denoising Diffusion Probabilistic Models. Adv Neural Inf Process Syst 2020;33:6840–51. Curran Associates, Inc.

57. Sharma G, Carter A. Artificial Intelligence and the Pathologist: Future Frenemies? Arch Pathol Lab Med 2017;141(5):622–3.

58. Allen TC. Regulating Artificial Intelligence for a Successful Pathology Future. Arch Pathol Lab Med 2019;143(10):1175–9.

59. Lennerz JK, Green U, Williamson DFK, et al. A unifying force for the realization of medical AI. Npj Digit Med 2022;5(1):1–3.

60. Marble HD, Huang R, Dudgeon SN, et al. A Regulatory Science Initiative to Harmonize and Standardize Digital Pathology and Machine Learning Processes to Speed up Clinical Innovation to Patients. J Pathol Inf 2020;11:22.

61. Pesapane F, Volonté C, Codari M, et al. Artificial intelligence as a medical device in radiology: ethical and regulatory issues in Europe and the United States. Insights Imaging 2018;9(5):745–53.

62. Borengasser M, Hungate WS, Watkins R. Hyperspectral Remote Sensing: Principles and Applications. CRC Press 2007.

63. Kefauver SC, Peñuelas J, Ustin SL. Applications of hyperspectral remote sensing and GIS for assessing forest health and air pollution. In: 2012. IEEE International Geoscience and Remote Sensing Symposium 2012;3379–82.

64. Leon R, Martinez-Vega B, Fabelo H, et al. Non-Invasive Skin Cancer Diagnosis Using Hyperspectral

Imaging for In-Situ Clinical Support. J Clin Med 2020;9(6):1662.

65. Sharma N. and Hefeeda M., Hyperspectral reconstruction from RGB images for vein visualization. *Proceedings of the 11th ACM multimedia systems conference. MMSys '20, 2020, Association for Computing Machinery*, New York, NY, 77–87 https://dl.acm.org/doi/proceedings/10.1145/3339825.

66. Zhang Y, Wu X, He L, et al. Applications of hyperspectral imaging in the detection and diagnosis of solid tumors. Transl Cancer Res 2020;9(2):1265–77.

67. Ortega S, Halicek M, Fabelo H, et al. Hyperspectral imaging and deep learning for the detection of breast cancer cells in digitized histological images. Proc SPIE-Int Soc Opt Eng 2020;11320: 113200V.

68. Akbari H, Halig LV, Schuster DM, et al. Hyperspectral imaging and quantitative analysis for prostate cancer detection. J Biomed Opt 2012;17(7): 076005.

69. Glaser AK, Reder NP, Chen Y, et al. Multi-immersion open-top light-sheet microscope for high-throughput imaging of cleared tissues. Nat Commun 2019;10(1): 2781.

70. Xie W, Reder NP, Koyuncu C, et al. Prostate Cancer Risk Stratification via Nondestructive 3D Pathology with Deep Learning-Assisted Gland Analysis. Cancer Res 2022;82(2):334–45.

71. Liu JTC, Glaser AK, Bera K, et al. Harnessing nondestructive 3D pathology. Nat Biomed Eng 2021; 5(3):203–18.

72. Gaba F, Tipping WJ, Salji M, et al. Raman Spectroscopy in Prostate Cancer: Techniques, Applications and Advancements. Cancers 2022;14(6):1535.

73. Grosset AA, Dallaire F, Nguyen T, et al. Identification of intraductal carcinoma of the prostate on tissue specimens using Raman micro-spectroscopy: A diagnostic accuracy case–control study with multi-cohort validation. PLoS Med 2020;17(8):e1003281.

Genomics and Artificial Intelligence: Prostate Cancer

Elyssa Y. Wong, BS, Timothy N. Chu, BS, Seyedeh-Sanam Ladi-Seyedian, MD*

KEYWORDS

• Genomics • Prostate cancer • Artificial intelligence • Machine learning

KEY POINTS

- Commercially available machine learning (ML)-based genomic classifiers are now incorporated into clinical guidelines and recommendations for the better management of patients with prostate cancer.
- The integration of artificial intelligence with traditional methods of genomic analysis can leverage the strengths of both, yielding a more robust and comprehensive assessment.
- ML-based approaches have the potential to enhance personalized medicine and allow for tailored interventions that optimize therapeutic outcomes.

INTRODUCTION

Management of patients with prostate cancer (PCa) is often challenging due to the difference in the biology of cancer between patients and the various genetic alterations involved in this cancer. Generally, transcriptome and genomic analysis have generated new information regarding PCa and the intracellular signaling pathways that regulate prostate carcinogenesis, thereby advancing our understanding of the disease's biology.[1] Increasing enthusiasm has greeted the incorporation of molecular profiling and genomic-based risk prediction models throughout the past decade.[2] Genetic research has used machine learning (ML) and artificial intelligence (AI) to uncover gene expression profiles for the construction of statistical models to predict clinical outcomes and pave the way for personalized therapy.[3]

Molecular signatures derived from gene expression profiling have become important risk-assessment tools to aid in therapeutic decision-making for PCa, such as identifying candidates for active surveillance, choosing the type and intensity of treatment, and determining the benefit of adjuvant therapy or multimodal therapy.

Decipher, Oncotype DX Genomic Prostate Score, and Prolaris are some of the commercially available ML-based genomic classifiers that are being incorporated into clinical guidelines and recommendations for the better management of patients with PCa.[4]

In this article, we aimed to provide an overview of recent discoveries in the fields of genomics of PCa and AI, which are expected to improve the clinical management of patients with PCa.

BIOLOGY OF PROSTATE CANCER

PCa oncogenesis involves complex interactions between inherited susceptibility, acquired somatic gene alterations, and microenvironmental and macroenvironmental factors. Localized PCa often has multiple foci with various genetic alterations that have different capacities for metastatic seeding and inherent treatment resistance.[5]

The adult human prostate is anatomically separated into 3 zones: central, transition, and peripheral. Most PCa develops in the outermost peripheral zone.[6] Genetically altered basal or luminal prostate epithelial cells can cause high-grade lesions that resemble adenocarcinomas.

Catherine & Joseph Aresty Department of Urology, Center for Robotic Simulation & Education, Norris Comprehensive Cancer Center, University of Southern California, Los Angeles, CA, USA
* Corresponding author. University of Southern California Institute of Urology, 1441 Eastlake Avenue Suite 7416, Los Angeles, CA 90089.
E-mail address: Sanam.Seyedian@med.usc.edu

Urol Clin N Am 51 (2024) 27–33
https://doi.org/10.1016/j.ucl.2023.06.006

Prostatic intraepithelial neoplasia seems as luminal epithelial cell hyperproliferation with decreased or loss of basal epithelium and is regarded to be a probable precursor to malignancy; it frequently co-occurs with prostate adenocarcinoma.[7,8] In high-grade prostatic intraepithelial neoplasia lesions, the multilayered luminal epithelium has various markers of transformation, including the loss of basal markers p63 (TP63), cytokeratin 5 (KRT5), and KRT14; the gain of luminal markers, such as KRT8 and KRT18; and the overexpression of the enzyme alpha methylacyl-CoA racemase, which is associated with adenocarcinoma.[6,9] TMPRSS2 gene has been linked to luminal differentiation. A gene fusion between TMPRSS2 and ERG, an oncogenic transcription factor, is the most common chromosomal aberration in PCa, causing carcinogenesis in more than 50% of cases.[6]

Early genomic aberrations include TMPRSS2-ERG fusions in 40% to 60% of patients, SPOP loss-of-function mutations in 5% to 15%, and FOXA1 gain-of-function mutations in 3% to 5%. PTEN deletions and TP53 mutations occur in 10% to 20% of localized PCas and more than 50% of advanced diseases.[10]

Changes in androgen receptor (AR) gene signaling are the major cause of resistance to androgen deprivation therapy. Metastatic castration-resistant prostate cancer (mCRPC) commonly has AR pathway alterations due to amplification or gain-of-function mutations, increased AR transcription, or enhanced AR signaling. Loss of dependence on AR signaling occurs in 15% to 20% of advanced, treatment-resistant, prostate tumors and can present as castration-resistant neuroendocrine PCa, which is highly treatment-resistant.[11] mCRPC progression is linked to the dysregulation of additional growth control and genetic stability genes. PIK3CA, PIK3CB, and AKT1 gain-of-function mutations account for 5% of mCRPC cases, whereas PTEN homozygous deletions and loss-of-function mutations account for more than 40%.[12] Twenty to 30% of mCRPC cases show WNT signaling pathway activation and MYC oncogene overexpression, and 20% to 50% have TP53 or RB1 mutations. RB1 deletion worsens mCRPC prognosis.[13,14]

DNA damage response (DDR) genes are also important in PCa. Men with inherited BRCA1 or BRCA2 mutations have a 3-fold to 8-fold increased lifetime risk of PCa, which can be aggressive due to additional MYC activation in combination with TP53 and PTEN inactivation.[15,16] PCa risk also increases with inherited mutations in MLH1, MSH2, and PMS2 (Eeles 2013).[17] Twenty three percent of metastatic prostate tumors have somatic aberrations in DDR gene (mostly BRCA2, ATM, BRCA1, CHEK2, CDK12, and PALB2).[18,19]

ARTIFICIAL INTELLIGENCE IN IDENTIFICATION OF GENOMIC ALTERATION SIGNATURES

ML algorithms can identify somatic gene signatures and clinically relevant patterns of genomic alterations that can predict PCa prognosis and provide an avenue for the development of novel therapeutic strategies. In a study by Liu and colleagues, ML models were applied to distinguish epitranscriptomic biomarkers in the periprostatic adipose tissue for predicting localized PCa and locally advanced PCa. They established a framework for evaluating the relationship between CpG methylation and gene expression levels in the periprostatic adipose tissue and recognized 30 genes with downregulation and hypermethylation in their promoter regions that can predict the metastasis and progression risk of patients with PCa. Among these 30 genes, which were enriched in DNA replication and cell regulation pathways, WRAP73 (WD Repeat Containing, Antisense to TP73) was significantly altered differently in metastatic patients versus primary patients. In addition to WRAP73, 5 other protein-coding genes were significantly differentially mutated between the primary and metastasis patients. These genes were POLR3K (RNA Polymerase III Subunit K), EEF1D (Eukaryotic Translation Elongation Factor 1 Delta), IGFALS (Insulin Like Growth Factor Binding Protein Acid Labile Subunit), H2AW (H2A.W Histone), and FASTK (Fas Activated Serine/Threonine Kinase).[20]

In another study by Xie and colleagues, ML was used to predict lymph node metastasis based on alternative splicing, which is a specific modality of gene expression and has an important role in gene expression regulation and gene mutation modulation. This study revealed that alternative splicing types in PCa without lymph node metastasis were distinct from those with lymph node metastasis. The model could detect lymph node metastasis before the surgery, which may optimize surgical planning and adjuvant treatments.[21] Lin and colleagues applied ML algorithms to next-generation sequencing of circulating cell-free DNA data to find targetable patterns of genomic alterations associated with the progression from metastatic castration-sensitive PCa to a castration-resistant state. The algorithms revealed repetitive patterns of genomic mutations in the RTK, PI3K, MAPK, and G1/S signaling pathways that were linked with metastatic castration-resistant PCa and could distinguish between samples from patients with metastatic castration-resistant PCa and samples of patients with metastatic castration-sensitive PCa. These findings demonstrated that the progression from castration-sensitive metastatic PCa to a castration-resistant state is accompanied by an accumulation of genetic changes in both MAPK and PI3K signaling. The detection of these alterations in cell-free DNA may alleviate the difficulties of obtaining tumor bone biopsies and enable the development of targeted therapies.[22]

ARTIFICIAL INTELLIGENCE-BASED GENOMICS IN DIAGNOSIS OF PROSTATE CANCER

Genomic analysis has revolutionized our understanding of PCa, revealing specific genetic alterations, mutations, and gene expression patterns associated with the disease. As genomics continues to evolve, the integration of AI, particularly ML and deep learning (DL), has emerged as a powerful tool for the diagnosis of PCa.

AI has shown promise in the analysis of pathogenic variants in patients with PCa. For instance, a study by AlDubayan and colleagues demonstrated the superior performance of a DL method over a standard germline detection method in identifying pathogenic variants.[23] Interestingly, the study found that the highest number of pathogenic variants were identified when both DL and standard methods were used together, suggesting that AI can complement, rather than replace, traditional methods. AI has also been instrumental in analyzing the genomic profile of tumor tissue or circulating tumor DNA, helping to identify potential biomarkers that distinguish PCa from normal tissue and other benign conditions. ML models offer the ability to analyze complex and high-dimensional genomic data while considering multiple genomic features simultaneously. This capability has been demonstrated in a study by Dong and colleagues, where a gene score calculated from the relative expression quantities of 30 key genes was used to predict normal prostate samples and PCa samples with high accuracy.[24]

The application of AI has also assisted with merging genomic analysis with the histopathological evaluation of prostate biopsy tissue, a mainstay of diagnosing PCa. Several studies have found that AI algorithms can successfully detect and grade tumors, reaching expert-level performance and agreement rates with expert uropathologists. Furthermore, the increased computational power of ML models has allowed for the integration of histologic imaging data with immunohistochemistry and molecular genetic techniques, reducing the need for additional, labor-intensive testing and potentially contributing to more accurate prognostic information.

The integration of AI with omics data, such as transcriptomics, epigenomics, and proteomics, is another promising area of research. For example, a study by Penney and colleagues used ML to predict PCa tumors versus normal tissues from metabolite profiles.[25] Similarly, Pachynski and colleagues used an AI-based algorithm to investigate the underlying molecular, cellular, and spatial differences between multiparametric MRI (mpMRI)-visible and mpMRI-invisible PCa, correlating these differences with multiomic data.[26]

In conclusion, AI has been instrumental in analyzing and understanding sequencing data, which holds promise for the development of personalized clinical strategies for PCa management. Because more genomic data become available and AI algorithms continue to evolve, we can expect to see significant advancements in this field. However, it is important to remember that ML models are dependent on the quality and quantity of the data they are trained on. Therefore, the integration of AI with traditional methods can leverage the strengths of both, yielding a more robust and comprehensive approach to genomic analysis in PCa.

ARTIFICIAL INTELLIGNCE-BASED GENOMICS IN PROGNOSIS OF PROSTATE CANCER

ML algorithms have also been used to develop predictive models that estimate the risk of disease progression, recurrence, or metastasis in patients with PCa. These models integrate genomic data with clinical variables, imaging, and other relevant information to generate personalized risk scores or treatment recommendations. For example, the Decipher Prostate genomic classifier and the P-NET artificial neural network have demonstrated accurate prediction of metastasis in patients with PCa based on their genomic profiles.[27] Zheng and colleagues focused on the development of a genomic-clinicopathologic nomogram for predicting lymph node invasion in PCa. Their nomogram combines a 37-gene-based support vector machine model based on the differential expression of genes between lymph node invasive and nonlymph node invasive PCa and combines this with Gleason grade.[28] In another study, Zhang and colleagues defined a risk prediction model using the methylation status of 6 CpG islands that were generated through ML. Their model was found to predict the prognosis of cancer-specific deaths or biochemical recurrences (BCRs) with AUCs of 0.823 at 3 years, 0.844 at 5 years, and 0.891 at 7 years.

Furthermore, the authors used their model to stratify the risk of patients.[29]

Cheng and colleagues used ML algorithms and identified a novel prognosis signature based on differentially expressed long noncoding RNA related to cuproptosis, a form of programmed cell death. The constructed signature was found to be closely associated with several clinical traits, immune cell infiltration, immune-related functions, immune checkpoints, gene mutation, tumor mutational burden, microsatellite instability, and drug sensitivity.[30] These findings could potentially be used to improve clinical outcomes for patients with PCa by providing a more personalized approach to treatment based on the patient's unique genomic profile.

Some studies used ML methodologies to identify specific prognostic genes related to PCa. Wang and colleagues used 3 ML-based algorithms (LASSO, random forest and boruta, XGboost) to select critical features from all cellular senescence genes. By using 5 cohorts of 1159 patients, 3 common genes were identified (SPAG 5, TACC3, TROAP), which they used to create a prognostic predictor that averaged an AUC of 0.7 for 1-year, 3-year, and 5-year progression of PCa.[31]

Other studies have looked at DNA-based prognostic biomarkers by using ML methods. For example, Shepherd and colleagues used a random forest approach to identify specific combinations of 5 mRNAs (CAV1, THBS1, CTGF, IMP2, and AKT1), which could distinguish between high (≥8) versus low (≤6) Gleason score PCa good accuracy. They applied this data to a progression-free survival model, which achieved an accuracy of 63.61% when combined with PSA data.[32] Liu and colleagues explored tRNA-derived fragments (tRFs) to determine the prognosis for PCa. Using ML, they identified 8 tRFs of interest, which they combined into one tRF score as a prognostic signature. They achieved an AUC of 0.792 for 5-year disease free and an AUC of 0.815 when combined with Gleason scores.[33] These studies show the utility of using ML to further explore the genes related to PCa to improve our ability to improve prognostic prediction for PCa especially when combined with traditional methods.

ARTIFICIAL INTELLIGENCE-BASED GENOMICS IN THE TREATMENT OF PROSTATE CANCER
Disease Monitoring and Treatment Response

Because genomic advances with the incorporation of AI, there has been a focus on predicting treatment responses for patients with PCa. By analyzing the genetic makeup of PCa cells and integrating it with AI models, urologists can gain objective data on the characteristics of prostate tumors. This has the potential to enhance personalized medicine and allow for tailored interventions that optimize therapeutic outcomes. Multiple studies have used genomic features to attempt and predict treatment responses to better tailor individualized therapeutic regimens for patients. Dejong and colleagues used an ML-based prediction model trained on data from the CPCT0-2 cohort to predict the response of mCRPC to enzalutamide and abiraterone with an AUC of 0.82.[34] Chawla and colleagues created a predictive ML model called Precily, which is meant to predict treatment responses using gene expression data and showed that their PTEN-negative LNCap PCa cell lines were more sensitive to PI3Kinase/mTOR signaling targeting drugs (iparasertib, afuresertib, and so forth).[35] Snow and colleagues trained a deep neural network targeting PCa cells with gain-of-function mutations in ARs to assess their response to therapy (darolutamide). Of 44 mutations, they correctly predicted that 12 mutations would be nonresponsive and 31 would be antagonized by darolutamide.[36]

AI has also been used to assess the genetic characteristics of PCa cells to better understand what factors may lead to different responses to treatment. Huang and colleagues used an eXtreme gradient Boosting model, which was used to assess robust replication stress signatures (RSS), which reflects DNA replication stress. Higher RSS scores were associated with Tp53, RB, and PTEN deletions, which were used to assess the therapeutic vulnerability of PCa.[37] Xie and colleagues used an artificial neural network to classify patients with PCa into 2 plasma molecular subtype categories that were used to predict response to immunotherapy. They observed that patients in their plasma cell group subtype 1 had a significantly lower chance of responding to immunotherapy compared with plasma cell subtype 2 group, $P < .001$.[38] These studies highlight the ability of AI-based genomics to identify various genetic signatures that can provide insight into improving therapeutic regimens, which will provide maximal clinical benefit for patients affected by PCa.

Recurrence

BCR of PCa remains one of the primary concerns for any clinician treating patients afflicted by this malignancy. Several studies have attempted to combine genomics with AI in an attempt to better understand potential drivers for BCR. Some studies have identified specific genes that were predictive of BCR. Fan and colleagues used an ML method trained on RNA-seq data from 327 patients with PCa with Cox regression analysis to construct an angiogenesis-related biosignature to predict BCR of PCa. They identified 3 key genes (NRP1, JAG2, and VCAN) in a training cohort and successfully validated these genes in 3 independent cohorts as prognostic factors with an AUC greater than 0.7 in their training set and greater than 0.65 in their validation set.[39] Vittrant and colleagues trained a random forest model trained on gene expression data from 3 RNA-seq data sets totaling 171 patients with PCa, which identified a 3 gene biomarker signature (JUN, HES 4, and PPDPF), which predicted BCR with better accuracy (74.2%) than clinicopathological variables (69.2%).[40]

AI has also been used to identify biomarkers of interest in the prediction of BCR. Huang and colleagues created an AI method using a deep convolutional neural network that identifies pathologic regions of interest trained on whole slide images (n = 243) from The Cancer Genome Atlas Prostatic Adenocarcinoma database, which was able to predict 3-year BCR with an AUC of 0.78. They subsequently performed a biomarker analysis using their DL method and identified TMEM173 as a biomarker of interest in terms of predicting BCR.[41] Pinckaers and colleagues developed a morphologic biomarker (DLS) using a DL system that was trained on a nested-case control study of 685 patients and validated their model on an independent cohort of 204 patients. The DLA marker was able to predict the speed of BCR with an odds ratio of 3.32 (CI 1.63–6.77; $P = .001$) from their test set.[42] One study used mRNA as a variable to predict BCR and developed a random survival forest model that was able to achieve AUC's of 0.824 and 0.772 for 2-year and 5-year BCR-free survival, respectively.[43] These studies reflect the potential that AI has in helping better predict BCR, which has important implications in the management and treatment of patients with PCa.

SUMMARY

The study of PCa from a genomic standpoint can benefit immensely from the computational power and pattern recognition offered by ML models. In today's clinics, Decipher, Oncotype DX Genomic Prostate Score, and Prolaris are some of the commercially available ML-based genomic classifiers that are being used to predict outcomes and guide management. These efforts continue to be expanded on because ML models are applied to

novel biomolecules to better define unique molecular signatures correlating with metastasis and disease progression.

By using AI to understand the genetic drivers of PCa, we will be able to better tailor treatment strategies based on an individual patient's genomic profile. Urologists can use this tool to make informed decisions regarding the best treatment strategies, surgical planning, as well as targeted therapies, which will maximize survivability and quality of life for patients being treated for PCa. Ultimately, these tools may facilitate a paradigm shift in the guideline-based treatment of PCa toward personalized and precise care for each individual patient.

CLINICS CARE POINTS

- In today's clinics, Decipher, Oncotype DX Genomic Prostate Score, and Prolaris are some of the commercially available ML-based genomic classifiers that are being used to predict outcomes and guide management.

DISCLOSURES

The authors declare no commercial or financial conflicts of interest or any funding sources.

FUNDING/SUPPORT

No funding.

REFERENCES

1. Ikeda S, Elkin SK, Tomson BN, et al. Next-generation sequencing of prostate cancer: genomic and pathway alterations, potential actionability patterns, and relative rate of use of clinical-grade testing. Cancer Biol Ther 2019;20(2):219–26.
2. Ross AE, D'Amico AV, Freedland SJ. Which, when and why? Rational use of tissue-based molecular testing in localized prostate cancer. Prostate Cancer Prostatic Dis 2016;19(1):1–6.
3. Libbrecht MW, Noble WS. Machine learning applications in genetics and genomics. Nat Rev Genet 2015;16(6):321–32.
4. Li R, Zhu J, Zhong WD, et al. Comprehensive evaluation of machine learning models and gene expression signatures for prostate cancer prognosis using large population cohorts. Cancer Res 2022;82(9): 1832–43.
5. Sandhu S, Moore CM, Chiong E, et al. Prostate cancer. Lancet 2021;398(10305):1075–90.

6. Rebello RJ, Oing C, Knudsen KE, et al. Prostate cancer. Nat Rev Dis Primers 2021;7(1):9.

7. Lee SH, Shen MM. Cell types of origin for prostate cancer. Curr Opin Cell Biol 2015;37:35–41.

8. Park JW, Lee JK, Phillips JW, et al. Prostate epithelial cell of origin determines cancer differentiation state in an organoid transformation assay. Proc Natl Acad Sci U S A 2016;113(16):4482–7.

9. Sfanos KS, Yegnasubramanian S, Nelson WG, et al. The inflammatory microenvironment and microbiome in prostate cancer development. Nat Rev Urol 2018;15(1):11–24.

10. Fraser M, Sabelnykova VY, Yamaguchi TN, et al. Genomic hallmarks of localized, non-indolent prostate cancer. Nature 2017;541(7637):359–64.

11. Quigley DA, Dang HX, Zhao SG, et al. Genomic hallmarks and structural variation in metastatic prostate cancer. Cell 2018;174(3):758–69.e9.

12. Carver BS, Chapinski C, Wongvipat J, et al. Reciprocal feedback regulation of PI3K and androgen receptor signaling in PTEN-deficient prostate cancer. Cancer Cell 2011;19(5):575–86.

13. Abida W, Cyrta J, Heller G, et al. Genomic correlates of clinical outcome in advanced prostate cancer. Proc Natl Acad Sci U S A 2019;116(23):11428–36.

14. Armenia J, Wankowicz SAM, Liu D, et al. The long tail of oncogenic drivers in prostate cancer. Nat Genet 2018;50(5):645–51.

15. Taylor RA, Fraser M, Rebello RJ, et al. The influence of BRCA2 mutation on localized prostate cancer. Nat Rev Urol 2019;16(5):281–90.

16. Taylor RA, Fraser M, Livingstone J, et al. Germline BRCA2 mutations drive prostate cancers with distinct evolutionary trajectories. Nat Commun 2017;8:13671.

17. Eeles R, Goh C, Castro E, et al. The genetic epidemiology of prostate cancer and its clinical implications. Nat Rev Urol 2014;11(1):18–31.

18. Robinson D, Van Allen EM, Wu YM, et al. Integrative clinical genomics of advanced prostate cancer. Cell 2015;161(5):1215–28.

19. Mateo J, Seed G, Bertan C, et al. Genomics of lethal prostate cancer at diagnosis and castration resistance. J Clin Invest 2020;130(4):1743–51.

20. Liu Q, Reed M, Zhu H, et al. Epigenome-wide DNA methylation and transcriptome profiling of localized and locally advanced prostate cancer: Uncovering new molecular markers. Genomics 2022;114(5):110474.

21. Xie P, Batur J, An X, et al. Novel, alternative splicing signature to detect lymph node metastasis in prostate adenocarcinoma with machine learning. Front Oncol 2022;12:1084403.

22. Lin E, Hahn AW, Nussenzveig RH, et al. Identification of somatic gene signatures in circulating cell-free DNA associated with disease progression in metastatic prostate cancer by a novel machine learning platform. Oncol 2021;26(9):751–60.

23. AlDubayan SH, Conway JR, Camp SY, et al. Detection of pathogenic variants with germline genetic testing using deep learning vs standard methods in patients with prostate cancer and melanoma. JAMA 2020;324(19):1957–69.

24. Dong H, Wang X. Identification of signature genes and construction of an artificial neural network model of prostate cancer. J Healthc Eng 2022;2022:1562511.

25. Penney KL, Tyekucheva S, Rosenthal J, et al. Metabolomics of prostate cancer gleason score in tumor tissue and serum. Mol Cancer Res 2021;19(3):475–84.

26. Pachynski RK, Kim EH, Miheecheva N, et al. Single-cell spatial proteomic revelations on the multiparametric mri heterogeneity of clinically significant prostate cancer. Clin Cancer Res 2021;27(12):3478–90.

27. Elmarakeby HA, Hwang J, Arafeh R, et al. Biologically informed deep neural network for prostate cancer discovery. Nature 2021;598(7880):348–52.

28. Zheng Z, Mao S, Gu Z, et al. A genomic-clinicopathologic nomogram for the prediction of lymph node invasion in prostate cancer. J Oncol 2021;2021:5554708.

29. Zhang E, Hou X, Hou B, et al. A risk prediction model of DNA methylation improves prognosis evaluation and indicates gene targets in prostate cancer. Epigenomics 2020;12(4):333–52.

30. Cheng X, Zeng Z, Yang H, et al. Novel cuproptosis-related long non-coding RNA signature to predict prognosis in prostate carcinoma. BMC Cancer 2023;23(1):105.

31. Wang X, Ma L, Pei X, et al. Comprehensive assessment of cellular senescence in the tumor microenvironment. Brief Bioinform 2022;23(3). https://doi.org/10.1093/bib/bbac118.

32. Shephard AP, Giles P, Mbengue M, et al. Stroma-derived extracellular vesicle mRNA signatures inform histological nature of prostate cancer. J Extracell Vesicles 2021;10(12):e12150.

33. Liu W, Yu M, Cheng S, et al. tRNA-derived rna fragments are novel biomarkers for diagnosis, prognosis, and tumor subtypes in prostate cancer. Curr Oncol 2023;30(1):981–99.

34. de Jong AC, Danyi A, van Riet J, et al. Predicting response to enzalutamide and abiraterone in metastatic prostate cancer using whole-omics machine learning. Nat Commun 2023;14(1):1968.

35. Chawla S, Rockstroh A, Lehman M, et al. Gene expression based inference of cancer drug sensitivity. Nat Commun 2022;13(1):5680.

36. Snow O, Lallous N, Ester M, et al. Deep learning modeling of androgen receptor responses to prostate cancer therapies. Int J Mol Sci 2020;21(16). https://doi.org/10.3390/ijms21165847.

37. Huang RH, Hong YK, Du H, et al. A machine learning framework develops a DNA replication stress model for predicting clinical outcomes and therapeutic vulnerability in primary prostate cancer. J Transl Med 2023;21(1):20.

38. Xie X, Dou CX, Luo MR, et al. Plasma cell subtypes analyzed using artificial intelligence algorithm for predicting biochemical recurrence, immune escape potential, and immunotherapy response of prostate cancer. Front Immunol 2022;13:946209.

39. Fan B, Wang Y, Zheng X, et al. A novel angiogenesis-related gene signature to predict biochemical recurrence of patients with prostate cancer following radical therapy. J Oncol 2022; 2022:2448428.

40. Vittrant B, Leclercq M, Martin-Magniette ML, et al. Identification of a transcriptomic prognostic signature by machine learning using a combination of small cohorts of prostate cancer. Front Genet 2020;11:550894.

41. Huang W, Randhawa R, Jain P, et al. A novel artificial intelligence-powered method for prediction of early recurrence of prostate cancer after prostatectomy and cancer drivers. JCO Clin Cancer Inform 2022; 6:e2100131.

42. Pinckaers H, van Ipenburg J, Melamed J, et al. Predicting biochemical recurrence of prostate cancer with artificial intelligence. Commun Med 2022;2:64.

43. O'Donnell A, Wolsztynski E, Cronin M, et al. Improving the post-operative prediction of bcr-free survival time with mrna variables and machine learning. Cancers 2023;15(4). https://doi.org/10.3390/cancers15041276.

Radiomics and Artificial Intelligence
Renal Cell Carcinoma

Alex G. Raman, MS[a,b], David Fisher, BS[a], Felix Yap, MD[c], Assad Oberai, PhD[d],
Vinay A. Duddalwar, MD, FRCR[a,d],*

KEYWORDS

- Renal carcinoma • Imaging • Artificial intelligence • Radiomics • Kidney • Deep learning

KEY POINTS

- Successful artificial intelligence (AI) algorithms have been built, from a research perspective, for kidney tumor segmentation, classification, grading, and staging.
- Radiomics metrics have been shown to have significant correlations with biological tumor markers and may serve as an additional tool for determining renal cell carcinoma treatment.
- Because there is currently no routinely used clinical AI model for renal cell carcinoma diagnosis, treatment, or prognosis, independent assessments of these models are essential to enable successful clinical integration.

INTRODUCTION
Overview for Clinical Need

Renal cell carcinoma (RCC) accounts for 90% of primary renal cancers and represents a significant cause of morbidity and mortality worldwide. Kidney cancer is the 14th most common cancer globally, with more than 431,000 new cases diagnosed and 179,000 deaths in 2020.[1] Kidney cancer is also a major health-care problem in the United States, with 81,800 estimated new cases and 14,890 estimated deaths in 2023.[2]

Most renal tumors are incidentally diagnosed on routine imaging, often as a small renal mass, which is defined as less than 4 cm. However, imaging appearance is not always diagnostic and there are often overlapping similarities in the appearances of both benign and malignant renal masses. As a result, accurate preoperative characterization of renal masses carries a significant error rate.[3,4] Moreover, 20% to 30% of renal tumors detected on imaging are benign following resection with the majority being less than 4 cm in diameter and identifying these patients beforehand could potentially spare them from unneeded surgery.[5]

Although percutaneous biopsy is playing an increasingly important role in confirming pathologic diagnosis in selected patients, biopsy can be prone to sampling error and life-threatening complications such as bleeding.[6] Imaging has become more frequent and more important as management of RCC has increasingly moved to a less-aggressive approach, with a larger role for active surveillance. Given these factors, there is a need for a robust and noninvasive biomarker to accurately characterize the histologic type of renal masses in a clinical setting.

In routine clinical practice, a combination of qualitative and semiquantitative techniques is used to classify a renal mass as a likely benign or malignant tumor. Visual assessments of the size, contour, attenuation, and tissue-enhancement characteristics are important for determining the probability of cancer.[7]

[a] Department of Radiology, University of Southern California, 1500 San Pablo Street, 2nd Floor, Los Angeles, CA 90033, USA; [b] Western University of Health Sciences, 309 East Second Street, Pomona, CA 91766-1854, USA; [c] Radiology Associates, San Luis Obispo, 1310 Las Tablas Road, Templeton, CA 93465, USA; [d] Viterbi School of Engineering, University of Southern California, 3650 McClintock Avenue, Los Angeles, CA 90089, USA
* Corresponding author. Norris Comprehensive Cancer Hospital, 1441 Eastlake Avenue, NET #2315, Los Angeles, CA 90033.
E-mail address: Vinay.Duddalwar@med.usc.edu

Urol Clin N Am 51 (2024) 35–45
https://doi.org/10.1016/j.ucl.2023.06.007
0094-0143/24/© 2023 Elsevier Inc. All rights reserved.

Finally, in contrast to tumor enhancement being a quantifiable parameter measured in Hounsfield units (HU) on CT, tumor shape in the kidney has typically been a qualitative assessment, often categorized under a binary system as either "regular" or "irregular." This makes visual shape analysis of a tumor contour subjective and susceptible to interobserver or intraobserver interpretation variability. All of these factors motivate the need for algorithms that can consider the large amount of available data in kidney cancer and provide accurate and trustworthy results, whether based on deep learning, radiomics, or other techniques (**Fig. 1**).

Overview for Machine Learning

Machine learning (ML), and in particular, deep learning (DL), now plays an important role in the detection, diagnosis, and prognosis of different types of diseases. This is especially true when these inferences are made using medical images as input. For these applications, the tremendous progress in computer vision algorithms has been brought to bear on medical tasks. Algorithms that were originally developed for automating tasks, such as driving, have now been adapted to medical applications. There are 2 broad classes of DL algorithms that work with medical images. These are algorithms that map images of one type to another type, and algorithms that map images to a single or multiple binary or real variables.

In algorithms that map images to images (**Fig. 2**A), the transformation is often achieved through a U-net architecture.[8] In this architecture, the input image is first successively passed through convolution layers and downsampled, reaching a bottleneck layer. The output of the bottleneck layer is passed through transpose convolutional layers, which successively upsample their input. The output of the downsampling branch is also directly passed to the upsampling branch through skip connections. This simple but highly effective architecture has been remarkably successful in a wide variety of medical imaging tasks that include image segmentation, image denoising, image deblurring, image enhancement, and image transformation and image harmonization.

In algorithms that map images to binary or other types of parameters (**Fig. 2**B), the input image is typically passed through a series of convolutional neural network (CNN) layers leading up to a latent code.[9] The latent code is then passed through several fully connected layers to produce the final output. This output can be a class (malignant/benign, stage), grade, or a parameter of interest (time to recurrence). It is worth noting that the part of the algorithm that maps the latent code to the parameter of interest is not required to be a neural network. Other ML algorithms such as support vector machines and decision trees can also be used for this task.

ML algorithms also play a role when images are first analyzed using radiomics (**Fig. 2**C). In this case, the radiomics analysis yields a set of

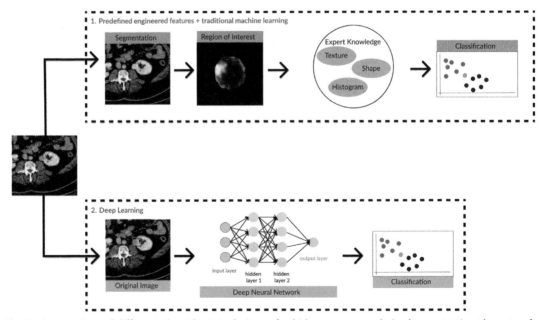

Fig. 1. An overview of different algorithmic techniques for kidney cancer analysis, demonstrating the setup for traditional machine learning as well as deep learning approaches.

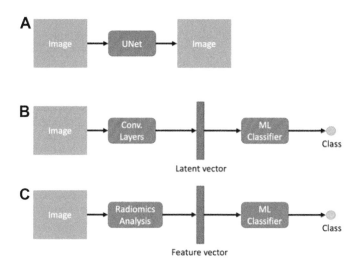

Fig. 2. (*A*) The UNet algorithm for image segmentation, (*B*) a neural network for image classification, and (*C*) a machine learning (ML) algorithm that uses radiomics features for classification.

features that are then used as input to an ML algorithm. Similar to the case discussed above, these algorithms can be neural networks, support vector machines, decision trees, or other classification and/or regression methods. The output of this algorithm is once again a parameter of clinical interest such as the diagnosis of a tumor, quantification of tumor grade, prediction of time to recurrence, and so forth.

DISCUSSION
Artificial Intelligence for Kidney and Tumor Segmentation

Fully automatic segmentation of both the kidney organ and tumor on CT imaging is often seen as a first step in ML-based cancer classification, staging, and treatment planning. The Kits19 and Kits21 challenges have provided an important baseline for the field that allow for the direct comparison of various algorithms on the task of kidney organ and tumor segmentation.[10,11] In each of these online challenges, teams were given access to training data that included CT scans of patients with kidney tumors as well as annotated, "ground truth" labels of where in the CT image the kidneys and tumors were located (**Fig. 3**). The goal of both challenges was to develop an algorithm that would achieve the best "score" on a hidden test dataset. The metric of choice used to judge these algorithms was the Sorenson-Dice coefficient; a measure of overlap between a ground truth and a predicted segmentation.[12]

The Kits19 dataset included preoperative CT imaging from a total of 300 patients who underwent radical or partial nephrectomy at the University of Minnesota between 2010 and 2018. Two hundred and ten patients were included in the training set

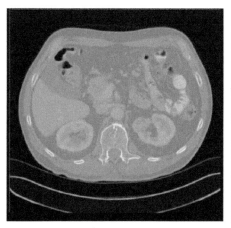
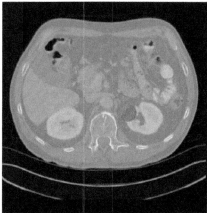

Fig. 3. An example patient from the Kits19 dataset. On the left is the original CT image. On the right is the CT image with kidney (*light blue*) and tumor (*red*) segmentations.

and 90 cases were included in the held-out test set. Tumor subtypes in this challenge included clear cell, clear cell/papillary, papillary, chromophobe, urothelial, multilocular-cystic, Wilms, oncocytoma, angiomyolipoma, mixed epithelial/stromal, spindle-cell neoplasm, and unclassified. Similarly, the Kits21 dataset included CT imaging from patients who underwent either radical or partial nephrectomy at either M Health Fairview or Cleveland Clinic and included 300 training cases (overlapping with Kits19), with an unknown number of held-out test cases. Of note, the Kits21 dataset included cases of kidney cysts in addition to kidney tumors. The top 5 winning teams of each of these challenges, along with their respective scores can be seen in **Table 1**, with the winning team in Kits19 achieving a kidney organ Dice score of 0.97, and a tumor Dice score of 0.85, and the winning team in Kits21 achieving a kidney/masses Dice score of 0.98 and a masses Dice score of 0.89.[13–22]

The top performing algorithm in 2019, nnUNet, served as the foundation for the 2021 winning algorithm as well.[23] The UNet is a well-known algorithm in 3D medical image segmentation, coined based on its "U-shaped" architecture that involves learning filters that can compress 3D images and reconstruct an output segmentation mask of the same size and shape as the original 3D image.[8] One of the main difficulties in developing robust medical imaging segmentation algorithms, even when using a network as efficient and broadly applicable as UNet, is determining optimal data augmentation, postprocessing steps, and hyperparameters of the network. The nnUNet algorithm helps solve these problems by automatically selecting preprocessing and postprocessing steps, as well as network hyperparameters based on a set of heuristic rules that consider various properties of a specific training dataset. The top performing Kits21 algorithm used an initial nnUNet model to generate a coarse location for the kidney + masses, and then essentially zoomed in on the kidney region, cropping out the abundant extraneous information contained within the rest of the CT image, and trained 3 separate nnUNets on the zoomed in data, for the tasks of kidney, tumor, and cyst segmentation.

In addition to the Kits challenges, several other authors have demonstrated promising outcomes in kidney and tumor segmentation.[24] For instance, one group trained a generative adversarial network on a training set of 70 cases with a validation set of 23 and test set of 20 cases and achieved a Dice score of 0.859 for segmentation of kidney tumors.[25] Another group used 90 training cases, and 50 test cases with a 3D fully connected network using pyramid pooling, achieving a kidney Dice score of 0.931 and a tumor Dice score of 0.802.[26] Finally, a group used 50 training, 8 validation, and 36 test subjects, along with a novel patching scheme in a CNN and achieved a tumor Dice score of 0.913.

Although it is difficult to compare these models trained on different datasets in order to establish what the state-of-the-art Dice metric is for the task of kidney organ and tumor segmentation, the Kits19 and Kits21 challenges succeed in helping to set this benchmark. These clever and sophisticated neural networks show promising results; however, more research is needed to determine if the models trained on Kits and other data are portable to outside institutions and can still achieve the same levels of accuracy and success as they do on their own test sets.

Artificial Intelligence for Kidney Tumor Classification, Staging, and Grading

Numerous studies have demonstrated effective artificial intelligence (AI) algorithms that can

Table 1
Top 5 scores from the Kits19 and Kits21 challenges

Kits 19		
Place Team	Kidney Dice	Tumor Dice
1 Fabian Isensee and Klaus H. Maier-Hein	0.974	0.851
2 Xiaoshuai Hou et al	0.967	0.845
3 Guangrui Mu et al	0.973	0.832
4 Yao Zhang et al	0.974	0.831
5 Jun Ma	0.973	0.825

Kits 21		
Place Team	Kidney + Masses Dice	Masses Dice
1 Zhongchen Zhao et al	0.977	0.886
2 Alex Golts et al	0.976	0.881
3 Yasmeen George	0.976	0.876
4 Xi Yang et al	0.973	0.874
5 Mengran Wu and Zhiyang Liu	0.970	0.863

classify kidney masses into malignant and benign classes. Such classifications are important, of course, for determining treatment choices as well as disease prognosis.[27] A study by Coy and colleagues[28] focused on differentiating clear cell RCCs from oncocytomas using DL with a cohort of 179 patients, achieving an accuracy of 0.754. Meanwhile, Xi and colleagues chose to differentiate between a larger variety of RCCs (clear cell, papillary, chromophobe, clear cell/papillary, multilocular cystic, and unclassified RCC) and various benign masses (oncocytoma, angiomyolipoma, mixed epithelial and stromal tumor, metanephric adenoma, and renal adenoma) using a ResNet. Their cohort consisted of 1162 renal lesions, and they used T2 and T1 MRI, as well as clinical variables as input, achieving an accuracy of 0.70, which was higher than the average predictive accuracy of experts in the study.[29] Another DL study by Oberai and colleagues[30] demonstrated the use of a CNN model to differentiate between benign masses (oncocytoma and lipid-poor angiomyolipoma) and malignant masses (clear-cell, papillary, and chromophobe). This model had an overall accuracy of 78% with an area under the curve (AUC) of 0.82. Study by Yap and colleagues demonstrated the use of radiomics for classification of benign and malignant renal masses.[31] In this study, a random forest classifier was used to achieve an AUC of 0.75. It was shown that shape metrics provided important predictive information, even when compared with more commonly used texture metrics. Interestingly, the addition of clinical history and demographic information, when added to radiomics features did not increase model performance in a similar task of differentiating benign from malignant renal masses.[32] Finally, Zhou and colleagues[33] differentiated between RCCs and cysts/angiomyolipomas, using a pretrained InceptionV3 model and a dataset

size of 192 patients, achieving an accuracy of 0.97. Each of these studies demonstrate the promise of ML in differentiating between different types of malignant and benign renal tumors using radiologic imaging, from an academic standpoint (**Table 2**). However, currently, there is no software that is routinely used clinically to assist radiologists in classifying renal tumors.

A similar task explored by AI researchers is renal cancer subtyping based on radiomics features, that is, classifying known malignant masses into the various RCC subtypes. A systematic review by Bhandari and colleagues[34] surveyed 4 studies that used CT-based radiomic features to differentiate between low-grade and high-grade clear cell RCC with AUCs of 0.82 to 0.978 as well as 8 studies that also used CT radiomics to classify RCCs into categories such as clear cell RCC, fat-poor angiomyolipoma, papillary, chromophobe, and oncocytoma with similarly good AUCs of 0.82 to 0.96. Useful predictors in these classification tasks included features such as texture, shape, intensity, and wavelet. A recent study demonstrated the usefulness of a radiomics based nomogram in the differentiation between clear cell and non–clear cell RCC.[35] The nomogram had a comparable performance to algorithms typically thought to be more sophisticated such as random forest and support vector machine classifiers, and achieved an accuracy of 0.911 on the test set. In addition, an SVM based on radiomics from corticomedullary and nephrographic phase CT images has been shown to have an excellent performance in discriminating between oncocytoma, chromophobe, and clear cell RCC, with an AUC of 0.935 in the test set.[36] This study also demonstrated a statistically significant correlation between the radiomics score and expression of Cytokeratin7 protein, a protein that has been implicated in various types of RCCs.[37] Furthermore, another

Table 2
Results of classification articles for differentiating malignant from benign renal masses

Authors	Study Purpose	Cohort Size	Result
Coy et al,[28] 2019	Differentiate ccRCC vs oncocytoma	179 patients	Accuracy 74.4%
Xi et al,[29] 2020	Differentiate RCC vs benign masses	1162 patients	Accuracy 70%
Oberai et al,[30] 2020	Differentiate RCC vs benign masses	143 patients	Accuracy 78%
Yap et al,[31] 2021	Differentiate RCC vs benign masses	735 patients	AUC 0.75
Zhou et al,[33] 2019	Differentiate RCC vs benign masses	192 patients	Accuracy 94%–96%

radiomics-based nomogram has been shown to classify papillary type 1 and type 2 RCCs well, with an AUC of 0.831.[38] This distinction is important because papillary type 1 tumors tend to be slow growing while type 2 tumors tend to be more aggressive. Thus, some of the latest research in differentiating between renal tumor subtypes based on imaging demonstrate that while sophisticated ML methods can have excellent discriminative abilities, well thought-out nomograms based on both clinical and radiomics data may also play an important role in achieving optimal algorithms that can be easier to understand for both physicians and patients. Of note, however, a validation study that looked at Radiomics Quality Scores of publications to determine their overall scientific quality and reporting demonstrated that many studies were suboptimal due to lack of certain parameters such as recording imaging protocols in detail, using multiple segmentations, and using multiple time points of images.[39] Thus, a careful analysis of all study methodologies should be performed when interpreting the results of radiomics research.

Tumor, nodes, metastases (TNM) staging is the most commonly used method for staging RCC, and radiologic imaging is important in assessing each of these 3 categories. However, a main weakness of this type of imaging is the difficulty in determining whether tumor invades landmarks such as the renal capsule or Gerota fascia, both of which are important considerations for Stage 3 and Stage 4 RCCs.[40] A relatively new area of study involves using radiomics to predict renal cancer staging automatically. One study used 159 cases from The Cancer Imaging Archive dataset to develop a classifier that could predict either low (Stage 1 or Stage 2) or high (Stage 3 or Stage 4) stages based on CT data alone.[41] This team used a novel imaging histogram-based classifier that inputs to a fully connected neural network for prediction and achieves an accuracy of 0.83. This accuracy was shown to be higher than the accuracy of other methods the team tested including SVM and Rest-Net50. Another group demonstrated the use of DL algorithms in predicting RCC staging by using mostly clinical variables such as sex, age, and symptoms, along with radiomic data such as tumor size and location.[42] The output of their prediction model was the tumor stage (1–4) and the best performing CNN received an AUC of 0.948. As mentioned previously, capsular invasion is an important component of staging. One study also used radiomics to predict which RCCs would have capsular invasion and which ones would not.[43] The authors tested 5 different ML classifiers, using morphological and texture features of the tumors as input, and the forward neural network model achieved the best result, with an AUC of 0.81. Study by Demirjian and colleagues[44] demonstrated the use of radiomics and texture features for predicting kidney tumor staging and grading. They used Random Forest, Adaboost, and ElasticNet models to achieve an AUC for predicting high-grade and low-grade clear cell RCC of 0.70 and an AUC for predicting high-stage and low-stage clear cell RCC of 0.80. These studies highlight the role of radiomics in kidney cancer staging as well as the importance of incorporating nonradiomic clinical variables in predictive models to achieve optimal model performance.

Significant work has gone into predicting pathologic tumor grade from radiologic images as well. There has been a particular focus on predicting The World Health Organization/International Society of Urological Pathology (WHO/ISUP) grade of clear cell RCC. One study aimed to predict either low-grade (Grade 1 or Grade 2) or high-grade (Grade 3 or Grade 4) clear cell RCC based on preoperative radiomics and clinical features.[43] This study of 406 patients used an SVM model to obtain an AUC of 0.887. Another study of 264 patients also aimed to predict high-grade and low-grade (with the same grading definitions as the previous study) clear cell RCC using so-called traditional features such as tumor size as well as preenhanced and postenhanced HU of the tumor, along with radiomic texture features.[45] This study demonstrated that an SVM constructed with both sets of these features performed better than SVMs constructed with either sets of features alone, achieving a maximum AUC of 0.91. Finally, the previously mentioned study by Wen-zhi and colleagues not only addressed staging of clear cell RCC but also addressed grading of tumors.[42] They developed a separate DL model to predict Grades 1 to 4, again based on clinical features and tumor characteristics on CT imaging. The highest AUC of the CNNs they developed was 0.771, with an accuracy of 63.7%. In each of these studies, prediction of clear cell RCC grade is performed with relatively high success based on clinical and radiomics features. From these studies it also seems, that, as expected, the 4-class problem of predicting each individual grade is more difficult than the binary classification of predicting low and high grades. Future research will likely expand to predicting more granular levels of tumor grading, as well predicting papillary RCC tumor grades.

Finally, a key area of focus for ML lies in developing algorithms that are easily explainable to humans. One proposed technique involves taking a human-centered design approach to building ML systems. This guideline involves following 6 key steps including specifying the "clinical scenario, constraints, requirements, and end users" as well as reporting "task performance of the ML systems" and determining "how to communicate with end users."[46] Each of these aspects of an ML system can help facilitate ease of use and understandability of algorithm results for patients, clinicians, and researchers. Kunapuli and colleagues used some of these underlying principles to develop a clinical decision support tool for renal mass classification. This study demonstrated the use of a Relational Functional Gradient Boosting model that could learn explainable rules to predict malignant and benign classes. The AUC of this model was 0.83 and serves as an example of how successful ML models that focus on explainability can be built.

Artificial Intelligence in the Treatment of Kidney Cancer

Scoring systems such as the "radius exophytic/endophytic nearness anterior/posterior location" (RENAL) nephrometry score, "preoperative aspects and dimensions used for an anatomic score" PADUA, and C-index, have all been used to guide surgical decision-making for the treatment of kidney tumors. RENAL score is based on 5 critical and reproducible anatomical features of solid renal masses—measuring the distance between the tumor and the edge of the kidney, the proximity of the tumor to the anterior or posterior renal surface, the exophytic or endophytic nature of the tumor, the anterior/posterior descriptor, and the location relative to the polar line.[47] PADUA score is calculated using tumor size in conjunction with a series of anatomical features—anterior or posterior face, longitudinal, and rim tumor location, involvement of the renal sinus or urinary collecting system, and percentage of tumor deepening into the kidney.[48] Meanwhile, C-index score is calculated as the distance between the center of the tumor to the center of the kidney, divided by the tumor radius.[49]

Motivated by a lack of data comparing the 3 scoring systems (SS), Sharma and colleagues compared the predictive value of the 3 SS by evaluating the correlation between RENAL, PADUA, and C-index scores in 50 patients. The authors also examined whether these scores were associated with positive or negative "trifecta outcomes," a metric defined in this study as having negative surgical margins, a warm ischemia time of less than 30 minutes, and minimal postoperative complications (Clavien-Dindo grades 0–2). The RENAL

and PADUA score did not correlate with any of the perioperative parameters, including operative time, estimated blood loss, Clavien-Dindo complications, and others, whereas the C-index had a significant correlation with operative time ($P = .02$) and trifecta outcomes ($P < .05$). C-index was found to have a lower reproducibility but correlated best with trifecta outcomes.

Heller and colleagues[50] have explored the fully automated computation of RENAL scores and its value in predicting oncologic and perioperative outcomes when compared with human-expert scores. Their method for score computation included the use of a deep neural network to segment the kidneys and tumors, with geometric algorithms used to estimate the components used for RENAL score. They found a significant agreement between the human-expert scores and the AI-scores (Lin's concordance correlation $\rho = 0.59$). Human scores and AI scores also successfully predicted outcomes such as presence of malignancy, necrosis, high-grade and stage disease ($P < .003$), surgical approach ($P < .004$) and specific perioperative outcomes ($P < .05$). Benidir and colleagues[51] also developed a method for automated PADUA score computation and subsequently compared their method to human-generated PADUA scores. Using a dataset of 300 patients with preoperative CT scans undergoing surgical excision for renal cancer, they developed a deep neural network approach coupled with a geometric algorithm to segment the kidney and tumor and estimate the components of PADUA. Both the automation-generated and human-generated PADUA scores were able to predict the need for partial nephrectomy ($P < .001$), as well as predict meaningful oncologic outcomes including the presence of malignancy, high-grade, and high-stage disease ($P < .004$).

In addition, Carlier and colleagues[52] evaluated how RENAL and PADUA scores would compare on kidney tumor segmentations that were done using a semiautomated method versus a fully automated method. First, they used a dataset of 210 patients CT scans and trained a DL algorithm for the automatic detection of RCC. Next, an operator determined RENAL and PADUA scores on a held-out test set of 41 cases that was segmented using the semiautomatic method and the fully automatic method. Concordances of RENAL and PADUA scores were above 80% for both segmentation methods.

In addition to its value in pretreatment assessment and prognosis prediction, radiomics plays a key role in posttreatment assessment. Khene and colleagues[53] developed an ML method to predict tumor response in patients who were treated with nivolumab for metastatic RCC, finding accuracy scores of 4 predictive models (K-nearest neighbor, random forest tree, logistic regression, and support Vector Machine) to be 0.82, 0.71, 0.91, and 0.81, respectively. AI also has the potential to play a significant role in predicting surgical complications in procedures such as robot-assisted laparoscopic partial nephrectomy (RALPN). By analyzing various patient data, including clinical factors like age, body mass index, and comorbidity index scores, along with tumoral and operative variables, AI algorithms can identify patterns and trends that may indicate a higher risk of postoperative complications. In the context of RALPN, AI can be particularly useful in assessing the impact of factors such as surgeon experience, blood loss, and opening of the collecting system on the occurrence of complications.[54]

Radiomics for predictive biomarkers

Research has also been performed regarding the use of radiomics features extracted from CT imaging to understand the tumor microenvironment of clear cell RCC. One retrospective study of 78 patients with localized clear cell RCC identified CT-based radiomics signatures for CD8 T-cell infiltration and programmed cell death ligand 1 (PDL1) expression.[55] This study found that radiomic features could differentiate between highly and nonhighly infiltrated tumors with moderate performance (AUC = 0.8) and between PDL1 positive and negative tumors with good performance (AUC = 0.8). Another study explored using radiomics features from CT images and correlating them with measurements from immunohistochemistry analysis including PDL1 expression and CD8-PD1 T cell to CD8T cell ratio.[56] The authors found that radiomics features could correlate with these biomarkers with AUCs ranging from 0.71 to 0.85. Overall, both studies suggest that radiomic features extracted from CT imaging could provide useful information for understanding the tumor microenvironment in clear cell RCC patients and may have the potential to predict prognosis and response to therapy.

Future Directions

Advances in AI and radiomics are paving the way for improved diagnosis, prognosis, and treatment of RCC. AI and radiomics are also expected to play a crucial role in personalized medicine for RCC. Algorithms can identify unique imaging signatures specific to individual patients, which can be used to develop tailored treatment plans and monitor disease progression in real time.[57] Another important direction of research is the integration of AI and radiomics with other biomarkers for RCC, including genomic and proteomics data. This approach could help in identifying new drug targets and developing more effective combination therapies. Additionally, AI algorithms may be helpful in identifying patients who are more likely to respond to particular types of treatment, enabling more efficient and targeted clinical trial designs.[58] Radiomics data can also be used as a surrogate endpoint for clinical trials, possibly reducing the need for invasive procedures and providing an alternative assessment for treatment response. Radiomics and AI have the potential to revolutionize the field of kidney cancer diagnosis and treatment by providing additional insight into tumor biology, predicting clinical outcomes, and developing personalized treatment plans. However, there are still many technical and clinical challenges that need to be addressed, including the lack of standardization of image acquisition and analysis, reproducibility of model results, and the need for large multicenter validation studies. Nonetheless, the future seems bright, and increasingly accurate and robust AI and radiomics models are being proposed, with the end goal, of course, being clinical utilization.

SUMMARY

Radiomics and AI algorithms have demonstrated significant potential in improving the diagnosis and treatment of kidney cancer. ML-based kidney organ and tumor segmentation, such as the nnUNet algorithm from the Kits19 and Kits21 challenges, has achieved high Dice scores, with further research needed to assess its portability and accuracy in real-world settings. Additionally, these algorithms have shown success in classifying kidney masses into malignant and benign classes, predicting oncologic and perioperative outcomes, and calculating scoring systems such as RENAL, PADUA, and C-index. With continued improvement in areas such as renal cancer subtyping, TNM staging, pathologic tumor grading, and developing easily explainable algorithms, radiomics holds promise as a noninvasive and robust method for enhancing patient treatment of RCC.

CLINICS CARE POINTS

- AI algorithms using radiomics will likely become clinically useful in the setting of renal cancer detection, classification, staging, and prognostication.

- These algorithms may also be useful in helping determine appropriate cancer treatment of patients.

- Radiomics metrics may serve as useful biomarkers for RCC.
- Careful independent evaluation and cross validation of algorithms will be necessary to ensure their optimal application to patient care.

DISCLOSURE

V.A. Duddalwar is a consultant to DeepTek, Cohere, and Radmetrix.

REFERENCES

1. Cancer Today. International Agency for Research on Cancer. 2020.
2. Society AC. Cancer Facts & Figures 2020. American Cancer Society; 2023.
3. Shin T, Duddalwar VA, Ukimura O, et al. Does computed tomography still have limitations to distinguish benign from malignant renal tumors for radiologists? Urol Int 2017;99(2):229–36.
4. Choudhary S, Rajesh A, Mayer NJ, et al. Renal oncocytoma: CT features cannot reliably distinguish oncocytoma from other renal neoplasms. Clin Radiol 2009;64(5):517–22.
5. Blute ML Jr, Drewry A, Abel EJ. Percutaneous biopsy for risk stratification of renal masses. Ther Adv Urol 2015;7(5):265–74.
6. Campbell SC, Clark PE, Chang SS, et al. Renal Mass and Localized Renal Cancer: Evaluation, Management, and Follow Up: AUA Guideline Part I. J Urol 2021;206:199.
7. Abou Elkassem AM, Lo SS, Gunn AJ, et al. Role of imaging in renal cell carcinoma: a multidisciplinary perspective. Radiographics 2021;41(5):1387–407.
8. Ronneberger O, Fischer P, Brox T. In, Computing and Computer Assisted Intervention, 2015. Springer International Publishing; Medical Image; 2015. p. 234–41.
9. LeCun Y, Boser B, Denker JS, et al. Backpropagation applied to handwritten zip code recognition. Neural Comput 1989;1(4):541–51.
10. Heller N, Isensee F, Maier-Hein KH, et al. The state of the art in kidney and kidney tumor segmentation in contrast-enhanced CT imaging: Results of the KiTS19 challenge. Med Image Anal 2021;67:101821.
11. Sathianathen NJ, Heller N, Tejpaul R, et al. Automatic segmentation of kidneys and kidney tumors: the KiTS19 international challenge. Frontiers Digital Health 2022;3:797607.
12. Dice LR. Measures of the amount of ecologic association between species. Ecology 1945;26(3):297–302.
13. Isensee F., Maier-Hein K., An attempt at beating the 3D U-Net. ArXiv. 2019;1:abs/1908.02182.
14. Hou X, Xie C, Li F, Nan Y. Cascaded Semantic Segmentation for Kidney and Tumor. University of Minnesota Libraries Publishing; 2019.
15. Mu G, Lin Z, Han M, et al. Segmentation of kidney tumor by multi-resolution VB-nets. University of Minnesota Libraries Publishing; 2019.
16. Zhang Y, Wang Y, Hou F, et al. Cascaded Volumetric Convolutional Network for Kidney Tumor Segmentation from CT volumes. University of Minnesota Libraries Publishing; 2019.
17. Ma J. Solution to the Kidney Tumor Segmentation Challenge 2019. University of Minnesota Libraries Publishing; 2019.
18. Liu S. In: Coarse to Fine Framework for Kidney Tumor Segmentation. Coarse to Fine Framework for Kidney Tumor Segmentation. 2019.
19. Golts A, Khapun D, Shats D, et al. An Ensemble of 3D U-Net Based Models for Segmentation of Kidney and Masses in CT Scans. Association for Computing Machinery 2022.
20. George YM. A Coarse-to-Fine 3D U-Net Network for Semantic Segmentation of Kidney CT Scans. International Challenge on Kidney and Kidney Tumor Segmentation. 2022.
21. Yang X, Jianpeng Z, Yong X. Transfer learning for KiTS21 Challenge. International Challenge on Kidney and Kidney Tumor Segmentation. 2022.
22. Wu M, Liu Z. Less is more. International Challenge on Kidney and Kidney Tumor Segmentation. 2022.
23. Isensee F, Jaeger PF, Kohl SAA, et al. nnU-Net: a self-configuring method for deep learning-based biomedical image segmentation. Nat Methods 2021;18(2):203–11.
24. Abdelrahman A, Viriri S. Kidney tumor semantic segmentation using deep learning: a survey of state-of-the-art. Journal of Imaging 2022;8(3):55.
25. Ruan Y, Li D, Marshall H, et al. MB-FSGAN: Joint segmentation and quantification of kidney tumor on CT by the multi-branch feature sharing generative adversarial network. Med Image Anal 2020;64:101721.
26. Yang G, Li G, Pan T, et al. Automatic Segmentation of Kidney and Renal Tumor in CT Images Based on 3D Fully Convolutional Neural Network with Pyramid Pooling Module. Paper presented at: 2018 24th International Conference on Pattern Recognition (ICPR); 20-24 Aug. 2018, 2018.
27. Kocak B, Kus EA, Yardimci AH, et al. Machine learning in radiomic renal mass characterization: fundamentals, applications, challenges, and future directions. Am J Roentgenol 2020;215(4):920–8.
28. Coy H, Hsieh K, Wu W, et al. Deep learning and radiomics: the utility of Google TensorFlow™ inception in classifying clear cell renal cell carcinoma and

oncocytoma on multiphasic CT. Abdom Radiol (NY) 2019;44(6):2009–20.

29. Xi IL, Zhao Y, Wang R, et al. Deep learning to distinguish benign from malignant renal lesions based on routine MR imaging. Clin Cancer Res 2020;26(8):1944–52.

30. Oberai A, Varghese B, Cen S, et al. Deep learning based classification of solid lipid-poor contrast enhancing renal masses using contrast enhanced CT. Br J Radiol 2020;93(1111):20200002.

31. Yap FY, Varghese BA, Cen SY, et al. Shape and texture-based radiomics signature on CT effectively discriminates benign from malignant renal masses. Eur Radiol 2021;31(2):1011–21.

32. Nassiri N, Maas M, Cacciamani G, et al. A radiomic-based machine learning algorithm to reliably differentiate benign renal masses from renal cell carcinoma. Eur Urol Focus 2022;8(4):988–94.

33. Zhou L, Zhang Z, Chen Y-C, et al. A deep learning-based radiomics model for differentiating benign and malignant renal tumors. Translational Oncology 2019;12(2):292–300.

34. Bhandari A, Ibrahim M, Sharma C, et al. CT-based radiomics for differentiating renal tumours: a systematic review. Abdom Radiol (NY) 2021;46(5):2052–63.

35. Cheng D, Abudikeranmu Y, Tuerdi B. Differentiation of clear cell and non-clear-cell renal cell carcinoma through CT-based Radiomics models and nomogram. Curr Med Imaging 2023;19(9):1005–17.

36. Yu Z, Ding J, Pang H, et al. A triple-classification for differentiating renal oncocytoma from renal cell carcinoma subtypes and CK7 expression evaluation: a radiomics analysis. BMC Urol 2022;22(1):147.

37. Trpkov K, Williamson SR, Gao Y, et al. Low-grade oncocytic tumour of kidney (CD117-negative, cytokeratin 7-positive): a distinct entity? Histopathology 2019;75(2):174–84.

38. Gao Y, Wang X, Wang S, et al. Differential diagnosis of type 1 and type 2 papillary renal cell carcinoma based on enhanced CT radiomics nomogram. Front Oncol 2022;12:854979.

39. Azadikhah A, Varghese BA, Lei X, et al. Radiomics quality score in renal masses: a systematic assessment on current literature. Br J Radiol 2022;95(1137):20211211.

40. Elkassem AA, Allen BC, Sharbidre KG, et al. Update on the role of imaging in clinical staging and restaging of renal cell carcinoma based on the AJCC 8th edition, from the AJR special series on cancer staging. Am J Roentgenol 2021;217(3):541–55.

41. Arafat Hussain M, Hamarneh G, Garbi R. Renal Cell Carcinoma Staging with Learnable Image Histogram-based Deep Neural Network. Paper presented at: Association for Computing Machinery; 2019, 2019.

42. Wen-Zhi G, Tai T, Zhixin F, et al. Prediction of pathological staging and grading of renal clear cell carcinoma based on deep learning algorithms. J Int Med Res 2022;50(11). 3000605221135163.

43. Yang L, Gao L, Arefan D, et al. A CT-based radiomics model for predicting renal capsule invasion in renal cell carcinoma. BMC Med Imaging 2022;22(1):15.

44. Demirjian NL, Varghese BA, Cen SY, et al. CT-based radiomics stratification of tumor grade and TNM stage of clear cell renal cell carcinoma. Eur Radiol 2022;32(4):2552–63.

45. Yi X, Xiao Q, Zeng F, et al. Computed tomography radiomics for predicting pathological grade of renal cell carcinoma. Front Oncol 2020;10:570396.

46. Chen H, Gomez C, Huang CM, et al. Explainable medical imaging AI needs human-centered design: guidelines and evidence from a systematic review. NPJ Digit Med 2022;5(1):156.

47. Kutikov A, Uzzo RG, The RENAL. nephrometry score: a comprehensive standardized system for quantitating renal tumor size, location and depth. J Urol 2009;182(3):844–53.

48. Ficarra V, Novara G, Secco S, et al. Preoperative aspects and dimensions used for an anatomical (PADUA) classification of renal tumours in patients who are candidates for nephron-sparing surgery. Eur Urol 2009;56(5):786–93.

49. Simmons MN, Ching CB, Samplaski MK, et al. Kidney tumor location measurement using the C index method. J Urol 2010;183(5):1708–13.

50. Heller N, Tejpaul R, Isensee F, et al, Computer-Generated R.E.N.A.L. Nephrometry scores yield comparable predictive results to those of human-expert scores in predicting oncologic and perioperative outcomes. J Urol 2022;207(5):1105–15.

51. Benidir T, Wood A, Abdallah N, et al. Predictive accuracy of computer-generated padua nephrometry scores based on continuous variables compared with categorical computer-generated scores and human-generated scores in predicting oncologic and perioperative outcomes. J Clin Oncol 2023;41(6_suppl):624.

52. Carlier M, Lareyre F, Lê CD, et al. A pilot study investigating the feasibility of using a fully automatic software to assess the RENAL and PADUA score. Prog Urol 2022;32(8–9):558–66.

53. Khene ZE, Mathieu R, Peyronnet B, et al. Radiomics can predict tumour response in patients treated with Nivolumab for a metastatic renal cell carcinoma: an artificial intelligence concept. World J Urol 2021;39(9):3707–9.

54. Mathieu R, Verhoest G, Droupy S, et al. Predictive factors of complications after robot-assisted laparoscopic partial nephrectomy: a retrospective multicentre study. BJU Int 2013;112(4):E283–9.

55. Varghese B, Cen S, Zahoor H, et al. Feasibility of using CT radiomic signatures for predicting CD8-T cell infiltration and PD-L1 expression in renal cell carcinoma. Eur J Radiol Open 2022;9:100440.

56. Alexander Te-Wei S, Steven Yong C, Bino V, et al. Bridging radiomics to tumor immune microenvironment assessment in clear cell renal cell carcinoma. Paper presented at: Proc.SPIE2023.

57. Liang W, Yang P, Huang R, et al. A combined nomogram model to preoperatively predict histologic grade in pancreatic neuroendocrine tumors. Clin Cancer Res 2019;25(2):584–94.

58. Negreros-Osuna AA, Ramírez-Mendoza DA, Casas-Murillo C, et al. Clinical-radiomic model in advanced kidney cancer predicts response to tyrosine kinase inhibitors. Oncol Lett 2022;24(6):446.

Artificial Intelligence in Pathomics and Genomics of Renal Cell Carcinoma

J. Everett Knudsen, BSE, Joseph M. Rich, BS, Runzhuo Ma, MD*

KEYWORDS

- Genomics • Pathomics • Artificial intelligence • Machine learning • Kidney neoplasms

KEY POINTS

- Artificial intelligence (AI) models, using techniques such as convolutional neural networks and logistic regressions, have shown promise in renal cell carcinoma diagnosis, grading, and subtyping.
- AI has outperformed traditional methods in identifying kidney cancer biomarkers and subtype classification, particularly in clear cell renal cell carcinoma.
- Despite progress, challenges remain, including the need for consensus on best practices, computational power for large-scale models, and the creation of a ground-truth training set for model development.

INTRODUCTION

Broadly defined, artificial intelligence (AI) is the ability of a computer to model some form of human interaction. AI as a concept can be traced as far back as third-century China with the invention of a humanlike machine that seemed as if it was meant to perform simple humanlike tasks.[1] Since the 1950s, AI has progressed at a blinding speed, as human innovation in the world of computers has skyrocketed. From social media to finance to sociology, AI has left a marked and profound impact on society. In the field of urology, AI (to its broadest definition) is in practice every day as surgeons perform prostatectomies and nephrectomies with surgical robots, but AI is also finding a home in the diagnosis, grading, treatment, and survival predictability of cancer.[1] In the United States alone, there were an estimated 81,800 cases of renal cell carcinoma (RCC), resulting in approximately 15,000 deaths.[2] On identification of a renal mass, physicians need accurate, reliable methods for determining tumor subtype, grade, stage, responsiveness to pharmaceutical treatment, and the likelihood of patient survival. Luckily, clinical applications of AI have resulted in the inception of genomics and pathomics—2 fields with broad, impactful applications in the diagnosis and treatment of RCC.

Genomics and pathomics arose when machine learning (ML) algorithms were applied to gene expression patterns and pathology images, respectively. Genomics can be broadly defined as the application of ML to expressions of genes and proteins within cells of interest. Useful outcomes of genomics include specific phenotype or genotype identification, patient stratification using ML-pinpointed biomarkers, understanding gene function, and mapping the temporal biochemical significance of gene expression over time.[3] Genomics in RCC is usually leveraged at a preoperative or postoperative time point to help physicians tailor treatment options or plan for upcoming surgeries. In a similar vein, pathomics emerged when AI and ML were applied to digital pathology images. Images are more than just visual objects—they can be quantified using color scales and filtered to generate numerically

Catherine & Joseph Aresty Department of Urology, USC Institute of Urology, Center for Robotic Simulation & Education, University of Southern California, Los Angeles, CA, USA
* Corresponding author. University of Southern California Institute of Urology, 1441 Eastlake Avenue Suite 7416, Los Angeles, CA 90089.
E-mail address: marunzhuo@gmail.com

Urol Clin N Am 51 (2024) 47–62
https://doi.org/10.1016/j.ucl.2023.06.002
0094-0143/24/© 2023 Elsevier Inc. All rights reserved.

determinate edge patterns. Similarly to gene expression data, quantified images can be fed into ML algorithms to predict patterns of interest. Pathomics can be thought of as computers learning to recognize patterns from whole-slide pathology images and then making useful predictions after viewing novel images.[4] The following review seeks to outline the progress and applications of genomics and pathomics in RCC.

ARTIFICIAL INTELLIGENCE IN RENAL CELL CARCINOMA PATHOMICS

Pathomics is the application of ML algorithms to digital pathology slides in order to extract patterns and understand relationships that might not be readily evident to human pathologists. Over the last few decades, computer hardware and software have become faster, more efficient, and capable of storing large volumes of digital information. Applied to the world of pathology, this means pathologists can now digitize whole-slide images (WSIs) and store them for later use. When digitized, images represent a wealth of quantifiable data in the form of color values, edge detection, pixel intensity, morphology, topology, and much more. Such information can then be fed into ML algorithms to assist pathologists in diagnosing and subtyping various clinical conditions[4] (**Fig. 1**). Pathomics specific to RCC includes determining specific subtypes, assigning a Furman grade to tumors, providing cancer staging for patients, and predicting survival outcomes in patients diagnosed with RCC (=**Table 1**).

Various models have been developed that seek to shed light on the aforementioned categories. A large number of these models are considered convolutional neural networks (CNNs), which, at their core, are multilayered data processing pipelines that allow computers to extract features from images.[5] Computer vision is the most commonly used AI modeling approach in pathomics because it allows computers to detect patterns of interest from image data. The differences between CNNs lie in the number of layers available, the sharing of information between layers, and the overall efficiency of the CNN itself.[6] Classic supervised models such as Random Forests (RFs), support-vector networks (SVNs), and logistical regressions have also been developed for use in pathomics. These models are reliant on human-labeled ground-truth examples.[1] RF models improve feature selection by allowing for further building of expandable decision trees in subspaces.[7] SVNs have also been developed for WSI image classification. These are more simplistic models that map nonlinear data onto a linear feature selection space to predict a binary outcome.[8] As such, these models are limited to diagnosis between benign and malignant lesions (ie, binary) rather than subtyping or Fuhrman grading (ie, multitier). Logistical regression modeling is a simple yet highly effective technique for classifying binary outcomes that can then be applied to novel data for classification of items of interest—in this case, benign versus malignant RCC.[9] There are also multiclass regression for subtyping or staging.

Artificial Intelligence Models for Renal Cell Carcinoma Subtyping

RCC is actually a collection of kidney neoplasms that arise from different parts of the nephron.

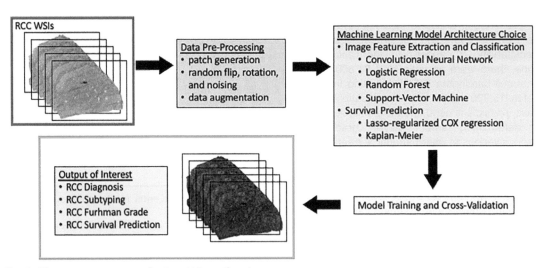

Fig. 1. The common process of using AI in pathomics.

Table 1
Summary of studies using artificial intelligence in renal cell carcinoma pathomics

Study	Application	Specific Aim(s)	Sample	Models	Performance Metrics
Azuaje et al,[79] 2019	Diagnosis	Connected H&E WSIs with protein expression using ML	WSIs: 783 (259 normal, 524 tumor); Prot: 194 (84 normal, 110 tumor)	RF, CNN, and FCNN	Accuracy Prot: 0.98 Accuracy WSIs: 095 AUC Prot: 0.99 AUC WSIs: 0.92
Chanchal et al,[22] 2023	Fuhrman Grading	Created shared residual channel (SRC)-CNN with better performance	3442 WSI patches	SRC CNN	Accuracy: 0.9014 F1 score: 0.8906
Cheng et al,[80] 2020	Diagnosis and Subtyping	Distinguished between TFE3-RCC and ccRCC WSIs using ML	148 WSIs from cases with TFE3-RCC or ccRCC	LR, SVM with linear kernel, SVM with Gaussian kernel, and RF	AUCs: LR: 0.873 RF: 0.848 SVM-L: 0.842 SVM-G: 0.894
Cheng et al,[81] 2018	Survival Prediction from Tumor Microenvironment	Examined tumor microenvironment in pRCC and predicted stage and risk index	190 TCGA samples 856 ROIs for model development	SSAE CNN	Binary outcome for 5-y survival: Stage: 0.63 Subtype: 0.66 Predicted risk index AUC: 0.78
Fenstermaker et al,[11] 2020	Diagnosis, Subtyping, and Grade	Created ML model to distinguish between normal tissue, ccRCC, pRCC, and cpRCC as well as assign Fuhrman grade	42 TCGA WSIs	CNN with 5 fully connected layers	Accuracy: Diagnostic: 0.994 Subtype: 0.975 Tumor Grade: 0.984 Diagnostic Sens.: 1.0 Diagnostic Spec.: 0.971 Diagnostic AUC: 0.98
Gondim et al,[15] 2023	Subtyping	Created a WSI patch classifier using Google AutoML Vision and deployed model on web-based API for clinical usage	252 WSIs (197 for path classifier and 55 for WSI-level tumor classification) 298,071 unique patches	Google AutoML Vision	AuPRC: 0.939

(continued on next page)

Table 1
(continued)

Study	Application	Specific Aim(s)	Sample	Models	Performance Metrics
Holbrook et al,[77] 2018	Fuhrman Grading	Created model to classify low- vs high-grade ccRCC	59 patients; 94 training WSIs, and 20 test WSIs	AdaBoost CNN feature detection; SVM for histogram polar gradient; AdaBoost for combined	F-scores ranged from 0.78 to 0.83
Kalra et al,[26] 2020	TCGA Search Function	Created ML-based TCGA WSI search function	30,000 TCGA image database covering 25 anatomic sites and 32 cancer subtypes	Yottixel image search algorithm	Accuracy: Bladder urothelial carcinoma 93% Kidney RCC 97% Ovarian serous cystadenocarcinoma 99% Prostatic adenocarcinoma 98% Skin cutaneous melanoma 99% Thymoma 100%
Khoshdeli et al,[19] 2018	Diagnosis and Grading	Compared performance of 2 different methods of CNN to determine subtype and grade of RCC	2461 images: 796 normal, 271 fat, 42 blood, 784 stroma, 84 low-grade tumors, 484 ccRCC	GoogLeNet CNN; Shallow CNN	GoogLeNet: Precision: 0.99 Recall: 0.98 F1-score: 0.99 Shallow CNN: Precision 0.94 Recall: 0.90 F1-score: 0.92
Kruk et al,[21] 2017	Fuhrman Grading	Used a wavelet transformation preprocessing step followed by ML modeling to assign Fuhrman grade to ccRCC WSIs	94 ccRCC images	SVM with Gaussian kernel; Breiman RF	Average Sens.: 94.3% Average Spec.: 98.6%

Author, Year	Application	Description	Dataset	Model	Results
Lu et al,[17] 2021	Subtyping	Developed a CLAM deep-learning model for subtyping RCC based on WSI-level labels. Adapted to smartphone microscopy	884 WSIs: 489 ccRCC, 284 pRCC, 111 cpRCC; BWH 135 WSIs-46 ccRCC, 46 pRCC, 43 cpRCC	CLAM deep-learning model	Average AUC: 0.991 ± 0.004 (sd.)
Ohe et al,[24] 2023	Phenotyping and Survival Prediction	Developed ALEXNET model to distinguish between clear and mixed/eosinophilic ccRCC and predict survival rate.	TCGA 435 WSIs, 95 WSIs for validation	Deep CNN called ALEXNET	Average AUC: 0.929 (95% CI 0.88–0.98) Average survival rate: Mixed/eosinophilic 54.3% Clear 80.9%
Tabibu et al,[13] 2019	Diagnosis, Subtyping, and Survival Prediction	Developed CNN ML model for RCC diagnosis and subtyping. Correlated these results for HR prediction	1027 ccRCC, 303 pRCC, 254 cpRCC, 379, 47, 83 normal slides from each subtype	CNN with DAG-SVM on the fully connected CNN layer; Lasso-regularized Cox for survival	Accuracy: ccRCC vs benign: 93.39% cpRCC vs benign: 87.34% Average accuracy for all subtyping 94.07% Lasso-Cox HR: 2.265 (95% CI 1.5343–3.343)
Tian el al,[20] 2019	RCC Grading and Survival Prediction	Developed Lasso-regularized Cox model to assign Fuhrman grade to ccRCC and predict HR	305 ccRCC WSIs from TCGA	Lasso regression model using linear regression with L1 regularization; Cox proportional hazard model for survival prediction	Accuracy: 83.3% grade prediction Sens.: 84.6% grade prediction Spec.: 81.3% grade prediction Avg. AUC: 0.84 HR: 2.05 (95% CI 1.21–3.47)

Abbreviations: CI, confidence interval; H&E, hematoxylin and eosin; HR, hazard ratio; SSAE, stacked sparse autoencoder.

Each subtype of RCC has distinct patterns of gene expression and histologic features. Of the subtypes of RCC, the 3 most common subtypes are clear cell RCC (ccRCC), papillary RCC (pRCC), and chromophobe RCC (cpRCC).[10] Besides the RCC subtypes, oncocytoma, metanephric adenoma, and fat-poor angiomyolipoma are benign conditions that present similarly to RCC. As such, physicians are interested in distinguishing between benign and malignant neoplasms and between RCC subtypes using histologic images. Research in pathomics has provided a variety of models targeted toward this very task.

Diagnosis of kidney cancer starts with a patient's presenting symptoms and subsequent medical imaging to look for kidney masses. After mass detection, neoplasms may be biopsied by a needle or, when appropriate, removed entirely with full or partial nephrectomy.[10] WSIs are then generated from biopsy or resected tumor samples. In the world of pathomics, Fenstermaker and colleagues created a CNN capable of distinguishing between normal renal parenchyma and malignant tissue. Data were obtained from 42 patients who had samples stored in the National Institutes of Health's The Cancer Genome Atlas Data Access Portal (TCGA), a WSI database used by many cancer researchers.[11,12] Tabibu and colleagues also created a CNN with support vector machine (SVM) layer to classify normal versus malignant kidney tissue.[13] In 2021, Zhu and colleagues created a CNN capable of classifying normal kidney parenchyma, oncocytoma, and RCC.[14] Gondim and colleagues then produced a model in Google AutoML Vision that could also distinguish metanephric adenoma from the aforementioned kidney tissue types.[15]

Besides distinguishing between benign and malignant neoplasms, subtyping of RCC has been a great focus in RCC pathomics. The previously mentioned CNNs created by Tabib and colleagues and Fenstermaker and colleagues were also capable of distinguishing between ccRCC, pRCC, and cpRCC.[13] Ghaffari Laleh and colleagues and Gondim and colleagues also produced models with similar subtyping capabilities.[15,16] Focusing on an extremely rare RCC subtype, Cheng and colleagues used logistic regression, SVM, and RF to distinguish between TFE3 Xp11.2 translocation RCC (TFE3-RCC) and ccRCC.

Finally, Lu and colleagues have developed a model that also uses deep learning but requires far less time by trained pathologists to label the training dataset. Using a method called clustering-constrained-attention multiple-instance learning (CLAM), WSIs are labeled at the image level rather than in smaller patches. These WSI labels then allow the model to look for regions of interest, which caused the pathologist to assign the label in the first place. Therefore, CLAM approaches reduce the time necessary to label slides in a spatial format and reduce noise in the training dataset. The model by Lu and colleagues was capable of binary normal versus malignant predictions and subtyping classification predictions and outperformed classic weakly supervised approaches.[17]

Artificial Intelligence Models for Renal Cell Carcinoma Fuhrman Grading

When diagnosed with RCC both patients and physicians are also concerned with grading of the tumor, which gives an idea of the aggressiveness associated with the specific neoplasm. The most widely used grading scale is the Fuhrman system, which assesses nuclear morphology as a prognostic indicator for RCC.[10] The Fuhrman scale assigns 4 grades, with a higher grade indicating a worse prognosis. Similar to RCC subtyping, Fuhrman grading models use a variety of model types including CNNs, logistic regressions, RFs, SVMs, multiple-instance learning models, and CLAM models. These models are, again, considered computer vision approaches because they allow the computer to "see" nuclear morphology and assess severity.

In 2014, Yeh and colleagues used a Kernel regression model to determine nuclear size variations and then correlate these size variations with Fuhrman grades. The model was able to distinguish between low- (Fuhrman grades 1 and 2) and high-grade (Fuhrman grades 3 and 4) with high accuracy.[18] Khoshdeli and colleagues created a shallow CNN and a deep CNN based on GoogLeNet to distinguish between normal tissue, low-, and high-grade ccRCC. They found that both models were capable of making such distinctions, but the GoogLeNet-based model outperformed the shallow CNN.[19] Tian and colleagues presented a Lasso model that was capable of predicting a 2-tiered Fuhrman grade for ccRCC based on 26 model features.[20] In 2017, Kruk and colleagues presented a model capable of assigning Fuhrman grades 1 to 4 rather than the high- and low-grade distinctions seen in previous studies. This model used wavelet transformation in a preprocessing step to reduce noise and improve edge detection. SVM and RF classifiers were then applied to the preprocessed WSIs to assign a Fuhrman grade to WSIs. High accuracy for both SVM and RF classifiers was achieved using only 11 model features.[21]

Fenstermaker and colleagues also presented a 4-tiered Fuhrman grading model in which they used a CNN with a learned first layer, a pixel compressor, and several further layers with full sharing of information.[11] Further, Chanchal and colleagues have also developed the Renal Cell Carcinoma Grading Network (RCCGNet), which is a CNN with a shared residual block that was trained on 722 RCC WSIs. The model assigns a 5-tiered grade in that it can distinguish between normal tissue as well as between Fuhrman grades 1 and 4.[22] Each advancement made by researchers in pathomics represents further advancement toward AI helping pathologists understand the severity of patients' disease with high confidence.

Artificial Intelligence Models for Renal Cell Carcinoma Survival Prediction

For patients with any form of neoplastic disease, prognosis is arguably the most important metric that they would like to understand. Survival prediction is, perhaps, the thing that is of utmost clinical relevance when it comes to pathomics and genomics. In RCC pathomics, several models have been developed that seek to assign a quantifiable value to survival likelihood with the hope that physicians can use these predictions to provide better counseling and support to their patients. For researchers in pathomics, development of a survival prediction algorithm is reliant on the collection of WSIs taken from resected or biopsied tumor specimens and on patient factors such as age, biological sex, treatment course, and postoperative survival outcomes. WSI and patient outcome information are then correlated to develop a model capable of predicting survival after viewing novel pathology images.[20]

As previously discussed, Tian and colleagues developed a Lasso model to predict and assign RCC Fuhrman grades from WSIs. The 160 WSI samples (42 training, 116 validation) used in this study were pulled from TCGA, which also includes deidentified patient information important for survival predictability. Tian and colleagues then constructed crude and adjusted Cox proportional hazard models and validated them using the additional 116 training WSIs. The Cox models were capable of predicting an overall survival percentage.[20] In a similar vein, Tabibu and colleagues also predicted survival using a similar approach as Tian and colleagues. Tabibu and colleagues created a CNN capable of determining RCC subtype, and this CNN detected several features of interest that were also useful for predicting survival. They calculated the risk index of each patient using lasso-regularized Cox modeling for each feature used in the subtyping classifier. Tumor shape and nuclei shape features were significantly associated with patient survival. Chen and colleagues took a different approach in which they used a digital pathology software called QuPath to select a variety of features based on cell morphology and create a ML-based pathomics signature (MLPS) for each WSI analyzed. They then used Cox survival regression analysis to predict disease-free survival[23]; this is the first instance of MLPS generation used to predict survival in a patient population. Ohe and colleagues also developed a survival prediction algorithm targeted toward predicting prognosis in clear versus eosinophilic subtypes of ccRCC. They created a deep CNN from 435 TCGA ccRCC WSIs that distinguished between clear and eosinophilic phenotypes in ccRCC and assigned an AI score to each phenotype. Kaplan-Meier survival analysis was able to predict worse survival rates in patients with mixed/eosinophilic-predominant subtypes versus subtypes. Patients with higher AI scores as determined by the deep CNN had worse survival prognosis, which was validated by real-world survival outcomes.[24] A final survival prediction model was developed by Cheng and colleagues. For this model, researchers focused on classifying the topographic features of the tumor microenvironment in pRCC. Historically, pRCC is not as studied as more common subtypes of RCC such as ccRCC, so this group hoped to shed more light on how the tissue surrounding the tumor affects prognosis. They used an unsupervised approach with a neural network called a stacked sparse autoencoder for feature extraction, then used K-means clustering and Delaunay triangulation for the identification of nuclei morphology patterns. Features from WSI images were then used to build a lasso-regularized Cox regression model to predict risk indices for patients. Certain tumor microenvironment topologies increased risk in pRCC.[25]

Clinical Applications of Artificial Intelligence in Renal Cell Carcinoma Pathomics

As discussed earlier, RCC pathomics has given physicians a wide variety of models capable of determining RCC subtype, grade, and survival prediction. However, it is essential that pathomics moves from theoretic exercises to real-world, clinical applications in order to be useful when it comes to treating patients. Of the models outlined earlier, a few have provided the first steps toward clinical applications beyond just the development of AI models. In addition to improved efficiency and applicability to binary and subtyping tasks, Lu and colleagues' CLAM model generated WSI heatmap overlays that were able to show pathologists the regions of interest that led the model to assign a specific subtype. These heatmaps are highly clinically relevant because they allow pathologists to quickly target areas of a slide that show abnormal cellular architecture or nuclear atypia, meaning pathologists' cognitive loads are reduced.[17] Lu and colleagues were also able to feed their model WSIs taken by smartphone cameras, with the model producing similar results to those taken by typical light microscopy. Applications such as these might be deployed in resource-limited areas where either expert pathologists or highly technical equipment is not readily available. Lu and colleagues imagine a scenario in which a physician in a rural area could submit a digitized biopsy specimen to an online application programming interface (API) and receive a subtype in a matter of seconds rather than sending it to be read by pathologist.[17] Web-hosted APIs for pathologic diagnostic aid could help pathologists efficiently and effectively assign diagnoses in the future.

Another clinical application that extends beyond RCC is a model developed by Kalra and colleagues that is capable of searching all the WSIs uploaded to TCGA. By building a WSI-based search function, pathologists might be able to pull WSIs from uploaded patient samples and compare them with a novel sample they are working with. In this way, they might be able to view other examples of specific subtypes or morphologies before assigning a diagnosis to a new patient case.[26]

ARTIFICIAL INTELLIGENCE IN RENAL CELL CARCINOMA GENOMICS

AI models have been used in a variety of genomic problems including gene expression analysis, transcription factor binding site identification, exon splicing patterns, finding disease-causing genetic variants, and predicting chromatin structure, among a wide array of additional applications.[27–31] Genomics lends itself nicely to ML approaches due to the availability of patterns in genomics data, large dataset sizes, and ability to combine model results with prior knowledge and/or experimental validation. Historically, linear models have had success in supervised (eg, regression, SVMs, RF) and unsupervised (eg, K-means, principal component analysis (PCA), t-distributed stochastic neighbor embedding [t-SNE]) learning tasks in bioinformatics due to their simplicity and robustness.[32–36] More recently,

with increasing advances in both biological data and computing power, deep learning has been gaining traction in this field as a means of uncovering complex genomic relationships.

Artificial Intelligence Models for Genomics

Some of the most popular deep-learning models for supervised learning in genomics include fully connected neural networks, convolutional neural networks, recurrent neural networks, and graph convolutional networks[3] (**Fig. 2**). Each architecture has pros and cons involving computational cost, invariance, interpretability, and prediction quality.

Fully connected networks are the standard feedforward neural network in which all nodes of each layer are connected to all nodes of each adjacent layer. In the context of genomics, the input for a neural network is the one-hot encoding of a DNA sequence. Nodes take as input the weighted average of all nodes from the previous layer, and the result is passed through a (likely) nonlinear activation function before the process is repeated for the following layer. The size of the final layer of the network corresponds to the value or number of classes being predicted. These networks have been used in a wide range of genomic applications including gene expression, splicing patterns, and sequence analysis.[27–29]

Convolutional neural networks pass small filters (ie, low-dimensional matrices) with shared parameters as sliding windows over input data, allowing for translation invariance (ie, relative position of a portion of data does not alter computation with the filter). The dot product between a portion of input data and the filter is performed, and then the filter slides to the next section of input data. Each filter represents a small pattern, which in genomics possesses input data comprised of genetic sequences, which could identify specific motifs. One of the main benefits of this sliding window approach includes saving on computational costs as a result of parameter sharing. Because these filters possess relatively understandable qualities to human interpretation, CNNs also possess a degree of explainability by visualizing the output of a filter, finding which sequence maximally activates a filter, or nullifying a filter and measuring the impact on the model's predictions.[37–39] The semantic value possessed by these filters allows domain knowledge to affect filter design, including cases where certain filters are intentionally initialized in order to seek out specific motifs. Some applications of CNNs include predicting transcription factor binding sites, DNA methylation states, microRNA (miRNA) targets, and pharmacogenomic properties.[6,40–43]

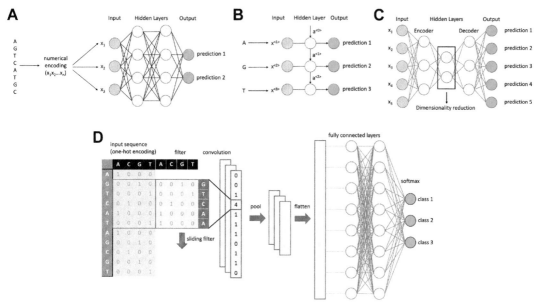

Fig. 2. Popular neural network architectures in genomics. (*A*) Fully connected feedforward neural network shows a genomic sequence as input data and binary classification output. Each input sequence is represented as a string of numbers through numerical encoding (eg, one-hot, binary, ordinal, learned embeddings), where each number serves as an input feature (x_1-x_n, where n is the number of features). Only the first 3 input features are shown. (*B*) Recurrent neural network shows individual nucleotides of a sequence as input data ($x^{<1>}$-$x^{<3>}$), with calculation of subsequent hidden layer (*N*) based on both input at that layer ($x^{<n>}$) and activation from the previous layer ($a^{<n-1>}$). (*C*) Autoencoder demonstrates encoding and decoding layers with potential for dimensionality reduction. (*D*) Convolutional neural network shows input data as (one-hot encoded) sequence with convolution operation, pooling layers, data flattening, and fully connected layers resulting in multiclass classification output. All figures show input layer (*orange*), hidden layers (*gray*), and output layer (*green*).

Recurrent neural networks pass information from temporally earlier information as input to the network trained for the subsequent data input value, thus allowing the network to possess memory. This memory property allows the network to retain time invariance (ie, is not the absolute position of an input sequence that determines prediction, but rather the context of the sequence in which the input appears). Some applications of RNNs include single-cell DNA methylation states,[44] retinol-binding protein binding,[45] and DNA accessibility.[46,47]

Graph convolutional networks apply deep learning to graphical input data. These networks apply convolution operations and subsequent nonlinear activation functions to neighboring groups of nodes to predict behaviors relating to interactions. Applications include protein-protein interaction modeling and gene expression network analysis.[48–50]

A popular deep-learning model for unsupervised learning includes autoencoders. These models use the same data as both input and output, with a hidden bottleneck layer that forces reproduction of input data with removal of redundant features. Autoencoders can be applied to impute missing data and for dimensionality reduction among other uses.[51–53]

To address problems of small or homogeneous datasets, 2 popular data augmentation techniques include transfer learning and generative models. Transfer learning involves pretraining a model with another dataset to provide initial parameter values, which may improve model predictions compared with random initialization.[54] Generally, the larger the transferred dataset and the more similar to the user's dataset, the better the predicted performance boost. Transfer learning has shown promise in biological image classification and sequence-based prediction of chromatin accessibility.[55,56] Generative models include variational autoencoders (VAEs) and generative adversarial networks (GANs). VAEs are autoencoders with probabilistic encoding, allowing for variations in decoding and data generation. VAEs have had success in RNA-seq analysis and predicting drug response.[57,58] GANs are designed adversarially, in which a generator tries to "trick" a discriminator into confusing generated data as being real. GANs have been used in sequence generation and scRNA-seq simulation.[59–61]

Model interpretability remains an ongoing challenge in deep learning due to the obscure meaning of each parameter's influence on model predictions. Genomics provides no exception to the difficulty of the interpretability problem, yet it underscores the problem's importance due to explainability of predictions often being essential to uncover biological meaning in relationships or pathways. Numerous approaches to interpretability have been explored in genomics. In addition to CNN-specific node-based strategies enumerated earlier, some architecture-agnostic methods for tackling interpretability include implementation of attention mechanisms to focus on regions of particular interest based on prior knowledge, in-silico mutagenesis (observing degree of change in model prediction based on induced point mutation in the data), motif-embedding (observing degree of change in model prediction after artificially embedding a motif in an unnatural location), gradient magnitude calculation (where higher magnitude indicates high degree of importance of that region), and feature interaction identification through simulated mutagenesis.[39]

In RCC in particular, AI has been used in a variety of ways. PCA has been used to cluster RCC by immune subtypes and weighted correlation network analysis with RF to predict gene expression of distinguishing hub genes.[62] Four supervised learning algorithms—J48, RF, SMO, and Naïve Bayes—could discern early versus late-stage ccRCC based on transcriptomic signature, and feature selection predicted 62 of the most important distinguishing genes between the 2 groups.[63] t-SNE analysis revealed a mitochondrial genetic signature that spanned histopathologic subgroups and predicted worse survival for patients with RCC.[64] The Min-Redundancy and Max-Relevance algorithm was used to pick a profile of 13 genes highly correlated with RCC patient outcomes.[65] Other combinations of supervised and unsupervised learning help predict unique genetic subtypes and gene signatures of patients with RCC, with the TCGA-KIRC population as a popular dataset for input.

Artificial Intelligence in Identifying Renal Cell Carcinoma Biomarkers

The application of AI has shown promising results, particularly in biomarker identification and subtype classification. Recent studies have proposed novel methods that leverage AI for kidney cancer biomarker identification and subtype classification, demonstrating superior performance compared with traditional methods.

Liu and colleagues presented a study on the use of bioinformatics tools and a neural network model

for identifying biomarkers in ccRCC.[66] The investigators used a 2-step approach. First, they identified differentially expressed genes (DEGs) between ccRCC and normal renal tissues using data from the Gene Expression Omnibus (GEO) database. They then constructed a protein-protein interaction network of the DEGs and screened for hub genes using cytoHubba. Ten hub genes were identified, including AURKB, CCNA2, TPX2, and NCAPG, which were found to be highly expressed in ccRCC compared with normal renal tissue. In the second step, the investigators used a neural network model to verify the relationship among these genes. The model was trained using data from 10 ccRCC tumor samples and 10 normal kidney tissues. The results from the neural network model showed strong correlations between the hub genes, validating their potential as biomarkers for ccRCC. The study demonstrated the potential of AI in enhancing the identification and verification of biomarkers in ccRCC.

AI was used to analyze DNA methylation and gene expression data as well. Malouf and colleagues used a supervised clustering approach to analyze promoter DNA methylation and gene expression using a 56 genes epi-signature in TCGA dataset of ccRCC and chromophobe samples.[67] This approach allowed them to identify distinct clusters based on the methylation patterns and gene expression profiles of the samples. Furthermore, unsupervised clustering was used to analyze DNA methylation using CpG sites located in promoter CpG islands and outside promoter CpG islands. This analysis revealed 2 epi-clusters with distinct characteristics. One cluster (C1) contained almost all tumors with benign potential, whereas the other cluster (C2) contained tumors with potential malignant behavior.

Pirmoradi and colleagues used miRNA data, which are often high-dimensional and contains many irrelevant and redundant features.[68] To address this, the researchers used a filter method for feature selection, specifically the Arithmetical Mean Geometric Mean measure. This method, with its low computational cost, effectively identifies the most discriminant miRNAs as significant features, thereby enhancing the performance of disease or subtype classification. Then the study introduces a self-organizing deep neuro-fuzzy system for the classification task. This system is designed to overcome common challenges in the field, such as the curse of dimensionality, low sample numbers, and unbalanced data. Remarkably, the proposed classifier achieved an average classification accuracy of 93.2%, sensitivity of 92.4%, and specificity of 98.1% in test data. These results indicate the system's ability to classify kidney cancer subtypes with high accuracy based on complex rules obtained using deep-learning algorithms. Another group applied the tensor decomposition (TD)-based unsupervised feature extraction method to analyze messenger RNA (mRNA) and miRNA expression profiles.[69] The AI-driven analysis identified miRNA signatures and their associated genes, which were found to be involved in cancer-related pathways. Moreover, 23 genes were significantly correlated with the survival of patients with ccRCC. The investigators demonstrated that the results are robust and does not highly depend on the databases selected. Compared with traditional supervised methods tested, TD achieves much better performance in selecting prognostic miRNAs and mRNAs; this suggests that integrated analysis using the TD-based unsupervised feature extraction technique is an effective strategy for identifying prognostic signatures in cancer studies.

Artificial Intelligence and Renal Cell Carcinoma Liquid Biopsy

Liquid biopsy is a noninvasive diagnostic tool that is gaining traction in the management of RCC. It involves the analysis of circulating tumor cells, circulating tumor DNA, and other biomarkers present in body fluids, such as blood. Liquid biopsy offers a real-time snapshot of the tumor's genetic landscape, allowing for early detection, monitoring disease progression, and assessing treatment response. Combining with AI, it holds significant promise for personalized medicine in RCC, enabling clinicians to tailor treatment strategies based on the unique molecular profile of each patient's tumor.

Iwamura and colleagues presented a study on the use of AI for diagnosing urologic diseases, including RCC, based on blood sample.[70] The study analyzed immunoglobulin N-glycan signatures from 100 serum subjects with RCC. The data were used in a supervised ML model to establish a scoring system that gave the probability of the presence of RCC. The results indicated that the RCC score could be a promising biomarker for the early diagnosis of RCC and for differentiating between invasive renal pelvis cancer and RCC. The score showed excellent diagnostic accuracy at any pathologic stage. However, further external validation trials are needed to validate the urologic disease-specific scoring system in routine clinical practice.

Manzi and colleagues used AI techniques in conjunction with lipidomics for the early detection of ccRCC.[71] The researchers developed an ML model that was trained to identify patterns in the lipid profiles of patients, which could potentially indicate the presence of ccRCC. The model was tested and validated using an independent set of patient data, demonstrating promising results in terms of accuracy, sensitivity, and specificity. The investigators also attempted to apply this model to other types of RCC, although the sample size for these types was limited. The results of this study suggest that this ML approach could be a valuable tool for early ccRCC diagnosis, pending further validation in larger and more diverse patient cohorts.

Artificial Intelligence and Renal Cell Carcinoma Staging

Bhalla and colleagues used AI techniques to classify early and late-stage patients of ccRCC based on gene expression data.[72] The study used ML for feature selection, reducing the number of features from 19,166 to 64 using a software package called Weka. They also developed prediction models using SVM and RFs and evaluated their performance using 10-fold cross-validation. The researchers also presented a Web platform called CancerCSP, where users could provide gene expression data and predict whether the cancer was in the early or late stage. This application of ML provided better insights to understand the mechanisms responsible for metastasis in various cancers.

Artificial Intelligence and Renal Cell Carcinoma Survival Prediction

Recent studies have demonstrated the use of AI in developing prognostic models for RCC. These models leverage large-scale genomic data to identify differentially expressed genes and signatures that can predict disease progression and patient survival.

Chen and colleagues used ML techniques to develop a prognostic model for patients ccRCC.[73] The researchers identified 333 DEGs between ccRCC and normal tissues from the GEO database. They used univariate Cox regression analysis to retrieve the survival-related DEGs and further used multivariate Cox regression with the LASSO penalty to identify potential prognostic genes. A 7-gene signature was identified, including APOLD1, C9orf66, G6PC, PPP1R1A, CNN1G, TIMP1, and TUBB2B. The seven-gene signature was evaluated in the training set, internal testing set, and external validation using data from the ICGC database. The Kaplan-Meier analysis showed that the high-risk group had a significantly shorter overall survival time than the low-risk group in the training, testing, and ICGC datasets. The researchers concluded that the 7-gene signature can serve as an independent biomarker for predicting prognosis in patients with ccRCC.

Singh and colleagues have developed a ML model to predict the progression of pRCC from early to late stages using RNA sequencing data.[74] The team used a ML pipeline incorporating different feature selection algorithms and classification models. They identified 80 genes that are consistently altered between stages by different feature selection algorithms, which are related to cellular components such as centromere, kinetochore and spindle, and biological process mitotic cell cycle. The AI model developed in this study demonstrates the potential of ML in providing valuable insights into the progression of pRCC.

THE INTERACTION BETWEEN PATHOMICS AND GENOMICS AND THE EMERGENCE OF MULTIOMICS

The integration of AI with multiomics data is revolutionizing the field of RCC. Recent studies have demonstrated the potential of ML and deep-learning techniques in extracting meaningful insights from complex biological data, including genomics, proteomics, and pathomics.

Singh and colleagues used AI techniques to investigate the methylation patterns of pRCC and their relationship with gene expression using multiomics data.[75] ML models were used to analyze gene expression (RNA), DNA methylation, and clinical information. AI techniques facilitated the analysis of various representations of methylation data and enabled functional enrichment analysis to uncover biological processes associated with PRCC. The findings highlight the potential of AI in enhancing our understanding of pRCC by integrating multiomics data.

Ning and colleagues focused on improving the prediction of prognosis in ccRCC using multiomics data.[76] They sought to address the limitations of traditional methods that relied on hand-crafted features and single-modal data. Drawing inspiration from the success of CNNs in medical image analysis, they proposed a novel framework that combines deep features extracted from computed tomography/histopathological images with eigengenes derived from functional genomic data. This approach outperformed models based on single-modality features, effectively stratifying patients into high- and low-risk subgroups. The study also explored the relationship between deep image features and eigengenes, offering insights into the interpretation of deep image features using genomic data.

Holdbrook and colleagues presented an automated image-based system that leveraged AI to classify ccRCC slides by quantifying nuclear pleomorphic patterns.[77] The system, which quantified nuclear patterns, was tested on tissue slides from 59 patients, with results correlating to a multigene assay-based scoring system. The AI used a "Fraction Value" (FV) score, with a high correlation found between the FV predicted and the multigene score.

Ing and colleagues developed an ML approach to identify latent vascular phenotypes that could predict the outcome of renal cancer.[78] They used a 2-step framework for quantitative imaging of tumor vasculature to derive a spatially informed, prognostic gene signature. The algorithms they developed classified endothelial cells and generated a vascular area mask in hematoxylin and eosin micrographs of ccRCC cases from TCGA. The investigators successfully applied digital image analysis and targeted ML to develop prognostic, morphology-based, gene expression signatures from the vascular architecture. This novel morphogenetic approach has the potential to improve previous methods for biomarker development.

Azuaje and colleagues used a deep-learning CNN to find prognostic correlations between patterns of protein expression and histopathology images.[79] They found that certain proteomics patterns cause visually appreciable changes in pathology slide findings; this is another step toward connecting gene and protein expression patterns with pathomics modeling and will help pathologists make faster, more robust diagnoses in the future.

These studies underscore the transformative potential of AI in RCC research, particularly in the realm of multiomics data integration and prognosis prediction. The application of AI in this context could significantly enhance diagnostic accuracy, enable personalized treatment strategies, and ultimately improve patient outcomes.

CHALLENGES AND FUTURE DIRECTION

In this narrative review, the authors have discussed a wide array of AI models and their various applications to problems in RCC. Both pathomics and genomics models can help diagnose malignant disease and predict survival in RCC, but there are still a few challenges to overcome. As demonstrated by the number of models outlined in this review, there are a wide variety of computational approaches to consider when undergoing model development. However, there is no consensus on the best approach—some models may offer slight performance edges over others, but these enhancements are not something that patients coming into the urology clinic will necessarily understand. To bridge this gap, researchers must make sure to ground the theory behind their work in practical clinical applications. The first steps are being made in the right direction, but we encourage researchers and physicians to work together to understand how theoretic models can be deployed in real-world scenarios to make greater impacts on patient care. Secondly, projects in pathomics and genomics also require an enormous amount of computing power to predict outcomes of interest. Institutions and hospital groups are often resource-limited and might lack the computational power necessary to deploy and maintain large-scale clinical models. Therefore, computational needs might be met by the use of commercially available servers such as Google AutoML Vision, which allows for the web-based development and deployment of clinical AI models.[15] Another limitation of AI modeling generally is the need to construct a ground-truth, human-verified training set for model development. For pathomics and genomics, this is a time- and labor-intensive task, especially as more and more tumor WSIs are generated and novel genes are discovered. In pathomics, approaches in WSI labeling with CLAM computing lighten the workload, but ground-truth training set development still represents a bottleneck.[17] Finally, the performance of AI models highly depends on the training data, which may result in unexpected bias. For example, in genomics, race may limit the generalizability of a fully trained AI model when applied to patients coming from a minority racial group. More diverse datasets can mitigate bias in this regard.

SUMMARY

The intersection of AI models with histopathology images and gene expression patterns has produced the rapidly expanding fields of pathomics and genomics, respectively. Applications of pathomics and genomics in RCC have given researchers and clinicians new tools for diagnosis and subtyping of kidney tumors. It has also allowed for the development of more robust survival prediction models that, in the future, can help patients and their families better understand the prognosis of a new RCC diagnosis. ML has also helped uncover new gene expression patterns specific to different subtypes and grades of RCC. These models are helping researchers better understand the biological origins of RCC as well as uncover potential avenues for treatment, particularly targeted medical therapies. Pathomics and genomics are also being used in combination, thanks to the ability of AI model to deal with multimodal data. With AI, patients and physicians should look forward to the future discoveries and innovations to come in the growing fields of pathomics and genomics, to shed light in the field of RCC.

CLINICS CARE POINTS

- AI has been used to assist in pathological renal cell carcinoma cancer diagnosis, subtyping, Fuhrman grading, and survival prediction in the research setting.
- A synergetic integration of AI and genetics assists basic science research in identifying renal cell carcinoma biomarkers, classifying genetic subtypes, and enabling multiomics. This powerful integration also holds promise in clinical application such as liquid biopsy.
- While AI carries substantial potential to support clinicians with the pathologic diagnosis and genomic classification of renal cell carcinoma, it is imperative to proceed with rigorous clinical trials and obtain FDA approval.

DISCLOSURES

The authors declare no commercial or financial conflicts of interest or any funding sources.

FUNDING/SUPPORT

No funding.

REFERENCES

1. Hamet P, Tremblay J. Artificial intelligence in medicine. Metab Clin Exp 2017;69:S36–40.
2. Siegel RL, Miller KD, Wagle NS, et al. Cancer statistics, 2023. CA Cancer J Clin 2023;73(1):17–48.
3. Eraslan G, Avsec Ž, Gagneur J, et al. Deep learning: new computational modelling techniques for genomics. Nat Rev Genet 2019;20(7):389–403.
4. Niazi MKK, Parwani AV, Gurcan M. Digital Pathology and Artificial Intelligence. Lancet Oncol 2019;20(5): e253–61.
5. Gu J, Wang Z, Kuen J, et al. Recent advances in convolutional neural networks. Pattern Recognit 2018;77:354–77.
6. Li Z, Liu F, Yang W, et al. A Survey of Convolutional Neural Networks: Analysis, Applications, and Prospects. IEEE Trans Neural Netw Learn Syst 2022; 33(12):6999–7019.
7. Ho TK. Random decision forests. Proceedings of 3rd International Conference on Document Analysis and Recognition 1995;1:278–82.

8. Cortes C, Vapnik V. Support-vector networks. Mach Learn 1995;20(3):273–97.

9. Subasi A. Machine learning techniques. Academic Press; 2020. p. 91–202.

10. Rini BI, Campbell SC, Escudier B. Renal cell carcinoma. Lancet 2009;373(9669):1119–32.

11. Fenstermaker M, Tomlins SA, Singh K, et al. Development and Validation of a Deep-learning Model to Assist With Renal Cell Carcinoma Histopathologic Interpretation. Urology 2020;144:152–7.

12. Grossman RL, Heath AP, Ferretti V, et al. Toward a Shared Vision for Cancer Genomic Data. N Engl J Med 2016;375(12):1109–12.

13. Tabibu S, Vinod PK, Jawahar CV. Pan-Renal Cell Carcinoma classification and survival prediction from histopathology images using deep learning. Sci Rep 2019;9(1):10509.

14. Zhu M, Ren B, Richards R, et al. Development and evaluation of a deep neural network for histologic classification of renal cell carcinoma on biopsy and surgical resection slides. Sci Rep 2021;11(1): 7080.

15. Gondim DD, Al-Obaidy KI, Idrees MT, et al. Artificial intelligence-based multi-class histopathologic classification of kidney neoplasms. J Pathol Inform 2023;14:100299.

16. Ghaffari Laleh N, Muti HS, Loeffler CML, et al. Benchmarking weakly-supervised deep learning pipelines for whole slide classification in computational pathology. Med Image Anal 2022;79: 102474.

17. Lu MY, Williamson DFK, Chen TY, et al. Data-efficient and weakly supervised computational pathology on whole-slide images. Nat Biomed Eng 2021;5(6): 555–70.

18. Yeh FC, Parwani AV, Pantanowitz L, et al. Automated grading of renal cell carcinoma using whole slide imaging. J Pathol Inform 2014;5(1):23.

19. Khoshdeli M, Borowsky A, Parvin B. Deep Learning Models Differentiate Tumor Grades from H&E Stained Histology Sections. In: 2018 40th annual international conference of the IEEE engineering in medicine and biology society. EMBC); 2018. p. 620–3.

20. Tian K, Rubadue CA, Lin DI, et al. Automated clear cell renal carcinoma grade classification with prognostic significance. PLoS One 2019;14(10): e0222641.

21. Kruk M, Kurek J, Osowski S, et al. Ensemble of classifiers and wavelet transformation for improved recognition of Fuhrman grading in clear-cell renal carcinoma. Biocybern Biomed Eng 2017;37(3): 357–64.

22. Chanchal AK, Lal S, Kumar R, et al. A novel dataset and efficient deep learning framework for automated grading of renal cell carcinoma from kidney histopathology images. Sci Rep 2023;13(1):5728.

23. Chen S, Jiang L, Gao F, et al. Machine learning-based pathomics signature could act as a novel prognostic marker for patients with clear cell renal cell carcinoma. Br J Cancer 2022;126(5): 771–7.

24. Ohe C, Yoshida T, Amin MB, et al. Deep learning-based predictions of clear and eosinophilic phenotypes in clear cell renal cell carcinoma. Hum Pathol 2023;131:68–78.

25. Cheng J, Mo X, Wang X, et al. Identification of topological features in renal tumor microenvironment associated with patient survival. Bioinforma Oxf Engl 2018;34(6):1024–30.

26. Kalra S, Tizhoosh HR, Shah S, et al. Pan-cancer diagnostic consensus through searching archival histopathology images using artificial intelligence. NPJ Digit Med 2020;3:31.

27. Xiong HY, Alipanahi B, Lee LJ, et al. The human splicing code reveals new insights into the genetic determinants of disease. Science 2015;347(6218): 1254806.

28. Jha A, Gazzara MR, Barash Y. Integrative deep models for alternative splicing. Bioinforma Oxf Engl 2017;33(14):i274–82.

29. Ezziane Z. Applications of artificial intelligence in bioinformatics: A review. Expert Syst Appl 2006; 30(1):2–10.

30. Quang D, Chen Y, Xie X. DANN: a deep learning approach for annotating the pathogenicity of genetic variants. Bioinforma Oxf Engl 2015;31(5):761–3.

31. Chen C, Hou J, Shi X, et al. DeepGRN: prediction of transcription factor binding site across cell-types using attention-based deep neural networks. BMC Bioinf 2021;22(1):38.

32. Liu S, Lu M, Li H, et al. Prediction of Gene Expression Patterns With Generalized Linear Regression Model. Front Genet 2019;10. Available at: https:// www.frontiersin.org/articles/10.3389/fgene.2019. 00120. Available at: Accessed May 29, 2023.

33. Byvatov E, Schneider G. Support vector machine applications in bioinformatics. Appl Bioinf 2003; 2(2):67–77.

34. Chen X, Ishwaran H. Random Forests for Genomic Data Analysis. Genomics 2012;99(6):323–9.

35. Wu FX. Genetic weighted k-means algorithm for clustering large-scale gene expression data. BMC Bioinf 2008;9(6):S12.

36. Kobak. The art of using t-SNE for single-cell transcriptomics | Nature Communications. Available at: https://www.nature.com/articles/s41467-019-13056-x Accessed May 30, 2023.

37. Alipanahi B, Delong A, Weirauch MT, et al. Predicting the sequence specificities of DNA- and RNA-binding proteins by deep learning. Nat Biotechnol 2015;33(8):831–8.

38. Luo X, Tu X, Ding Y, et al. Expectation pooling: an effective and interpretable pooling method for

predicting DNA–protein binding. Bioinformatics 2020;36(5):1405–12.

39. Novakovsky G, Dexter N, Libbrecht MW, et al. Obtaining genetics insights from deep learning via explainable artificial intelligence. Nat Rev Genet 2023;24(2):125–37.

40. Vaz JM, Balaji S. Convolutional neural networks (CNNs): concepts and applications in pharmacogenomics. Mol Divers 2021;25(3):1569–84.

41. Abdeltawab H, Khalifa F, Ghazal M, et al. A pyramidal deep learning pipeline for kidney whole-slide histology images classification. Sci Rep 2021;11(1):20189.

42. Schulte-Sasse R, Budach S, Hnisz D, et al. Integration of multiomics data with graph convolutional networks to identify new cancer genes and their associated molecular mechanisms. Nat Mach Intell 2021;3(6):513–26.

43. Zhang Z, Park CY, Theesfeld CL, et al. An automated framework for efficiently designing deep convolutional neural networks in genomics. Nat Mach Intell 2021;3(5):392–400.

44. Angermueller C, Lee HJ, Reik W, et al. DeepCpG: accurate prediction of single-cell DNA methylation states using deep learning. Genome Biol 2017; 18(1):67.

45. Pan X, Rijnbeek P, Yan J, et al. Prediction of RNA-protein sequence and structure binding preferences using deep convolutional and recurrent neural networks. BMC Genom 2018;19(1):511.

46. Quang D, Xie X. DanQ: a hybrid convolutional and recurrent deep neural network for quantifying the function of DNA sequences. Nucleic Acids Res 2016;44(11):e107.

47. Quang D, Xie X. FactorNet: A deep learning framework for predicting cell type specific transcription factor binding from nucleotide-resolution sequential data. Methods San Diego Calif 2019; 166:40–7.

48. Barabási AL, Gulbahce N, Loscalzo J. Network medicine: a network-based approach to human disease. Nat Rev Genet 2011;12(1):56–68.

49. Zhang XM, Liang L, Liu L, et al. Graph Neural Networks and Their Current Applications in Bioinformatics. Front Genet 2021;12. Available at: https://www.frontiersin.org/articles/10.3389/fgene.2021.690049. Available at: Accessed May 30, 2023.

50. Wang K, Li Z, You ZH, et al. Adversarial dense graph convolutional networks for single-cell classification. Bioinformatics 2023;39(2):btad043.

51. Tangherloni A, Ricciuti F, Besozzi D, et al. Analysis of single-cell RNA sequencing data based on autoencoders. BMC Bioinf 2021;22(1):309.

52. Doncevic D, Herrmann C. Biologically informed variational autoencoders allow predictive modeling of genetic and drug induced perturbations. biorxiv 2022. https://doi.org/10.1101/2022.09.20.508703.

53. Talwar D, Mongia A, Sengupta D, et al. AutoImpute: Autoencoder based imputation of single-cell RNA-seq data. Sci Rep 2018;8(1):16329.

54. Weiss K, Khoshgoftaar TM, Wang D. A survey of transfer learning. J Big Data 2016;3(1):9.

55. Guo C, Wei B, Yu K. Deep Transfer Learning for Biology Cross-Domain Image Classification. J Control Sci Eng 2021;2021:e2518837.

56. Agarwal A, Chen L. DeepPHiC: predicting promoter-centered chromatin interactions using a novel deep learning approach. Bioinformatics 2023;39(1): btac801.

57. Rampášek L, Hidru D, Smirnov P, et al. Dr.VAE: improving drug response prediction via modeling of drug perturbation effects. Bioinformatics 2019; 35(19):3743–51.

58. Grønbech CH, Vording MF, Timshel PN, et al. scVAE: variational auto-encoders for single-cell gene expression data. Berger B. Bioinformatics 2020; 36(16):4415–22.

59. Lan L, You L, Zhang Z, et al. Generative Adversarial Networks and Its Applications in Biomedical Informatics. Front Public Health 2020;8. https://doi.org/10.3389/fpubh.2020.00164.

60. Wang X, Ghasedi Dizaji K, Huang H. Conditional generative adversarial network for gene expression inference. Bioinformatics 2018;34(17): i603–11.

61. Viñas R, Andrés-Terré H, Liò P, et al. Adversarial generation of gene expression data. Bioinformatics 2022;38(3):730–7.

62. Wang Z, Chen Z, Zhao H, et al. ISPRF: a machine learning model to predict the immune subtype of kidney cancer samples by four genes. Transl Androl Urol 2021;10(10):3773–86.

63. Jagga Z, Gupta D. Classification models for clear cell renal carcinoma stage progression, based on tumor RNAseq expression trained supervised machine learning algorithms. BMC Proc 2014;8(Suppl 6):S2.

64. Marquardt A, Solimando AG, Kerscher A, et al. Subgroup-Independent Mapping of Renal Cell Carcinoma—Machine Learning Reveals Prognostic Mitochondrial Gene Signature Beyond Histopathologic Boundaries. Front Oncol 2021;11. Available at: https://www.frontiersin.org/articles/10.3389/fonc.2021.621278. Available at: Accessed May 27, 2023.

65. Terremätte P, Andrade DS, Justino J, et al. A Novel Machine Learning 13-Gene Signature: Improving Risk Analysis and Survival Prediction for Clear Cell Renal Cell Carcinoma Patients. Cancers 2022; 14(9):2111.

66. Liu B, Xiao Y, Li H, et al. Identification and Verification of Biomarker in Clear Cell Renal Cell Carcinoma via Bioinformatics and Neural Network Model. BioMed Res Int 2020;2020:6954793.

67. Malouf GG, Su X, Zhang J, et al. DNA Methylation Signature Reveals Cell Ontogeny of Renal Cell Carcinomas. Clin Cancer Res Off J Am Assoc Cancer Res 2016;22(24):6236–46.

68. Pirmoradi S, Teshnehlab M, Zarghami N, et al. A self-organizing deep neuro-fuzzy system approach for classification of kidney cancer subtypes using miRNA genomics data. Comput Methods Programs Biomed 2021;206:106132. https://doi.org/10.1016/j.cmpb.2021.106132.

69. Ng KL, Taguchi YH. Identification of miRNA signatures for kidney renal clear cell carcinoma using the tensor-decomposition method. Sci Rep 2020; 10(1):15149.

70. Iwamura H, Mizuno K, Akamatsu S, et al. Machine learning diagnosis by immunoglobulin N-glycan signatures for precision diagnosis of urological diseases. Cancer Sci 2022;113(7):2434–45.

71. Manzi M, Palazzo M, Knott ME, et al. Coupled Mass-Spectrometry-Based Lipidomics Machine Learning Approach for Early Detection of Clear Cell Renal Cell Carcinoma. J Proteome Res 2021;20(1):841–57.

72. Bhalla S, Chaudhary K, Kumar R, et al. Gene expression-based biomarkers for discriminating early and late stage of clear cell renal cancer. Sci Rep 2017;7:44997.

73. Chen L, Xiang Z, Chen X, et al. A seven-gene signature model predicts overall survival in kidney renal clear cell carcinoma. Hereditas 2020;157(1):38.

74. Singh NP, Bapi RS, Vinod PK. Machine learning models to predict the progression from early to late stages of papillary renal cell carcinoma. Comput Biol Med 2018;100:92–9.

75. Singh NP, Vinod PK. Integrative analysis of DNA methylation and gene expression in papillary renal cell carcinoma. Mol Genet Genomics 2020;295(3): 807–24.

76. Ning Z, Pan W, Chen Y, et al. Integrative analysis of cross-modal features for the prognosis prediction of clear cell renal cell carcinoma. Bioinforma Oxf Engl 2020;36(9):2888–95.

77. Holdbrook DA, Singh M, Choudhury Y, et al. Automated Renal Cancer Grading Using Nuclear Pleomorphic Patterns. JCO Clin Cancer Inform 2018;2: 1–12.

78. Ing N, Huang F, Conley A, et al. A novel machine learning approach reveals latent vascular phenotypes predictive of renal cancer outcome. Sci Rep 2017;7(1):13190.

79. Azuaje F, Kim SY, Perez Hernandez D, et al. Connecting Histopathology Imaging and Proteomics in Kidney Cancer through Machine Learning. J Clin Med 2019;8(10):1535.

80. Cheng J, Han Z, Mehra R, et al. Computational analysis of pathological images enables a better diagnosis of TFE3 Xp11.2 translocation renal cell carcinoma. Nat Commun 2020;11(1):1778. https://doi.org/10.1038/s41467-020-15671-5.

81. Cheng J, Mo X, Wang X, et al. Identification of topological features in renal tumor microenvironment associated with patient survival. Bioinformatics 2018;34(6):1024–30. https://doi.org/10.1093/bioinformatics/btx723.

Bladder Cancer and Artificial Intelligence
Emerging Applications

Mark A. Laurie, MS[a,b,c,d], Steve R. Zhou, MD[a], Md Tauhidul Islam, PhD[b],
Eugene Shkolyar, MD[a,c], Lei Xing, PhD[b], Joseph C. Liao, MD[a,c],*

KEYWORDS

- Artificial intelligence • Urology • Bladder cancer • Deep learning • AI-assisted diagnosis
- Image processing • Treatment planning • Outcome prediction

KEY POINTS

- Bladder cancer is a costly, highly recurrent disease that requires lifetime surveillance after initial diagnosis, and its early detection is critical to optimize patients' expected survival and quality of life.
- Several studies have investigated the potential for AI to improve the effectiveness of the bladder cancer clinical workflow in its detection and treatment phases.
- Significant effort remains to validate the effectiveness of AI for bladder cancer clinical decision support.

INTRODUCTION

Bladder cancer (BC) is the sixth leading cancer diagnosed in the United States and the fourth among males.[1] In 2022, there were an estimated 81,180 new cases in the United States and 17,100 deaths. More than 95% of BC is urothelial carcinoma and at diagnosis approximately 75% of cases are non–muscle invasive BC (NMIBC), with the remainder being muscle invasive BC (MIBC) or metastatic disease.[2,3] BC has one of the highest lifetime treatment costs per patient and represents a significant challenge in oncology given its wide range of disease risks, management options, and prognoses.[4]

NMIBC recurrence rates are 70% at 3 years, and up to 20% progress to MIBC, driving intensive surveillance schedules and high cost.[4] Numerous guidelines have stratified patients by their risk of recurrence and progression based on clinical and pathologic factors.[3] These risk groups are used as the basis for surveillance scheduling and decision making regarding treatment. Appropriate risk stratification, however, remains challenging because of heterogenous groupings and variable quality of surgical resections. Such issues present a particular issue to clinicians in counseling patients on their disease risks, selecting appropriate adjuvant intravesical therapies, and deciding when to pursue radical surgery. Therefore, tools that aide in cancer detection, risk stratification and prognostication, improvement of the quality of care, and in decision making are needed to improve the overall quality of NMIBC management.

In MIBC, prognosis depends on stage of disease at time of treatment. For years, the mainstay of management consisted of neoadjuvant, platinum-based chemotherapy followed by radical cystectomy (RC) with urinary diversion.[5] This strategy itself represents a challenge to providers because of poor tolerability of platinum chemotherapies by a significant subset of patients with BC, unknown

a Department of Urology, Stanford University School of Medicine, 453 Quarry Road, Mail Code 5656, Palo Alto, CA 94304, USA; b Department of Radiation Oncology, Stanford University School of Medicine, 875 Blake Wilbur Drive Room G204, Stanford, CA 94305-5847, USA; c Veterans Affairs Palo Alto Health Care System, Palo Alto, CA 94304, USA; d Institute for Computational and Mathematical Engineering, Stanford University School of Engineering, Stanford, CA 94305, USA
* Corresponding author. 453 Quarry Road, Mail Code 5656, Palo Alto, CA 94304.
E-mail address: jliao@stanford.edu

Urol Clin N Am 51 (2024) 63–75
https://doi.org/10.1016/j.ucl.2023.07.002
0094-0143/24/Published by Elsevier Inc.

benefit in variant histology, and the morbidity associated with RC. To combat this, there has been an uptake in trimodal therapy for MIBC, which consists of radical transurethral resection of bladder tumor (TURBT) combined with chemotherapy and radiation.[5,6] Initially limited to small, solitary, fully resected lesions, the use of trimodal therapy has grown to capture a larger swath of patients who are poor surgical candidates. Ideal patient selection remains uncertain and represents a key unmet need in urology. Likewise, the selection of patients most likely to benefit from neoadjuvant chemotherapy, or selection between different agents as they become available, represents another challenge in MIBC. In metastatic disease, identification of patients at high risk of recurrence, early detection of metastasis, and selection of systemic treatment regimens and sequencing of these regimens remain challenging.

In recent years, artificial intelligence (AI) and machine learning (ML) have emerged as potentially powerful tools in clinical medicine, particularly in medical image analysis and genomics.[7,8] AI and ML are poised to play a major role in addressing the unmet needs in BC, including diagnostic cystoscopy, pathologic diagnosis, molecular biomarkers, risk stratification, treatment assessment, and outcome prediction. In this review, we discuss new and emerging applications of AI in BC (**Fig. 1**).

Artificial Intelligence Background

There is growing interest in the development of AI as a tool to address some of the challenges in BC.[9] Rooted in the disciplines of optimization, cognitive science, probability theory, and statistical learning theory, AI uses computer science principles and large datasets to solve problems.[10] Subsumed by AI is the field of ML, a domain specifically focused on the development and optimization of intelligent, computer-run algorithms trained on large datasets that are designed to accomplish a wide variety of tasks.[11] ML itself subsumes deep learning, which is most relevant as a potential decision aid for the management of BC. Like ML, deep learning uses large datasets and computer-run algorithms to solve a wide variety of problems.[12] Deep learning differs from other subfields of ML in that it directly learns features from raw data. Although conventional ML methods require the development of feature extractors that convert raw data to representative embeddings, deep learning performs this representation learning step implicitly in its formulation.

At its core, deep learning is composed of a series of artificial neural networks (ANNs) that extract relevant features from data to generate a desired output.[13] Many deep learning models are optimized using gradient descent, an iterative algorithm that uses the model's prediction and data sample's corresponding label to optimize its weights in a supervised setting. Deep learning models have been developed and applied to process and represent a wide variety of data modalities, including but not limited to tabular data, text, images, and videos.[14] Of particular interest to BC is the development of deep learning algorithms for image processing called convolutional neural networks (CNNs).[15] Designed to "see" semantic objects in images by representing complex, recognizable image features as compositions of representations of simpler features, CNNs have demonstrated success in numerous image processing tasks, such as image classification, object detection, instance segmentation, and semantic segmentation.[16,17]

AI has the potential to be used in BC detection, treatment, and outcome prediction. Detection is further subdivided into imaging-based tumor identification and tissue/molecular biomarker-based assessment of cancer grade, stage, and risk stratification. Promising applications of AI for BC imaging include integration with cystoscopy, CT, MRI, and ultrasound to identify and localize bladder tumors. AI has also been used to assess tumor stage and grade using molecular biomarkers and cytology samples. For treatment and outcome prediction, AI has demonstrated potential for prediction of postoperative outcomes after RC, radiation therapy treatment planning, and recurrence likelihood prediction. However, such challenges as generalizability, interpretability, and overdiagnosis remain to be addressed. In the following sections, we review and highlight the current state for each of these applications.

ARTIFICIAL INTELLIGENCE FOR BLADDER CANCER DETECTION: IMAGING ANALYSIS
Cystoscopy

Initial detection of BC most commonly occurs with diagnostic cystoscopy during evaluation for hematuria. Several studies have investigated integration of deep learning models during cystoscopy (**Table 1**).[18–21] The availability of carefully annotated imaging datasets of pathologically confirmed bladder tumors (**Fig. 2**) is an important starting point for model training.[18] In 2019, Shkolyar and colleagues[18] reported CystoNet developed to detect bladder tumors during cystoscopy and TURBT. The model was trained on 611 manually annotated images containing pathologically confirmed BC, and then validated on a dataset of more than 7000 frames of confirmed BC derived

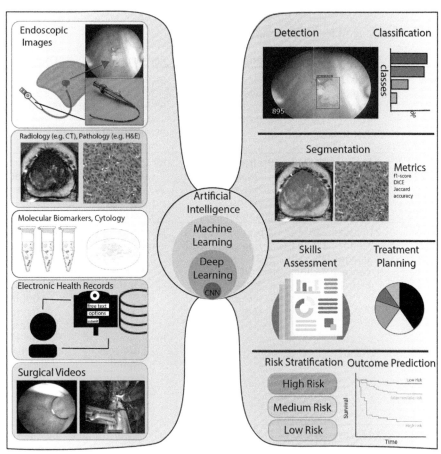

Fig. 1. Application of artificial intelligence for bladder cancer diagnosis and outcome prediction. AI can be used for bladder cancer diagnosis and outcome prediction. Subapplications of bladder cancer diagnosis include tumor detection, staging, grading, and segmentation. For outcome prediction, prediction of recurrence, survival, and chemotherapy response have also been investigated using AI. Challenges to be addressed before integration into the clinical workflow include ensuring that AI models be generalizable, interpretable, and specific enough to not overburden the existing health care system with false-positive diagnoses. CT, computed tomography; H&E, hematoxylin-eosin.

from 44 tumors and 26 unique cases; and more than 50,000 frames of normal/benign urothelium from 31 cases. The overall per frame sensitivity and specificity were 90.9% and 98.6%, respectively.[18] On a per-tumor basis, 39 out of 41 papillary tumors were detected and three out of three flat lesions were detected, yielding a final per-tumor sensitivity of 95.5%.[18] More recently, Chang and colleagues[22] implemented CystoNet in a real-time setting during TURBT and demonstrated initial feasibility of intraoperative integration.

Ikeda and colleagues[19] developed and applied a CNN to classify a cystoscopy dataset consisting of 2102 images. In this dataset, 1671 images contained normal tissue, and 431 images contained pathology-confirmed BC with a range of stages, grades, and morphologies. Here, a CNN pre-trained on the ImageNet dataset[23] (GoogLeNet[24])

was fine-tuned with their cystoscopy dataset. On the unseen test data, this transfer learning approach achieved an area under the receiver operating characteristic score of 0.98, a sensitivity of 89.7%, and a specificity of 94.0%. Similar studies have been performed that arrive at similar conclusions. Eminaga and colleagues[25] validated the performance of seven computer vision models with cystoscopy images originating from a digital atlas, and Yoo and colleagues[21] demonstrated the benefit of using tumor color as an engineered feature to predict bladder tumor presence and grade.

Another study described the use of frame-based deep learning models to predict bladder tumor grade and stage using blue-light cystoscopy images sourced from multiple centers.[20] Blue-light cystoscopy is a widely used enhanced cystoscopy

Table 1
Overview of studies using AI for bladder cancer detection

Study	Data (Validation)	Model	Performance	Comments
Shkolyar et al,[18] 2019	57 cases; 44 tumors; 59,515 frames (7542 tumor, 51,973 normal)	CNN with overlayed object detection RPN	90.9% per-frame sensitivity 95.5% per-tumor sensitivity 98.6% per-frame specificity	39 of 41 papillary tumor detected 3 of 3 flat tumors detected
Ikeda et al,[19] 2020	124 cases; 431 tumors; 431 frames (87 tumor, 335 normal)	Pretrained GoogleNet with fine-tuned cystoscopy dataset	89.7% per-frame sensitivity 94.0% per-frame specificity 0.98 AUC	Tumor frame distribution: 61.5% elevated 17.6% flat 20.9% mixed
Ali et al,[20] 2021	216 cases; 216 tumors; 216 BLC images (all cancer); 4 clinic centers	4 pretrained CNNs fine-tuned with BLC images: VGG16 ResNet50 InceptionV3 MobileNetV2	Benign vs malignant: 95.8% per-frame sensitivity 87.84% per-frame specificity Invasiveness: 88.0% per-frame sensitivity 96.56% per-frame specificity	Performance obtained via L10PO-CV Best-performing models exhibited superior performance over 2 board-certified urologists
Wu et al,[27] 2022	1427 cases; 647 tumors; 5752 frames (647 tumor, 5105 normal), 4 clinical centers	Pretrained pyramid-scheme parsing network fine-tuned with cystoscopy dataset	95.0% per-frame sensitivity 98.7% per-frame specificity	Best-performing models exhibited superior performance over 9 urologists with varying degrees of experience

Abbreviations: AUC, area under the curve; BLC, blue-light cystoscopy; RPN, recurrent proposal network.

technology that involves intravesical instillation of an imaging agent, hexaminolevulinate, which causes cancerous urothelium to selectively fluoresce under blue light.[26] The study compared tumor staging, grading, and malignancy status using four CNNs with two clinicians. Although limited by small sample size of clinicians, the results suggest that deep learning has the potential to improve prediction of tumor stage and grade at the time of visual inspection. Findings from Wu and colleagues[27] support this claim whereby their model detected lesions with a much higher sensitivity than that of trainee, competent, and expert urologists. As an alternative to frame-based models described previously, video processing deep learning models that use sequential images for model training may offer improved performance in real-world settings.[28]

Computed Tomography, MRI, and Ultrasound

CT, MRI, and ultrasound are widely used in urology and specifically in BC, ranging from initial diagnosis and staging to treatment response assessment and surveillance. AI may improve the performance of these imaging modalities, including automation of time-consuming tasks, tumor segmentation, classification, and treatment planning.[29,30] Furthermore, AI may enhance the identification of subtle imaging features and facilitate the surveillance of disease progression and treatment response.

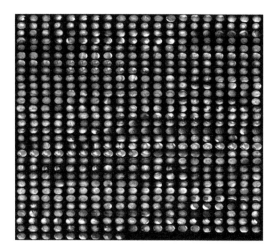

Fig. 2. Representative sample of the types of bladder tumors encountered during TURBT overlayed with expert-verified annotations. Here one can observe the wide variety of tumor morphologies, locations, and sizes, along with various pathologic assessments (not pictured).

CT scans are widely used for the initial evaluation and staging of BC. They may provide information about the tumor's location, size, and regional lymph node involvement.[31,32] Contrast-enhanced CT scans are particularly useful in detecting metastasis. Traditional CT image analysis methods rely on manual interpretation, which is time-consuming and prone to human error. However, with the advent of deep learning, computer algorithms can be trained to accurately segment and classify lesions seen on CT images.

MRI provides detailed soft tissue contrast, making it particularly useful for assessing muscle involvement and staging.[33,34] MRI holds promise in differentiating between NMIBC and MIBC, and identifying the involvement of adjacent structures, such as the prostate or pelvic sidewall.[35] By combining various MRI sequences, including T2-weighted, diffusion-weighted, and dynamic contrast-enhanced imaging, radiologists can obtain comprehensive information about tumor characteristics. Deep learning algorithms applied to MRI data can automate tumor segmentation, aid in identifying suspicious regions, and provide quantitative analysis of tumor features, with such methods demonstrating promise for other organ systems, such as the brain.[36,37]

Deep learning techniques, such as CNNs and recurrent neural networks, have shown potential in improving BC imaging.[31–34] By training these algorithms on large datasets of annotated images, complex patterns and features can be discerned. Deep learning models can accurately segment

bladder tumors, classify them according to malignancy, and predict patient outcomes based on imaging features. These models can also be integrated into computer-aided diagnosis systems,[38] which assist radiologists in their interpretation of CT and MRI scans, reducing diagnostic errors and improving overall efficiency. Furthermore, deep learning algorithms can aid in the identification of subtle changes in tumor size, shape, or enhancement patterns over time, enabling better monitoring of treatment response and early detection of disease recurrence, with successful findings demonstrated for other organ systems.[39]

Ultrasound is a noninvasive and safe imaging modality that uses high-frequency sound waves to generate images of the body's internal structures.[40,41] Ultrasound can be used repeatedly without significant risks[42,43] and has been investigated for BC screening and surveillance.[44,45] Transabdominal ultrasound may be useful for tumor detection and assessment of size and location in some instances.[46,47] In contrast to cystoscopy, it can evaluate surrounding structures to check for tumor spread. Although not routinely used, transrectal ultrasound can provide detailed images of the bladder lumen, especially for tumors near the bladder neck or urethra.[48,49] Contrast-enhanced ultrasound improves visualization of vascularized bladder tumors.[50,51] Recent advances in three-dimensional and four-dimensional ultrasound offer volumetric images that enhance visualization and assessment of tumor characteristics.[52] Application of deep learning to enhance ultrasound imaging of BC is at an early stage. Deep neural networks have been trained on annotated ultrasound images to recognize tumor features and differentiate between benign and malignant lesions. Recent work has shown that deep learning is promising in automating tumor segmentation, identifying suspicious regions, and assisting in treatment planning.[52]

ARTIFICIAL INTELLIGENCE FOR BLADDER CANCER DIAGNOSIS: GRADING, STAGING, AND MOLECULAR BIOMARKERS
Cytology, Pathology, and Risk Stratification

Urine cytology plays an important role in the diagnosis and surveillance of BC given its noninvasive nature. Numerous studies have used ML to accurately identify and classify cancerous cells, achieving high sensitivity and specificity.[53–56] This AI-based cytology analysis holds potential for enhancing the speed and accuracy of BC diagnosis. Pathologic examination of resected tumor tissue is the recognized standard in cancer diagnosis and risk stratification.[57–59] AI-powered pathology tools offer promise in improving diagnostic accuracy and aiding in risk stratification for patients with BC, which is essential for guiding treatment decisions and prognostication.[60–62] Numerous groups have developed deep learning models that predict disease progression in patients with BC based on clinical and pathologic features.[60,61,63,64] These AI-based risk stratification models may enable clinicians to identify high-risk patients who require more aggressive treatment or modified surveillance schedules. The integration of AI with cytology, pathology, and risk stratification processes offers promising avenues for enhancing BC management and improving patient outcomes.

Molecular Biomarkers and Gene Signatures

There has been significant effort aimed at identifying molecular biomarkers and gene signatures that can aid in the diagnosis, prognosis, and treatment of BC.[65–69] One of the most extensively studied molecular biomarkers in BC is the fibroblast growth factor receptor 3 (FGFR3) gene.[70,71] Mutations in the FGFR3 gene are prevalent in NMIBC and have been associated with a favorable prognosis. Another important biomarker is the telomerase reverse transcriptase (TERT) gene promoter mutation.[72] TERT promoter mutations are found in a significant proportion of BC cases and have been associated with aggressive tumor behavior and poor prognosis. Gene expression profiling is a powerful tool for identifying gene signatures associated with BC. Several studies have used high-throughput gene expression technologies, such as microarrays and RNA sequencing, to identify gene expression patterns that can predict disease outcomes and treatment responses.[67,68,73] One of the well-known gene signatures in BC is the Lund Taxonomy,[74,75] which classifies tumors into different molecular subtypes based on gene expression profiles. Gene signatures derived from the analysis of specific gene sets or pathways have also been investigated in BC. For example, the P53 pathway signature is associated with poor prognosis in BC.[75,76] Other gene signatures, such as those related to cell cycle regulation, DNA repair mechanisms, and immune response pathways, have shown potential as prognostic and predictive markers.

Deep learning–based gene signatures are increasingly being used for the prediction and prognosis of BC.[77,78] This approach leverages AI to analyze large-scale genomic data, identifying unique gene expression patterns associated with BC. These gene signatures, often composed of multiple genes, can serve as biomarkers for the disease, aiding in early detection, prediction of disease progression, and personalization of treatment strategies. The use of deep learning algorithms allows for the processing of complex, high-dimensional data, uncovering intricate relationships between genes and disease phenotypes that may not be readily apparent through traditional analysis methods.

ARTIFICIAL INTELLIGENCE FOR BLADDER CANCER TREATMENT AND OUTCOME PREDICTION
Predicting Postoperative Morbidity and Mortality

Although many cases of BC are managed via endoscopic resection with or without intravesical therapy, extirpative surgery remains the intervention of choice in patients with NMIBC at high risk for progression and in MIBC.[3,79,80] However, RC mortality rates are 1% to 3% at large centers.[81] More than 60% of patients experience at least one complication within 90 days of cystectomy, with 13% being grade 3 or higher.[82] Perioperative comorbidity indices, such as the adjusted Charlson Comorbidity Index (aCCI), American Society of Anesthesiology classification system (ASA), and National Surgical Quality Improvement Program risk calculator, are poor at predicting postoperative morbidity after RC.[83,84] Several recent studies have proposed supervised ML models that use preoperative variables to improve RC risk assessment and optimize patient selection for RC.

Klén and colleagues[85] trained a logistic regression (LR) classifier with Least Absolute Shrinkage and Selection Operator (LASSO) regularization to predict early death after RC. LASSO is a powerful and well-established method of pruning weakly predictive variables out of a linear model. This allowed the investigators to use a variety of preoperative factors (comorbidities and their indices, patient demographics, laboratory values) with a lower risk of overfitting their model. They trained their model on 733 patients from 16 different hospitals and reported an area under the curve (AUC) of 0.73 in an independent test set of 366 patients. Congestive heart failure, ASA class, and chronic pulmonary disease were the strongest predictors of postoperative mortalities.[85]

This approach, the well-established LR classifier with LASSO regularization, remains one of the most effective models in comparison with more complex ML algorithms. In a larger comparative study of 7557 patients from the National Surgical Quality Improvement Program risk calculator database who underwent RC, Taylor and colleagues[86] developed several supervised ML models for predicting adverse events, extended hospital course, and discharge to higher level of care. They carried out model training and 10-fold cross-validation using 80% of the dataset to show excellent model stability and minimal overfitting with a similarly expansive set of preoperative inputs. Selected algorithms included a generalized additive model, a neural network, a random forest model, and LASSO. LASSO outperformed all other models in the reserved test set. AUC was 0.63 for predicting adverse events, 0.68 for extended hospital stay, and 0.75 for discharge to a higher level of care.

Supervised ML outperforms individual comorbidity indices in predicting morbidity after RC. A 2022 study of 392 patients directly compared the predictive power of several supervised ML models with aCCI, ASA, and Gagne's combined comorbidity Index (GCI). AUC for comorbidity indices were 0.6 (aCCI), 0.63 (ASA), and 0.58 (GCI). In contrast, the AUC for LR was 0.763, second only to the Gaussian Naive Bayes model, which performed with an AUC of 0.794. Both the neural network and random forest also outperformed comorbidity indices with AUCs of 0.741 and 0.748, respectively.[87]

A handful of studies explore ML models with more novel inputs. Ying and colleagues[88] deployed a CNN to automatically segment and compute skeletal muscle volume on preoperative CT before RC. Cox regression analysis in their cohort of 299 patients showed independent association with overall survival (hazard ratio, 1.62; 95% confidence interval, 1.07–2.44; P = .022). Schuettfort and colleagues[89] built a LASSO model to predict various oncologic outcomes based on systemic inflammatory response biomarkers in 4199 patients. AUC was 0.673 for predicting lymph node involvement, 0.73 for predicting greater than or equal to pT3 stage, and 0.658 for upstaging to muscle-invasive cancer on final pathology.

Predicting Postcystectomy Survival and Cancer Control

Long-term cancer control after RC is poor. Even with negative margins, 5-year overall survival rates without neoadjuvant chemotherapy are approximately 47%.[90] Accurate prognostication can help determine surveillance schedules and candidacy for adjuvant systemic therapy after primary resection. Postoperative cancer control is currently prognosticated primarily by pathologic staging.[3,79,80] A recent retrospective multicenter study of 9000 patients reported a concordance index of 0.68 when standard American Joint Committee on Cancer TNM staging was used to predict 5-year progression-free probability after RC. The authors were able to improve the index to 0.75 using a Cox proportional hazards model to build a nomogram, although this was not based on an external test set.[91] Several studies have sought to improve prognostication with ML techniques.

Early efforts began in the early 2000s to train ANNs to predict RC outcomes using standard perioperative clinical data including pathologic stage, other adverse surgical pathologic findings (eg, lymphatic invasion), age, gender, and surgical approach. The results were equivocal. In 2006 Bassi and colleagues[92] developed an ANN to predict 5-year overall survival after RC and compared its predictive accuracy with an LR classifier developed from the same population (n = 369). The simple regression model performed just as well as the ANN (75.9% vs 76.4% concordance index). In 2013 Buchner and colleagues[93] used a population of 2111 patients to train an ANN to predict recurrence, cancer-specific mortality, and all-caused death. A Cox regression model was developed from the same population for comparison. The ANN was 74% accurate at predicting recurrence, 69% for cancer-specific mortality, and 69% for all-caused death. The Cox regression model was only less accurate by 4.7% (P < .001) at predicting cancer-specific mortality and 3.5% (P = .007) for predicting all-caused death. There was no difference in accuracy at predicting recurrence. Results were also reported without the use of a test set to demonstrate external validity.[93]

Later studies used various other supervised ML models, also with mixed results. In 2009 Catto and colleagues[94] used 609 patients with localized BC to train a neuro-fuzzy model to predict recurrence after RC based on standard clinicopathologic factors. They applied two published nomograms to predict recurrence in their cohort as a comparator. The model was 84% accurate, compared with 72% and 74% with the two nomograms. Although the authors did report performance using a held-out test set, the nomograms were developed from a different study population entirely, thus introducing selection bias and decreasing external validity in favor of the neuro-fuzzy model.[94] In 2015 Wang and colleagues[95] used data from 117 patients to train seven supervised ML methods to predict 5-year survival after RC. The accuracy of these ML models ranged from 70% to 80%, compared with 63.3% using a published nomogram. However, results were once again reported based on the same study cohort used to train the ML algorithms but not the nomogram. Although the authors did use 10-fold cross-validation to report misclassification probability (standard deviation for mean accuracy among folds approached $\pm 8\%$), no external test set was used, which all but guarantees that the nomogram will perform worse.[95]

In 2019, Hasnain and colleagues[96] published the largest study to date applying supervised ML algorithms to predict recurrence and survival after RC (n = 3499). This study notably used a more expansive set of input variables including medical comorbidities, neoadjuvant chemotherapy, surgical metrics and methods, and various other perioperative variables beyond pathologic stage and other standard clinicopathologic variables. ML models were stacked into "meta-classifiers" using various summation methods, such as "mixture-of-experts" and hard-voting. As a comparator, recurrence and survival were also predicted using pT stage in a univariate model. The meta-classifier was 70% sensitive and 70.2% specific in predicting 5-year recurrence. In comparison, isolated pT stage was 74.4% sensitive and 61.1% specific. Results were reported using nested cross-validation (10 outer folds, 5 inner folds), but not with a held-out test set.[96]

Sonpavde and colleagues[97] recently published the results of a study that trained an ANN with whole exome sequencing of tumor and normal tissue using RNA-Seq. The classifier predicted recurrence with an accuracy of 94% using test sets. The study is small (n = 117), but the preliminary results are promising.[97]

Limitations of the Existing Body of Work

Compared with standard regression models, such as LR classifiers, ANNs decrease the transparency of analysis by incorporating one or more hidden layers of nonlinear activation functions. Other nonlinear supervised ML models have a similar black box effect. This forfeits the benefit of an exploratory analysis, which would otherwise provide odds ratios for isolated variables to help inform a clinician's decision-making process. Granted, the strategy of AI and ML is to sacrifice a mechanistic understanding of the prediction problem in favor of an effective black box solution. This trade-off is reasonable, provided that a study formally states its goal to be predictive rather than exploratory, and a study takes strict measures to validate and test the black box. ANNs and more complex ML models are at higher risk of overfitting the data, especially without rigorous methodology to report misclassification probability and appropriate performance metrics.[98]

In this respect, limitations remain in the existing body of literature in regards to methodology. Many studies either lacked a held-out test set or reported performance using a test set from the same population that trained the ML algorithm but not the comparator. Existing studies in this space also tend to report accuracy as the primary performance metric, which is less representative of true performance when there is class imbalance. In the absence of neoadjuvant chemotherapy, about 80.9% of patients have disease recurrence within 2 years of RC.[90] Additional statistics, such as the AUC and the F1 score, are often better-suited but not always used.[99] The choice of model is often also suboptimal. More complex supervised ML models are designed to elucidate a network of nonlinear, nonintuitive relationships between a large array of inputs. They provide minimal benefit when given a simple set of a few clinicopathologic variables.[98] Indeed when proper methods were deployed, they were often outperformed by simple logistic-regression-based models, such as LASSO.[86,87] The latest studies have begun demonstrating appropriate model selection and proper methodology, but further prospective study is needed to demonstrate clinical value.[87,88,90]

A final major obstacle to deploying effective AI solutions in this space is the issue of "decaying relevance." Training ML models requires large swaths of clinical data to iteratively home in on a solution. It takes many years to generate the requisite volume of survival and recurrence data after RC. Chen and colleagues[100] demonstrated that predicting future inpatient orders is vastly more accurate with models trained on just 1 month of recent data than with 12 months of older but higher volume data. This is because of the speed at which clinical practice patterns evolve. For example, many patients with MIBC today receive neoadjuvant chemotherapy or radiotherapy, whereas most studies to date exclude patients who received any presurgical treatment. This severely limits the relevance of these AI tools on today's cystectomy candidates.

Application of Artificial Intelligence for Radiation-Based Treatment of Bladder Cancer

Radiation therapy is an important treatment modality in patients with MIBC.[101–103] Radiation therapy is used as a primary treatment of BC in cases where surgical intervention (ie, RC) is not possible or preferred by the patient,[104,105] or as palliative treatment to alleviate symptoms and improve the quality of life for patients with advanced or metastatic disease.

One of the challenges of radiation therapy for BC is minimizing the radiation dose to healthy surrounding organs, such as the bowel and rectum. Modern external beam radiation therapy,[106] including intensity-modulated radiation therapy, and image-guided radiation therapy allow for better sparing of healthy tissues, reducing the risk of complications and improving patients' overall tolerance to treatment.

Deep learning–based radiation therapy is emerging as a promising approach for the treatment of BC. This technique uses AI to optimize the planning and delivery of radiation therapy, aiming to maximize the dose to the tumor while minimizing exposure to surrounding healthy tissues.[107,108] Deep learning models can be trained to automatically segment the bladder and other critical structures in imaging data, a task that is traditionally time-consuming and prone to interobserver variability.[109,110] These models can also predict the movement and deformation of the bladder during treatment, allowing for more precise targeting of the radiation dose. Although at an early stage, deep learning has the potential to improve more precise delivery of radiation therapy for BC.

SUMMARY

AI holds strong potential to guide decision-making for BC diagnosis and treatment and to integrate such models into the current clinical workflow. This review summarizes the emerging AI applications for BC, including diagnostic cystoscopy, radiologic imaging, pathologic diagnosis, molecular biomarkers, risk stratification, treatment assessment, and outcome prediction.

Moving forward, several areas of development and integration of AI systems are needed: (1) curation of large, multicenter, multidimensional datasets for training and validation; (2) standardization of reporting and data management to facilitate communication; and (3) design of prospective clinical trials to validate the utility of these models in key timepoints of cancer management from screening, diagnosis, treatment, and surveillance. The myriad of data modalities collected in the BC clinical workflow, from clinical history, cystoscopy, cross-sectional imaging, laboratory data, and histopathology, can be effectively used in new multimodal deep learning models. The recent advent of artificial general intelligence and large language models, such as ChatGPT have sparked their application for writing and reasoning tasks in clinical and surgical specialites.[111]

Successful execution of the previously mentioned aims will have wide-reaching implications for patients, providers, and health care systems. The integration of AI into the current BC management clinical workflow will serve as a personalized decision support system for patients and clinicians throughout its detection, treatment, and downstream management, and will ultimately result in improved patient outcomes and quality of life.

DISCLOSURE

The authors declare no known competing financial interests or personal relationships that could have appeared to influence the work reported in this article.

FUNDING

The authors gratefully acknowledge research support from NIH R01 CA260426 (J.C.L. and L.X.), Department of Veterans Affairs BLR&D I01 BX005598 (J.C.L.), and the Urology Care Foundation (E.S.).

REFERENCES

1. Siegel RL, Miller KD, Fuchs HE, et al. Cancer statistics, 2022. CA Cancer J Clin 2022;72(1):7–33.
2. Sylvester RJ, Van Der Meijden APM, Oosterlinck W, et al. Predicting recurrence and progression in individual patients with stage Ta T1 bladder cancer using EORTC risk tables: a combined analysis of 2596 patients from seven EORTC trials. Eur Urol 2006;49(3):466–77.
3. Chang SS, Boorjian SA, Chou R, et al. Diagnosis and treatment of non-muscle invasive bladder cancer: AUA/SUO Guideline. J Urol 2016;196(4): 1021–9.
4. Yeung C, Dinh T, Lee J. The health economics of bladder cancer: an updated review of the published literature. Pharmacoeconomics 2014; 32(11):1093–104.
5. Chang SS, Bochner BH, Chou R, et al. Treatment of non-metastatic muscle-invasive bladder cancer: AUA/ASCO/ASTRO/SUO Guideline. J Urol 2017; 198(3):552–9.
6. Verghote F, Van Praet C, De Maeseneer D, et al. Radiotherapy use in muscle-invasive bladder cancer: review of the guidelines and impact of increased awareness in patient referral at a tertiary center in Belgium. Cancer Manag Res 2023;15:511–21.
7. Gomes B, Ashley EA. Artificial intelligence in molecular Medicine. N Engl J Med 2023;388(26): 2456–65.
8. Rajpurkar P, Lungren MP. The current and future state of AI interpretation of medical images. N Engl J Med 2023;388(21):1981–90.
9. Chang TC, Seufert C, Eminaga O, et al. Current trends in artificial intelligence application for endourology and robotic surgery 2021;48:151–60.

10. Vapnik VN. An overview of statistical learning theory. IEEE Trans Neural Netw 1999;10(5):988–99.

11. Nichols JA, Herbert Chan HW, Baker MAB. Machine learning: applications of artificial intelligence to imaging and diagnosis. Biophys Rev 2018;11(1):111–8.

12. LeCun Y, Bengio Y, Hinton G. Deep learning. Nature 2015;521(7553):436–44.

13. Alzubaidi L, Zhang J, Humaidi AJ, et al. Review of deep learning: concepts, CNN architectures, challenges, applications, future directions. J Big Data 2021;8(1):53.

14. Ian Goodfellow YB. Deep learning. MIT Press; 2017.

15. Ajit A, Acharya K, Samanta A. A review of convolutional neural networks. In: 2020 International conference on emerging trends in information technology and engineering. Ic-ETITE); 2020. p. 1–5. https://doi.org/10.1109/ic-ETITE47903.2020.049.

16. Zhao ZQ, Zheng P, Xu S tao, Wu X. Object detection with deep learning: a review. Published online April 16, 2019. http://arxiv.org/abs/1807.05511. Accessed July 3, 2023.

17. Liu D, Soran B, Petrie G, & Shapiro LG. A Review of Computer Vision Segmentation Algorithms. 2012. Available at: https://api.semanticscholar.org/CorpusID:14000252.

18. Shkolyar E, Jia X, Chang TC, et al. Augmented bladder tumor detection using deep learning 2019;76:714–8.

19. Ikeda A, Nosato H, Kochi Y, et al. Support system of cystoscopic diagnosis for bladder cancer based on artificial Intelligence. J Endourol 2020;34:352–8.

20. Ali N, Bolenz C, Todenhöfer T, et al. Deep learning-based classification of blue light cystoscopy imaging during transurethral resection of bladder tumors 2021. Published online.

21. Yoo JW, Koo KC, Chung BH, et al. Deep learning diagnostics for bladder tumor identification and grade prediction using RGB method. Sci Rep 2022;12(1):17699.

22. Chang TC, Shkolyar E, Del Giudice F, et al. Real-time detection of bladder cancer using augmented cystoscopy with deep learning: a pilot study. J Endourol 2023. https://doi.org/10.1089/end.2023.0056.

23. Alex Krizhevsky IS. ImageNet classification with deep convolutional neural networks. NeuriPS; 2012.

24. Christian Szegedy WL. Going deeper with convolutions. In: ; 2015.

25. Eminaga O, Eminaga N, Semjonow A, et al. Diagnostic classification of cystoscopic images using deep. convolutional neural networks 2018;2:1–8.

26. Daneshmand S, Schuckman AK, Bochner BH, et al. Hexaminolevulinate blue-light cystoscopy in non-muscle-invasive bladder cancer: review of the clinical evidence and consensus statement on appropriate use in the USA. Nat Rev Urol 2014;11(10):589–96.

27. Wu S, Chen X, Pan J, et al. An artificial intelligence system for the detection of bladder cancer via cystoscopy: a multicenter diagnostic study. J Natl Cancer Inst 2022;114(2):220–7.

28. Sequential modeling for cystoscopic image classification. https://www.spiedigitallibrary.org/conference-proceedings-of-spie/12353/123530B/Sequential-modeling-for-cystoscopic-image-classification/10.1117/12.2649334.short. Accessed July 3, 2023.

29. Bandyk MG, Gopireddy DR, Lall C, et al. MRI and CT bladder segmentation from classical to deep learning based approaches: current limitations and lessons. Comput Biol Med 2021;134:104472.

30. Zhang G, Wu Z, Xu L, et al. Deep learning on enhanced CT images can predict the muscular invasiveness of bladder cancer. Front Oncol 2021;11. https://www.frontiersin.org/articles/10.3389/fonc.2021.654685. Accessed July 10, 2023.

31. Lee MC, Wang SY, Pan CT, et al. Development of deep learning with RDA U-Net network for bladder cancer segmentation. Cancers 2023;15(4):1343.

32. Cha KH, Hadjiiski L, Chan HP, et al. Bladder cancer treatment response assessment in CT using radiomics with deep-learning. Sci Rep 2017;7(1):8738.

33. Li R, Chen H, Gong G, et al. Bladder wall segmentation in MRI images via deep learning and anatomical constraints. In: 2020 42nd annual international conference of the IEEE engineering in medicine & biology society. EMBC); 2020. p. 1629–32.

34. Dolz J, Xu X, Rony J, et al. Multiregion segmentation of bladder cancer structures in MRI with progressive dilated convolutional networks. Med Phys 2018;45(12):5482–93.

35. Li J, Qiu Z, Cao K, et al. Predicting muscle invasion in bladder cancer based on MRI: a comparison of radiomics, and single-task and multi-task deep learning. Comput Methods Programs Biomed 2023;233:107466.

36. Saeedi S, Rezayi S, Keshavarz H, et al. MRI-based brain tumor detection using convolutional deep learning methods and chosen machine learning techniques. BMC Med Inform Decis Mak 2023;23:16.

37. Raut G, Raut A, Bhagade J, et al. Deep learning approach for brain tumor detection and segmentation. In: 2020 International conference on convergence to digital world - quo vadis. ICCDW); 2020. p. 1–5.

38. Trinh TW, Glazer DI, Sadow CA, et al. Bladder cancer diagnosis with CT urography: test characteristics and reasons for false-positive and false-negative results. Abdom Radiol N Y 2018;43(3):663–71.

39. Bove S, Fanizzi A, Fadda F, et al. A CT-based transfer learning approach to predict NSCLC recurrence: the added-value of peritumoral region. PLoS One 2023;18(5):e0285188.

40. Wang X, Yang M. The application of ultrasound image in cancer diagnosis. J Healthc Eng 2021;2021: 8619251.

41. Islam MT, Tang S, Liverani C, et al. Non-invasive imaging of Young's modulus and Poisson's ratio in cancers in vivo. Sci Rep 2020;10(1):7266.

42. Islam MT, Tang S, Tasciotti E, et al. Non-invasive assessment of the spatial and temporal distributions of interstitial fluid pressure, fluid velocity and fluid flow in cancers in vivo. IEEE Access 2021;9: 89222–33.

43. Islam MT, Tasciotti E, Righetti R. Non-invasive imaging of normalized solid stress in cancers in vivo. IEEE J Transl Eng Health Med 2019;7:1–9.

44. Gharibvand MM, Kazemi M, Motamedfar A, et al. The role of ultrasound in diagnosis and evaluation of bladder tumors. J Fam Med Prim Care 2017; 6(4):840–3.

45. Stamatiou K, Papadoliopoulos I, Dahanis S, et al. The accuracy of ultrasonography in the diagnosis of superficial bladder tumors in patients presenting with hematuria. Ann Saudi Med 2009;29(2):134–7.

46. Malone PR. Transabdominal ultrasound surveillance for bladder cancer. Urol Clin North Am 1989;16(4):823–7.

47. Caruso G, Salvaggio G, Campisi A, et al. Bladder tumor staging: comparison of contrast-enhanced and gray-scale ultrasound. Am J Roentgenol 2010;194(1):151–6.

48. Fabiani A, Filosa A, Piergallina M, et al. The potential role of transrectal ultrasound as a tool for diagnosis or recurrence detection in bladder cancer. Two cases report. Arch Ital Urol Androl Organo Uff Soc Ital Ecogr Urol E Nefrol 2012;84(3):161–4.

49. Oktem GC, Kocaaslan R, Karadag MA, et al. The role of transcavitary ultrasonography in diagnosis and staging of nonmuscle-invasive bladder cancer: a prospective non-randomized clinical study. SpringerPlus 2014;3:519.

50. Gupta VG, Kumar S, Singh SK, et al. Contrast enhanced ultrasound in urothelial carcinoma of urinary bladder: an underutilized staging and grading modality. Cent Eur J Urol 2016;69(4):360–5.

51. Nicolau C, Bunesch L, Peri L, et al. Accuracy of contrast-enhanced ultrasound in the detection of bladder cancer. Br J Radiol 2011;84(1008):1091–9.

52. Shao C, Sun A, Xue H, et al. Three-dimensional ultrasound images in the assessment of bladder tumor health monitoring under deep learning algorithms. Comput Math Methods Med 2022;2022: 9170274.

53. Tsuneki M, Abe M, Kanavati F. Deep learning-based screening of urothelial carcinoma in whole slide images of liquid-based cytology urine specimens. Cancers 2022;15(1):226.

54. Sanghvi AB, Allen EZ, Callenberg KM, et al. Performance of an artificial intelligence algorithm for reporting urine cytopathology. Cancer Cytopathol 2019;127(10):658–66.

55. Sullivan PS, Chan JB, Levin MR, et al. Urine cytology and adjunct markers for detection and surveillance of bladder cancer. Am J Transl Res 2010;2(4):412–40.

56. Critical Evaluation of Urinary Markers for Bladder Cancer Detection and Monitoring - PMC. https:// www.ncbi.nlm.nih.gov/pmc/articles/PMC2483317/. Accessed July 12, 2023.

57. Compérat E, Oszwald A, Wasinger G, et al. Updated pathology reporting standards for bladder cancer: biopsies, transurethral resections and radical cystectomies. World J Urol 2022;40(4):915–27.

58. Compérat E, Varinot J, Moroch J, et al. A practical guide to bladder cancer pathology. Nat Rev Urol 2018;15(3):143–54.

59. Mazzucchelli R, Marzioni D, Tossetta G, et al. Bladder cancer sample handling and reporting: pathologist's point of view. Front Surg 2021;8: 754741.

60. Barrios W, Abdollahi B, Goyal M, et al. Bladder cancer prognosis using deep neural networks and histopathology images. J Pathol Inform 2022; 13:100135.

61. Mundhada A, Sundaram S, Swaminathan R, et al. Differentiation of urothelial carcinoma in histopathology images using deep learning and visualization. J Pathol Inform 2022;14:100155.

62. Shkolyar E, Bhambhvani H, Tiu E, et al. 1773P Prediction of neoadjuvant chemotherapy response in muscle-invasive bladder cancer: a machine learning approach. Ann Oncol 2022; 33:S1348.

63. Harmon SA, Sanford TH, Brown GT, et al. Multiresolution application of artificial intelligence in digital pathology for prediction of positive lymph nodes from primary tumors in bladder cancer. JCO Clin Cancer Inform 2020;4:367–82.

64. Wu S, Hong G, Xu A, et al. Artificial intelligence-based model for lymph node metastases detection on whole slide images in bladder cancer: a retrospective, multicentre, diagnostic study. Lancet Oncol 2023;24(4):360–70.

65. Poirion OB, Chaudhary K, Garmire LX. Deep Learning data integration for better risk stratification models of bladder cancer. AMIA Jt Summits Transl Sci Proc AMIA Jt Summits Transl Sci 2018; 2017:197–206.

66. Malinaric R, Mantica G, Lo Monaco L, et al. The role of novel bladder cancer diagnostic and surveillance biomarkers—what should a urologist really know? Int J Environ Res Public Health 2022;19(15):9648.

67. Islam MT, Xing L. Cartography of genomic interactions enables deep analysis of single-cell expression data. Nat Commun 2023;14(1):679.

68. Islam MT, Wang JY, Ren H, et al. Leveraging data-driven self-consistency for high-fidelity gene expression recovery. Nat Commun 2022;13(1):7142.

69. Batista R, Vinagre N, Meireles S, et al. Biomarkers for bladder cancer diagnosis and surveillance: a comprehensive review. Diagnostics 2020;10(1):39.

70. van Rhijn BWG, van Tilborg AAG, Lurkin I, et al. Novel fibroblast growth factor receptor 3 (FGFR3) mutations in bladder cancer previously identified in non-lethal skeletal disorders. Eur J Hum Genet EJHG 2002;10(12):819–24.

71. Ascione CM, Napolitano F, Esposito D, et al. Role of FGFR3 in bladder cancer: treatment landscape and future challenges. Cancer Treat Rev 2023;115:102530.

72. Wan S, Liu X, Hua W, et al. The role of telomerase reverse transcriptase (TERT) promoter mutations in prognosis in bladder cancer. Bioengineered 2021;12(1):1495–504.

73. Islam MT, Xing L. A data-driven dimensionality-reduction algorithm for the exploration of patterns in biomedical data. Nat Biomed Eng 2021;5(6):624–35.

74. Höglund M, Bernardo C, Sjödahl G, et al. The Lund taxonomy for bladder cancer classification: from gene expression clustering to cancer cell molecular phenotypes, and back again. J Pathol 2023;259(4):369–75.

75. Marzouka NAD, Eriksson P, Bernardo C, et al. The Lund molecular taxonomy applied to non-muscle-invasive urothelial carcinoma. J Mol Diagn JMD 2022;24(9):992–1008.

76. Liao Y, Tang H, Wang M, et al. The potential diagnosis role of TP53 mutation in advanced bladder cancer: a meta-analysis. J Clin Lab Anal 2021;35(5):e23765.

77. Wu Z, Wang M, Liu Q, et al. Identification of gene expression profiles and immune cell infiltration signatures between low and high tumor mutation burden groups in bladder cancer. Int J Med Sci 2020;17(1):89–96.

78. Lucas M, Jansen I, van Leeuwen TG, et al. Deep learning-based recurrence prediction in patients with non-muscle-invasive bladder cancer. Eur Urol Focus 2022;8(1):165–72.

79. Flaig TW, Spiess PE, Abern M, et al. NCCN Guidelines® Insights: Bladder Cancer, Version 2.2022: Featured Updates to the NCCN Guidelines. J Natl Compr Canc Netw 2022;20(8):866–78.

80. Babjuk M, Burger M, Compérat EM, et al. European Association of Urology guidelines on non-muscle-invasive bladder cancer (TaT1 and carcinoma in situ): 2019 Update. Eur Urol 2019;76(5):639–57.

81. Quek ML, Stein JP, Daneshmand S, et al. A critical analysis of perioperative mortality from radical cystectomy. J Urol 2006;175(3):886–90.

82. Shabsigh A, Korets R, Vora KC, et al. Defining early morbidity of radical cystectomy for patients with bladder cancer using a standardized reporting methodology. Eur Urol 2009;55(1):164–76.

83. Williams SB, Kamat AM, Chamie K, et al. Systematic review of comorbidity and competing-risks assessments for bladder cancer patients. Eur Urol Oncol 2018;1(2):91–100.

84. Golan S, Adamsky MA, Johnson SC, et al. National Surgical Quality Improvement Program surgical risk calculator poorly predicts complications in patients undergoing radical cystectomy with urinary diversion. Urol Oncol Semin Orig Investig 2018;36(2):77.e1–7.

85. Klén R, Salminen AP, Mahmoudian M, et al. Prediction of complication related death after radical cystectomy for bladder cancer with machine learning methodology. Scand J Urol 2019;53(5):325–31.

86. Taylor J, Meng X, Renson A, et al. Different models for prediction of radical cystectomy postoperative complications and care pathways. Ther Adv Urol 2019;11. 175628721987558.

87. Wessels F, Bußoff I, Adam S, et al. Comorbidity scores and machine learning methods can improve risk assessment in radical cystectomy for bladder cancer. Bladder Cancer 2022;8(2):155–63.

88. Ying T, Borrelli P, Edenbrandt L, et al. Automated artificial intelligence-based analysis of skeletal muscle volume predicts overall survival after cystectomy for urinary bladder cancer. Eur Radiol Exp 2021;5(1):50.

89. Schuettfort VM, D'Andrea D, Quhal F, et al. A panel of systemic inflammatory response biomarkers for outcome prediction in patients treated with radical cystectomy for urothelial carcinoma. BJU Int 2022;129(2):182–93.

90. Sonpavde G, Khan MM, Lerner SP, et al. Disease-free survival at 2 or 3 years correlates with 5-year overall survival of patients undergoing radical cystectomy for muscle invasive bladder cancer. J Urol 2011;185(2):456–61.

91. Postoperative nomogram predicting risk of recurrence after radical cystectomy for bladder cancer. J Clin Oncol 2006;24(24):3967–72.

92. Bassi P, Sacco E, De Marco V, et al. Prognostic accuracy of an artificial neural network in patients undergoing radical cystectomy for bladder cancer: a comparison with logistic regression analysis. BJU Int 2007;99(5):1007–12.

93. Buchner A, May M, Burger M, et al. Prediction of outcome in patients with urothelial carcinoma of the bladder following radical cystectomy using artificial neural networks. Eur J Surg Oncol EJSO 2013;39(4):372–9.

94. Catto JWF, Abbod MF, Linkens DA, et al. Neuro-fuzzy modeling to determine recurrence risk following radical cystectomy for nonmetastatic urothelial carcinoma of the bladder. Clin Cancer Res 2009;15(9):3150–5.

95. Wang G, Lam KM, Deng Z, et al. Prediction of mortality after radical cystectomy for bladder cancer by machine learning techniques. Comput Biol Med 2015;63:124–32.

96. Hasnain Z, Mason J, Gill K, et al. Machine learning models for predicting post-cystectomy recurrence and survival in bladder cancer patients. In: Katoh M, editor. PLoS One 2019;14:e0210976.

97. Sonpavde GP, Sadler L, Ravi A, et al. Neural network analysis of tumor and germline profiling to predict survival of muscle-invasive bladder cancer following radical cystectomy: an analysis of the Cancer Genome Atlas (TCGA). J Clin Oncol 2023;41(6_suppl):546.

98. Schwarzer G, Vach W, Schumacher M. On the misuses of artificial neural networks for prognostic and diagnostic classification in oncology. Stat Med 2000;19(4):541–61.

99. Sokolova M, Japkowicz N, Szpakowicz S. Beyond accuracy, F-score and ROC: a family of discriminant measures for performance evaluation. In: Sattar A, Kang B, editors. *AI 2006: Advances in artificial intelligence*. Vol 4304. Lecture notes in computer science. Springer Berlin Heidelberg; 2006. p. 1015–21.

100. Chen JH, Alagappan M, Goldstein MK, et al. Decaying relevance of clinical data towards future decisions in data-driven inpatient clinical order sets. Int J Med Inf 2017;102:71–9.

101. Huang C, Vasudevan V, Pastor-Serrano O, et al. Learning image representations for content-based image retrieval of radiotherapy treatment plans. Phys Med Biol 2023;68(9):095025.

102. Vasudevan V, Shen L, Huang C, et al. Neural representation for three-dimensional dose distribution and its applications in precision radiation therapy. Int J Radiat Oncol Biol Phys 2022;114(3):e552.

103. Vasudevan V, Shen L, Huang C, et al. Implicit neural representation for radiation therapy dose distribution. Phys Med Biol 2022;67(12):125014.

104. James ND, Hussain SA, Hall E, et al. Radiotherapy with or without chemotherapy in muscle-invasive bladder cancer. N Engl J Med 2012;366(16):1477–88.

105. Giacalone NJ, WU Shipley, Clayman RH, et al. Long-term outcomes after bladder-preserving trimodality therapy for patients with muscle-invasive bladder cancer: an updated analysis of the Massachusetts General Hospital experience. Eur Urol 2017;71(6):952–60.

106. Moschini M, Zaffuto E, Karakiewicz PI, et al. External beam radiotherapy increases the risk of bladder cancer when compared with radical prostatectomy in patients affected by prostate cancer: a population-based analysis. Eur Urol 2019;75(2):319–28.

107. Nguyen D, Long T, Jia X, et al. A feasibility study for predicting optimal radiation therapy dose distributions of prostate cancer patients from patient anatomy using deep learning. Sci Rep 2019;9(1):1076.

108. Lei Y, Wang T, Tian S, et al. Male pelvic multi-organ segmentation aided by CBCT-based synthetic MRI. Phys Med Biol 2020;65(3):035013.

109. Shen C, Nguyen D, Chen L, et al. Operating a treatment planning system using a deep-reinforcement learning-based virtual treatment planner for prostate cancer intensity-modulated radiation therapy treatment planning. Med Phys 2020;47(6):2329–36.

110. Kiljunen T, Akram S, Niemelä J, et al. A deep learning-based automated CT segmentation of prostate cancer anatomy for radiation therapy planning: a retrospective multicenter study. Diagn Basel Switz 2020;10(11):959.

111. Janssen BV, Kazemier G, Besselink MG. The use of ChatGPT and other large language models in surgical science. BJS Open 2023;7(2):zrad032.

Surgical Artificial Intelligence: Endourology

Zachary E. Tano, MD*, Andrei D. Cumpanas, MD, Antonio R.H. Gorgen, MD, Allen Rojhani, MD, Jaime Altamirano-Villarroel, MD, Jaime Landman, MD

KEYWORDS

- Artificial intelligence • Machine learning • Endourology • Kidney stone • PCNL • Ureteroscopy
- Benign prostatic hyperplasia

KEY POINTS

- Artificial intelligence (AI) is composed of machine learning that can be supervised with known algorithms and deep learning that creates undisclosed methodologies to find complex patterns in data.
- AI seems most promising in the near term for kidney stone volume detection and volume measurement. Other kidney stone-related assessments as well as endoscopic tissue diagnosis and benign prostatic hyperplasia management decisions are blossoming areas of research.
- Urologists must become familiar with AI assessment, and programs must be shared and criticized to further implement this technology into clinical practice.

INTRODUCTION

Artificial intelligence (AI) is best known to the general public through science fiction books and films, but AI has become a focus on practical interest and has been operationally implemented into many aspects of society, including medicine, urology, and endourology. The endourologic surgeon encounters many diagnostic and therapeutic decisions. These decisions affect medical and surgical management ranging from the diagnosis of benign and malignant disease, classifying theses diagnoses, predicting surgical outcomes to determine optimal treatment, and predicting temporizing or prevention outcomes to determine if active intervention is warranted. These questions are increasingly multifactorial, complex, and are difficult to assess even with the most advanced traditional statistical models due to isolating the proper predictive factors and finding the relationship between these factors. AI has the capability to assist surgeons and statisticians in this regard, but some forms of AI are intrinsically "black box" data processing where humans lose the ability to control input and evaluation methods. As such, it is essential for critical review of these algorithms before clinical implementation. Herein, the authors present a summary of the current state of AI and its applicability for the endourologic surgeon.

TYPES OF ARTIFICIAL INTELLIGENCE

Although commonly used interchangeably, AI and machine learning (ML) are different concepts.[1] ML is an AI process through which algorithms can incorporate large data sets, analyze them, and learn from the observed patterns, while also using them to make predictions.[2,3] ML can be "supervised," in which the input data set is already labeled (ie, CT scans preprocessed by a radiologist into a "stone" or "no-stone group) or "unsupervised," in which the input data set is unlabeled (ie, the algorithm is fed a sample of CT scans without preprocessing).[4] Commonly used ML algorithm's include support vector machine (SVM), decision trees, random forest, K-nearest

The authors have no commercial or financial conflicts of interest to disclose.

Department of Urology, University of California, Irvine, 3800 West Chapman Avenue, Suite 7200, Orange, CA 92868, USA

* Corresponding author.

E-mail address: ztano@hs.uci.edu

urologic.theclinics.com

neighbor (KNN), naïve Bayes classification, and linear and logistic regression (LR) models (**Fig. 1**).[3]

SVMs analyze labeled data sets with the purpose of maximizing the separation of data into two groups. This demarcation is achieved by determining the optimal cutoff between the groups, termed a "hyperplane." Once trained, the ML algorithm classifies new data to one side of the hyperplane[5] (see **Fig. 1**). In practice, data often do not conform to a simple binary classification scheme of "yes" or "no." As such, classical decision trees that rely on Boolean logic and have binary outcomes may not accurately capture the complex and ambiguous nature of real-world data. To overcome these limitations, fuzzy decision trees have been developed.[6,7] These trees are based on the concept of three-way decision proposed by Yao and colleagues.[6] The fundamental idea behind fuzzy trees is to allow for the partial membership of variables to multiple branches of the original Boolean logic tree, in recognition of the fact that variables may have uncertain or ambiguous values.[6,7] Random forest plots incorporate multiple decision trees that are linked together within an ML algorithm. The output of each decision tree is weighted equally, and the most common output prevails. This type of model limits bias by ensuring that the final output is not influenced by a single decision tree but is determined by a "majority vote" between multiple trees (see **Fig. 1**). Other methods used by ML algorithms are data nearness calculation or computing the object–group belonging probability as is the case of KNN and naïve Bayes classification.[8]

A subtype of ML, termed deep learning (DL) is usually associated with a more complex architecture, with AI units connected, like neurons in a multiple functional layer system (hence "deep" learning).[1] This computational web with multiple, interconnected feedback loops allows for the analysis of large data sets with apparently no visible connection between them, teaching themselves the "rules of the game" and performing complex tasks such as data classification, regression analysis, object detection, and image segmentation.[1,9] A visual representation of ML and DL is shown in **Fig. 1**.

STONE DETECTION AND CHARACTERIZATION
Simple Detection of Renal Stones

According to Hall and colleagues, there has been an approximately 50% increase in the prevalence of kidney stone disease over the past 2 decades.[10] If this trend continues, it is likely that urologists will face an increase in emergency department visit consultations, clinic consultations, and surgical procedures. Because a non-contrast CT (NCCT) scan is typically required for most of these visits to assess the stone burden, radiologists may also face time constrains when interpreting medical images. In the long run, this could have detrimental effects on diagnostic accuracy, treatment selection, and patient safety. As published by Sokolovskaya and colleagues, reducing the time required to read an abdominal NCCT scan takes to between 5 to 10 minutes has been associated with an increased error rate of 10% to 26%.[11] To address these challenges, multiple studies have suggested using AI algorithms to assist the NCCT screening for kidney stone burden, which may offer a time-efficient, accurate, and precise way to facilitate proper medical diagnosis and reduce the interobserver variability previously seen with maximum linear stone measurements assessment.[12–16]

Noise Reduction: Differentiating Ureteral Stones from Phleboliths

Although it may be feasible for most AI algorithms to diagnose kidney stones based on Hounsfield unit (HU) thresholds within a renal label map, differentiating ureteral stones from vascular calcifications (phleboliths) within the renal pelvis poses a significantly more complex challenge. The successful differentiation of ureteral stones from phleboliths relies heavily on the ability to accurately locate the calcification's relation to the ureter, specifically within or outside its lumen, which can be difficult due to the removal of surrounding anatomic landmarks when using an automatic HU threshold selection for analysis.[17] It has been proposed to include radiological signs, such as the "soft tissue rim sign" or the "comet sign," but those characteristics were insufficient for providing a clear diagnosis.[16,18] Thus, it is crucial to train AI algorithms to identify fine patterns such as pixel disperseness, skewness, and radiopacity histogram distribution, which may not be distinguishable to the naked human eye.[19] De Perrot and colleagues developed an ML algorithm that distinguished ureteral stones from phleboliths with an accuracy of 85.1%, a positive predictive value (PPV) of 81.5% and an negative predictive value (NPV) of 90% on low dose NCCT scans. The area under the curve for the algorithm was 0.902(16). Similarly, using a 2.5-dimensional convoluted neural network (CNN), Jenderberg and colleagues managed to differentiate ureteral stones from phleboliths (sensitivity 94%, specificity 90%, accuracy 92%, and area under the curve [AUC] 0.95).[16,18] Interestingly, when

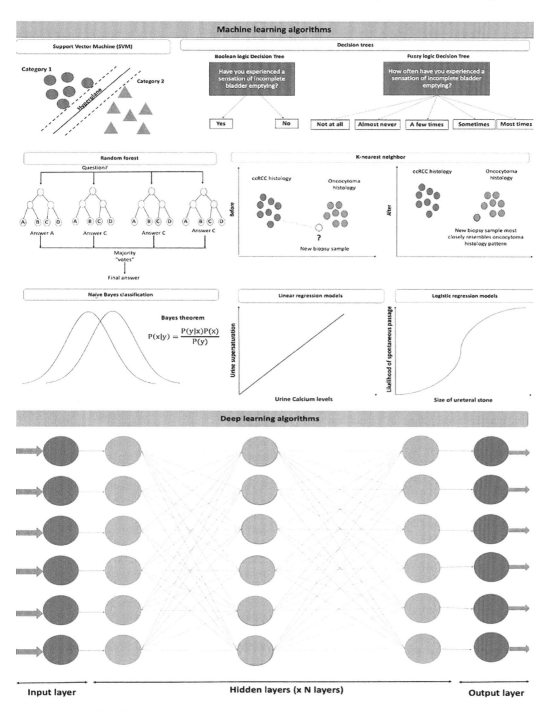

Fig. 1. Overview of artificial intelligence algorithms. (*A*) Support vector machines are designed to find the optimal cutoff, or a hyperplane, for two group classifications. (*B*) Decision trees use a series of repeated questions to arrive at a conclusion that can be binary versus nonbinary or Boolean logic versus Fuzzy logic, respectively. (*C*) Random forest models form a consensus based on the equally weighted output of multiple decision trees. (*D*) K-nearest neighbor algorithms cluster data points together into groups based on similarity to one another. (*E*) Naïve Bayes classification algorithms classify data based on the assumption that the presence of a certain criteria alone is unrelated to any other feature. (*F, G*) Linear and logistic regression models assess the relationship between a continuous variable and either a continuous or categorical variable, respectively. (*H*) Deep learning algorithms consist of multiple AI units that interact with each other in multiple layers.

compared with a group of radiologists, the CNN algorithm outperformed the radiologists (CNN vs radiologists; 93% vs 85%, $P = .03$).[18]

Calculating Stone Burden: Stone Volume Characterization

Although the accuracy of ML and DL algorithms in detecting renal calculi within the collecting system ranges from 85% to 99%, it is the overall stone burden and stone location rather than the mere presence or absence of kidney stones on NCCT scans that is the primary interest from the urologist's perspective.[13–16] Although still used by the American and European associations of urology as a threshold for recommending a certain surgical approach, linear measurements have been deemed unreliable in accurately quantifying the stone burden compared with the actual stone volume.[12,20,21] Thus, of particular importance is building an AI algorithm with an architecture that permits accurate characterization of the true stone burden volume. To date, only two studies have assessed such algorithms.[22,23]

Babajide and colleagues reported the use of an improved DL algorithm, previously used in brain MRI image analysis, for the identification and volumetric quantification of renal calculi on NCCT scans.[22] Although the algorithm demonstrated a perfect agreement in detecting stones, with both sensitivity and specificity reaching 100%, there was considerable discrepancy between the volume of stones determined by the algorithm and the "ground truth" volume at the voxel level.[22] The Dice 3D spatial overlap score, measuring the agreement of the algorithm with the reference standard, was reported to be 0.66(22). In contrast, Elton and colleagues used a 13-layer CNN to evaluate the volume of renal calculi on noisy, low-dose computed tomography (CT) scans and validated the algorithm's performance using an external data set of 6185 CT scans.[23] The algorithm exhibited high sensitivity (0.88) and specificity (0.91) in detecting the presence of renal calculi, with an area under the operator curve of 0.95 and a strong correlation between the AI-determined stone volume and the "ground truth" measurements (R = 0.974).[23]

Stone Composition

In recent decades, laser lithotripsy, specifically using the holmium yttrium aluminum garnet (Ho: YAG) laser and thulium fiber laser, has emerged as a primary surgical treatment modality for renal and ureteral calculi due to its high effectiveness and relatively favorable safety profile.[24–26] Nonetheless, the selection of laser settings remains largely dependent on the surgeon's subjective evaluation of ablation efficiency and desired fragment size. Typically, higher energies are used for "dusting," whereas lower energies are used for generating fragments intended for subsequent basket extraction.[27] This approach is highly variable between kidney stone centers sometimes even within the same center and lacks standardization. Stone composition has been demonstrated to affect laser efficiency, indicating the need for the development of an AI algorithm that can accurately and precisely predict intraoperative stone findings.[28] This represents the next logical step toward laser setting optimization and a faster, more efficient laser stone ablation. Multiple studies have sought to train AI software to predict stone composition preoperatively. They can be categorized into three main groups: those that used clinical and paraclinical data[29,30]; those that relied on CT imaging[31–33]; and those that relied on endoscopic visualization of the stone surface.[34,35]

When weighing different individual classifiers, such as patient demographics, relevant past medical history and social history, laboratory values, and physical examination findings, Kazemi and colleagues managed to design an ensemble learning data mining model that displayed a robust accuracy, achieving 97.1% accuracy in predicting the kidney stone type.[29] In contrast, Abrahams and colleagues' ML algorithm did not only consider patient-specific demographics and clinical findings but also included 24-h urine analyte variables for stone composition prediction.[30] The aim of their study was to compare the boosted decision tree algorithm (XG) ML algorithm's efficiency to an LR model in answering both a binary (calcium or non-calcium stones) and a multiple-choice stone composition question (calcium oxalate, hydroxyapatite, uric acid, or other).[30] The XG ML algorithm had a higher accuracy (91% vs 79%) but lower sensitivity (46% vs 26%) than the LR model when determining if the stone was calcium-based,[30] but for defining the exact subtype of chemical composition, the XG algorithm displayed both a lower sensitivity (LR vs XG; 0.64 vs 056) and accuracy (AUC: LR vs XG; 0.79 vs 0.59).[30]

In contrast to the non-CT AI assessments used to assess stone composition as previously described, Krieghauser and colleagues used preoperative CT scans to determine stone composition. The group assessed stones greater than 5 mm with different multiparametric algorithms, ranging from artificial neural networks to naïve Bayes tree software.[31] They found that although the algorithms were 100% accurate in distinguishing uric acid stones from non-uric acid stones on single-source dual-energy CT scans, the accuracy dropped to 75% when trying to distinguish between the different subtypes of non-uric acid stones, more specifically struvite, cystine, or calcium oxalate monohydrate.[31] Similarly, Zhang and colleagues' SVM classifiers incorporated the use of CT texture analysis, a novel imaging technique that relies on voxel distribution and pixel spatial interconnection to assess the heterogenous stone surface.[32] The SVM CT texture analysis's ability to predict the stone type was confirmed by comparing the output with the "ground truth" stone composition, as assessed by *ex vivo* Fourier transform infrared spectroscopy.[32] In fact, the SVM use of CT texture analysis proved to be an accurate (88%–92%) means of uric acid stone differentiation, with 94.4% sensitivity and 93.7% specificity.[32] More recently, Hokamp and colleagues reported the successful use of an ML protocol with 91.1% accuracy in identifying the main chemical component of a stone, regardless of the CT dosage (ie, normal or low-dose CT).[33]

Preoperative assessment of stone type can be important in planning procedures; however, there is a role in intraoperative identification of stone composition given findings that efficient lithotripsy might be related to stone type and that many stones are not homogenous.[28,35,36] Traditionally, endoscopic identification of stone composition depends on the observer's skill in predicting the stone composition during the fragmentation process. The learning curve for identifying commonly encountered stones such as pure calcium oxalate and uric acid stones is relatively short, as they exhibit distinctive visual characteristics; however, rarer stones such as brushite or cystine stones lack these features and are therefore subject to greater interobserver variability.[34,37,38] In addition, the major challenge in stone composition determination is that most of the stones encountered in clinical practice are of mixed composition, and thus the number of specific different "stone composition types" is exponentially increased.[35]

Black and colleagues developed a DL CNN that was capable to identify the composition of 63 *ex vivo* kidney stones based on digital photographs, with an overall recall of 85%.[34] Of note, the algorithm's efficiency differed with the stone composition—the most easily recognized stones were composed of uric acid (94%), calcium oxalate monohydrate (90%), and struvite (86%), whereas cystine (75%) and brushite (71%) were more difficult to distinguish.[34] This study successfully managed to lay the foundation of endoscopy live stone composition characterization, but it is not without limitations because stones are rarely of pure composition.[34] In fact, during laser

fragmentation, it is often possible to observe the "history" of the stone, with the outer layer of the stone's surface being distinct from the nucleus of the stone.[37,39] Moreover, the stones were placed in a controlled environment, without the interference of motion, breathing or different spectrums of illumination that could potentially impact the algorithm's efficiency when used in an *in vivo* setting.[34,35,39] As such, further studies have sought to determine whether endoscopic *in vivo* video-based stone composition characterization would be possible and Estrade and colleagues have successfully managed to train a DL CNN to automatically recognize the hidden morphologic characteristics of different kidney stone types with an accuracy ranging from 90% to 99% for pure stones and 87% to 98% for stones of mixed composition.[35] With regard to stone treatment, active real-time determination of stone composition as a procedure proceeds would be of extraordinary value as it would facilitate real time feedback to the laser (or other ablative modality) for operational optimization. Specifically, understanding the nature of the stone and specific ablative settings could result in very accurate fragmentation metrics (fragment size and shape) such that fragment extraction could be optimized to the technique being applied.

KIDNEY STONE TREATMENT OUTCOMES

When managing kidney stones, urologists are confronted with the decisions of whether to treat the stones, when to treat the stones, and how to maximize stone-free rate to avoid retreatment,[40] cited as 23% for ureteroscopy (URS) and 36% for percutaneous nephrolithotomy (PCNL) in the first year,[41] all while balancing patient morbidity with complications ranging from 3.5% for URS[42] to 15% for PCNL.[43] Current evidence-based guidelines serve as a touchstone with regard to treatment selection, but there have been multiple AI studies that have sought to confirm what is known or explore new outlets to aid the urologist in improving stone disease management with regards to predicting stone-free rate, reducing complications, predicting stone passage without treatment, and stone prevention.

Percutaneous Nephrolithotomy

PCNL AI studies have focused on stone-free rate, transfusion requirement, and automation of renal access. As previously described, predicting stone-free rate after PCNL is an important consideration when deciding on a procedure or when counseling patients on what kind of outcome they can expect. Two generally accepted stone-free rate predictive models are Guy's Stone Score (GSS)[44] and Clinical Research Office of the Endourologic Society (CROES) nomogram.[45] A stone-free rate prediction SVM model was recently compared with GSS and the CROES nomogram. The study was composed of 146 patients undergoing PCNL for stones 451 ± 227 m^2 in area accessed with a 26 Fr access sheath that resulted in a 73% stone-free rate based on NCCT evaluation with less than 4 mm residual stone to be considered stone-free. After "learning" for 2 years, the AI software had an accuracy ranging between 80% and 95% and outperformed the perineal stone-free prediction models (AUC: software vs GSS vs CROES; 0.915 vs 0.615 vs 0.621, $P < .001$). The next step for the investigators is to incorporate the software into clinical practice to assist with decision-making.[46] A second study sought to assess which preoperative patient factors might predict stone-free rate before PCNL through three ML platforms that all performed similarly (accuracies: LR vs XGBoost Regressor vs Random Forests; 71.4% vs 74.5% vs 75%), and they found that the most important predictive factors of stone-free rate were stone size, stone type, hemoglobin, and serum creatinine.[47]

Another important consideration for urologists and patients performing and undergoing PCNL, respectively, are complications and predicting those complications would be highly desirable for surgeons to choose a procedure with the highest benefit to risk ratio. Two studies highlighted AI that could predict the need for transfusion due to blood loss anemia or the need for stent due to urine leak. The AI platforms consisted of a ML decision support model consisting of sequential forward selection, Fischer's discriminate analysis, and a multiple classifier scheme in one study,[48] and an artificial neural network (ANN) in another.[49] Shabaniyan and colleagues predicted a transfusion requirement with the sensitivity, specificity, and accuracy of 85%, 85%, 85%, respectively, and a stent requirement with the sensitivity, specificity, accuracy of 71%, 90%, and 85% respectively.[48] Aminsharifi and colleagues predicted a transfusion requirement with a true positive rate, false positive rate, and accuracy of 85%, 25%, 86%, respectively, and a stent requirement with a true positive rate, false positive rate, and accuracy of 81%, 32%, 81%, respectively. Interestingly, the investigators also used the model to predict the type of procedure a patient would undergo if they failed PCNL (repeat PCNL, extracorporeal shockwave lithotripsy [ESWL], or URS) with all true positive rates and accuracies over 90% but with false positive rates of 39%, 12%, and 32% for PCNL, ESWL, and URS, respectively.[49]

Finally, the percutaneous access portion of the PCNL has been known to have a steep learning curve[50] and might be preventative for many urologists to perform the procedure. Technology to address this is an area of active research but one study incorporated AI into a device that assists urologists performing PCNL intraoperatively. Taguchi and colleagues introduced an automated needle targeting with x-ray (ANT-X) device, which uses AI calculations to correctly align a needle trajectory so a surgeon can more easily perform the bull's-eye technique for percutaneous access. The specific details regarding the AI were not mentioned in the article or references; however, the outcomes were favorable. In a randomized, single-blind study of 71 patients (35 ultrasound, 36 robot-assisted fluoroscopic [RAF] guidance), the ANT-X improved the primary outcome of puncture success rate (RAF vs ultrasound [US]; 1.82 vs 2.51, $P = .025$) as well as a secondary outcome of median puncture time (RAF vs US; 5.5 minute vs 8.0 minute, $P = .049$); there was not a difference in stone-free rate by abdominal x-ray 3 months after surgery (RAF vs US; 83.3% vs 70.6%, $P = .26$), complication rate, or fluoroscopy time.[51]

Ureteroscopy

There was a paucity of manuscripts that used AI in URS. However, Wang and colleagues compared four neural networks using CT scans from 1989 patients to predict the ability of the ureter to accommodate the semirigid ureteroscope and found that the DenseNet3D neural network performed best (AUC receiver operatorating characteristic [ROC] score of 0.884). The study has clinical implications of assisting the surgeon in deciding whether to passively dilate the ureter with a stent or actively dilate the ureter at the time of surgery as well as counseling the patient ahead of the surgery of those requirements.[52] With URS now the reigning champion of stone procedures by volume, more work will certainly be done in the near future to optimize retrograde intrarenal surgery using AI.

Extracorporeal Shockwave Lithotripsy

Just as with PCNL or URS, stone-free rate is a measure of success with ESWL. Several AI models have been used to predict stone-free rate through decision tree analysis[53] and an ANN[54–57] and all of them boasted a high level of accuracy with one study reporting that the AI predictions outperformed traditional statistical methods.[54] Predictive factors of stone-free rate after ESWL included stone characteristics such as volume,[53] length,[53,54] and HUs,[53] physiologic factors such as dynamic stone transport,[55] or treatment factors such as stent placement.[54] In a rare critical assessment in the form of a 2021 meta-analysis that examined eight papers and included 3264 patients, Rice and colleagues found that ML had at least equal efficacy compared with traditional statistical methods in predicting stone-free rate following ESWL with a true positive rate of 79%, a false positive rate of 14%, and an AUC of 0.90. The investigators mentioned that some studies had overtraining of their models (exemplified by high accuracy in the training set and a sharp drop off in the test set), lack of comparison between ML and typical statistical techniques, and lack of access to models to be either further evaluated on future data sets or applied to clinical practice. The need for prospective studies to obtain better evidence for the use of AI in clinical practice for ESWL was also cited.[58]

Investigators have reached beyond examining stone-free rate as an outcome for ESWL. In a study of 98 patients followed for at least 1 year, Michaels and colleagues described a feed-forward neural network (sensitivity 91%, specificity 92%, AUC 0.964) that outperformed discriminate function analyses and used the neural network to determine if residual stone increases the risk for *de novo* stone formation. Residual fragments were not found to be predictive of increasing stone burden,[59] which might be met with skepticism given the small patient numbers, short follow-up, and lack of metabolic data.[59] Muller and colleagues explored technical ESWL factors in a theoretic model developed by a CNN and found that ESWL hit rate, defined as the stone being greater than 50% in the focal zone on US that was used as a surrogate for the percentage of shockwaves hitting the stone, could be improved by 75%.[60] Finally, an ANN was used to find predictive factors that lead to emergency department visits for patients within 1 week of being treated by ESWL and the three most predictive factors consisted of a history of emergency department visits before the ESWL treatment, stone shape (long to short axis ratio), and stone burden with a training set AUC of 0.87 and a validation set AUC of 0.66.[61]

Postprocedure Sepsis Prediction

Postoperative sepsis has been reported to be as high as 4.7% for PCNL[62] and is one of the main goals of urologists but investigators have begun looking to AI for assistance to identify patients that have a high risk for developing sepsis. One study examined 1469 patients who underwent PCNL or URS with a postoperative sepsis incidence of 5.9%, of which 847 made inclusion criteria (50 cases in sepsis group and 747 in non-sepsis group), comparing a propensity score matched radiomics model that incorporated NCCT data and 26 other variables to a two-layer deep neural network (DNN). The investigators found that the DNN was a superior sepsis predictor in the internal (AUC: regression vs DNN; 0.881 vs 0.920) and external (AUC: regression vs DNN; 0.783 vs 0.874) validation data sets. The investigators did not include clinical risk factors after propensity score matching to control for confounders but did mention that females had sepsis more often than males.[63]

Trial of Passage

The decision to allow a patient to undergo a trial of passage has traditionally been limited to control of pain, ability to tolerate an oral diet, and lack of signs and symptoms of infection in combination with the urologist's judgment that the stone will pass based on stone size. Several AI models that include ANN,[64–66] SVM, and linear programmed SVM (LP-SVM),[66] 3D-CNN,[67] and multilayer perception with Keras framework[68] have shown the ability to predict the rate of spontaneous stone passage. The largest study conducted by Dal Moro and colleagues compared an ANN, SVM, and LP-SVM to linear regression when evaluating 1163 patients for spontaneously passing a stone based on NCCT and nine clinical factors. They found that SVM outperformed ANN and LR in terms of sensitivity (LR vs ANN vs SVM; 90.3% vs 95% vs 84.5%) and specificity (LR vs ANN vs SVM; 70% vs 63% vs 87%). Predictive factors for a successful trial of spontaneous passage were stone size, stone composition, stone position, and duration of symptoms before presentation; interestingly, previous stone expulsion and previous urologic treatment were second and third tier of importance, respectively.[66] In the most recent study done by Katz and colleagues, the 3D-CNN outperformed a model that only considered the largest linear stone measurement, similar to what is encountered in clinical practice in terms of sensitivity (3D-CNN vs stone size model; 95% vs 80%), specificity (3D-CNN vs stone size model; 77% vs 63%), accuracy (3D-CNN vs stone size model; 82% vs 72%), and AUC (3D-CNN vs stone size model; 0.95 vs 0.76). The investigators highlighted that the 3D-CNN identified patients that require intervention (NPV 96%), but the PPV, or correct prediction that the patient would pass the stone, was 72% so the model requires patients undergoing a trial of passage to have close follow-up.[67]

Kidney Stone Monitoring and Prevention

Stone disease effects 11% of Americans[69] and is projected to cost $4.57 billion by 2030.[70] Identifying patients that are at risk for developing stones and finding ways to prevent stone disease from ever occurring or a reduction in symptomatic stone disease can reduce patient morbidity and reduce costs. Several authors researched the role of AI in this quest. The relationship between genetic polymorphisms and environmental factors was analyzed by a discriminative analysis (DA) and an ANN in 151 patients with calcium oxalate stone disease and 105 control patients. The systems performed similarly when considering genetics alone (properly classified patients with genetics alone: DA vs ANN; 64% vs 65%); however, the ANN outperformed DA when adding environmental factors (properly classified patients with genetics and environment: DA vs ANN; 74% vs 89%). The investigators found that the VEGF genetic polymorphism and consumption of water or milk were associated with having calcium oxalate stone disease.[71] Dussol and colleagues also used an ANN to determine metabolic risk factors for calcium oxalate stone disease in an all-male population. The investigators chose an all-male study because the ANN showed that calcium oxalate stone disease was primarily due to calcemia in females and that endocrine factors may play a larger role than metabolic factors in this patient population. In the male population, the ANN found that the most discriminate variables were calcium oxalate supersaturation (CaOX SS) and 24-h urine urea (AUC: CaOX SS, 24-h urine urea; 0.73, 0.72). The ANN also found cutoffs at which patients became higher risk than controls for developing calcium oxalate stone disease: CaOX SS greater than 8.9 and 24-h urine urea greater than 22 g/day (or protein > 0.9 g/kg/day for the median body weight in the study). The investigators also created a clinically useful heat map to evaluate a patient's risk for calcium oxalate stone formation based on CaOx SS and 24 hour urine urea data.[72]

Predicting the 24-h Urine Changes

Both the American and European urologic associations have acknowledged the utility of 24-h urine testing in the clinical evaluation of patients undergoing metabolic stone disease workup.[73,74] The implementation of this noninvasive test in clinical practice has demonstrated significant benefits in guiding pharmacologic and dietary therapies as well as further reducing the recurrence of stone disease.[73] However, despite these indisputable advantages, recent data indicates that the utilization of 24-h urine analyte testing in the high-risk kidney stone population is low, with only 7.4% of patients receiving this test.[75] This may be attributed to a range of factors, including limited access to such testing in certain health care settings, cost, inadequate insurance coverage, physician difficulty in interpreting the testing results or poor patient urine collection.[76,77]

More recently, Kavoussi and colleagues developed a ML model from retrospective electronic health record for predicting 24-h urine abnormalities; they compared a boosted decision tree (XGBoost) model, LR, and a combination of the two methods. The XG Boost algorithm exhibited superior performance compared with an LR model in predicting abnormalities in diuresis, uric acid, and sodium levels. However, the LR model demonstrated higher accuracy in predicting changes in urinary citrate and pH levels. To enhance the performance of the XGBoost model, a model that combined the strengths of the gradient boosted decision tree and the LR model was developed. The strongest predictors of abnormal 24-h urine, in order of importance, were body mass index (BMI), age, male gender, and calcium oxalate stone composition. Although these findings hold promise, further optimization and validation of the XG Boost algorithm are necessary before its widespread implementation in a clinical setting.[76]

Artificial Intelligence and Malignancy for the Endourologist

Although many endourologists perform robotic oncologic procedures, AI in urologic oncology is best served in a dedicated discussion and there are no current studies that specifically address decision-making regarding biopsy of small renal masses or ablative procedures for the kidney or prostate. However, the endourologist is often confronted with cancer diagnosis during cystoscopy and URS and there have been several studies describing AI assistance in identifying tumors under direct vision during cystoscopy.

Artificial Intelligence Cancer Diagnosis Under Direct Endoscopic Vision

All urologists may find themselves observing potential malignancy under direct vision in the upper or lower collecting systems. For bladder cancer, the Cystoscopy Artificial Intelligence Diagnostic System built on a pyramid scene parsing network and trained with 69,204 cystoscopy-derived images from 10,729 patients across six hospitals had near-perfect bladder cancer diagnostic accuracy of 0.977 (95% CI = 0.974–0.979) and in a study with 260 urologists, outperformed all of them (sensitivity: trainees vs competent urologists vs expert urologists vs AI; 0.508 vs 0.562 vs 0.754 vs 0.954); moreover, the NPV range was 0.989 to 0.999, outperforming expert urologists, and the PPV ranged from 0.819 to 0.977, which was similar to expert urologists. The overall results are impressive but not perfect; in a supplemental subgroup analysis, there was a misdiagnosis of carcinoma in situ (CIS) 12% of the time.[78]

Another study highlights similar challenges with CIS that arise with endoscopic AI. A dilated U-Net AI network was trained with 1790 cystoscopic images of histologically confirmed bladder cancer from 120 patients who underwent transurethral resection of bladder tumor (TURBT) with overall sensitivity, specificity, PPV, and dice similarity coefficient were 84.9%, 88.5%, 86.7%, and 83.0%, respectively; however, the dice similarity coefficient dropped to 57.3% when evaluating CIS. The investigators are hopeful that this network can prevent overlooked tumors[79] but the current performance with CIS may be preventative and further studies are required as CIS can often be found via cytology.

Yoo and colleagues report the first time an AI has been tested to diagnose bladder cancer based on tumor color using the red/green/blue (RGB) components of white light imaging. In this retrospective study, 10,991 images of suspicious bladder tumors from cystoscopy were used to train and test a mask region-based CNN. According to the RGB value, the performance of their AI system, in terms of sensitivity, specificity, and diagnostic accuracy was ≥ 98% for the diagnosis of benign versus low- and high-grade tumors and greater than 90% for diagnosing nonspecific inflammation versus carcinoma in situ. Of note, the investigator found these results to outperform narrow band imaging.[80]

With regard to recognition of benign bladder lesions, one team led by Iwaki and colleagues was able to develop a DL CNN that showed, via Gradient-weighted Class Activation Mapping Software, that vessel clustering toward or around the lesion of interest might be responsible for the CNN identification of Hunner lesions. Their system had an accuracy of 0.912, a mean sensitivity of 81.9%, and a specificity of 85.2%.[81]

OTHER USES OF ARTIFICIAL INTELLIGENCE IN ENDOUROLOGY
Benign Prostatic Hyperplasia

Benign prostatic hyperplasia (BPH) is a very common disease affecting most men after 60 years of age.[82] However, despite being very common, the management and choice of treatment is indeed complex, as there are many options such as observation, an array of drugs, and a variety of surgical treatment such as transurethral resection of the prostate (TURP), endoscopic laser enucleation of the prostate, Aquablation, Rezūm, UroLift, and simple prostatectomy.[83] In that sense, one could see the application of AI in assisting with making a diagnosis, monitoring of BPH, or in decision-making. However, despite the potential of its use, there is a paucity of studies on AI for BPH. So far, AI has been studied in four scenarios: prostatic volume measurement, assessing the need for urodynamics, treatment response, and helping clinical decision-making.

Volume Measurement

For prostatic volume measurement, AI has been used to automatically segment prostates based on MRI. Habes and colleagues compared the AI with a 3D-segmented prostate by a radiologist (ground truth) and the ellipsoid formula (the most commonly tool for measurement prostatic volume in clinical practice) and showed that the AI had a very high correlation to the radiologist segmentation, or ground truth (intraclass correlation coefficient [ICC] 0.98) and was far greater than the ellipsoid formula (ICC 0.51).[84] Rouviere also achieved similar results, with AI having a high precision (dice score 0.97) and within the inter-reader variability of different radiologists (dice score 0.96).[85] Both studies were mainly designed for prostate cancer management, but they could potentially be used for BPH for helping to monitor prostate size, assess medication response (ie, inhibitor of 5-alpha reductase prostate volume reduction) and surgical planning.

Requirement for Urodynamic Assessment in Benign Prostatic Hyperplasia

In 2000, an ANN was able to assess patients' need for urodynamics in the setting of bladder outlet obstruction with a sensitivity of 94% and specificity of 91%, which could potentially reduce the number of patients undergoing urodynamics by 44%. The model couldn't predict the outcome though, and therefore, could not replace urodynamics for all patients.[86]

Management Decisions for Benign Prostatic Hyperplasia

AI was also developed for BPH decision-making with regard to assisting the urologist in choosing between observation, medical therapy, or surgical treatment. In 2014, a fuzzy intelligent system was able to correctly assess BPH severity in all 44 patients and in 90% of those patients was able to correctly determine the treatment recommendation compared with a panel of urologist experts (theoretic decision-making).[87] However, more recently in 2022, an ML algorithm performed poorly when using preoperative patient data and disease-related characteristics to predict the type of surgical treatment: monopolar or bipolar TURP versus bipolar transurethral vaporization. The poor results were due to BPH treatment being more related to a patient or surgeon preference or technological availability in the hospital rather than related to objective input parameters.[88]

Benign Prostatic Hyperplasia Medical and Surgical Outcomes

For response to medication use, there is only one study which assessed treatment response to tadalafil for BPH. However, the AI was not accurate enough to predict outcomes.[89] For surgery, an AI algorithm was developed which outperformed clinical algorithm on predicting outcomes after TURP with a correlation of 0.90 for international prostate symptom score (IPSS) score and 0.97 for maximum flow rate.[90]

ENVIRONMENTAL IMPACT OF ARTIFICIAL INTELLIGENCE

From medicine to agriculture to vehicles, AI networks are becoming increasingly implemented to improve industries. Most of these networks rely on exceptionally large data sets and computational power to train the AI during multiple iterations. On a large scale, this can have an adverse environmental impact due to energy consumption. Strubell and colleagues[91] highlight a few of these considerations and report that using conventional methods, training a single AI model with a neural architecture produces the same amount of carbon emissions as five cars throughout the lifetime of the car. Fortunately, researchers such as Sivasubramani and colleagues are working to fix this issue of energy consumption and have designed low-power nanomagnetic powered chips that can be used to construct AI systems.[92] Another team published a study in Nature Nanotechnology revealing their work that proves networks made of nanomagnets can be used to accomplish AI-like processing, which tremendously reduces energy consumption compared with current methods.[93]

SUMMARY

Based on the number of studies explored here alone, one can see that AI is a very active subject of research in endourology. The potential benefit should impart a sense of excitement in the urologic field; however, AI should be met with cautious optimism. The mechanisms of ML and DL are complex and in the case of DL, unsupervised with regard to input and evaluation techniques. Similar to complex traditional statistical methods, urologists can rely on computer scientist interpretation of AI, as they rely on statisticians, to an extent. Urologists must familiarize themselves with AI for continued protection of patients by serving as the bridge between technologic innovation and clinical practice. Most of the AI studies are retrospective and theoretic; the ability for critical appraisals by urologists is the keystone to validating theoretic models and designing prospective studies for the benefits of AI to be realized in clinical practice.

REFERENCES

1. Aung YYM, Wong DCS, Ting DSW. The promise of artificial intelligence: a review of the opportunities and challenges of artificial intelligence in healthcare. Br Med Bull 2021;139(1):4–15.
2. Yang B, Veneziano D, Somani BK. Artificial intelligence in the diagnosis, treatment and prevention of urinary stones. Curr Opin Urol 2020;30(6):782–7.
3. Dai JC, Johnson BA. Artificial intelligence in endourology: emerging technology for individualized care. Curr Opin Urol 2022;32(4).
4. Choi RY, Coyner AS, Kalpathy-Cramer J, et al. Introduction to Machine Learning, Neural Networks, and Deep Learning. Transl Vis Sci Technol 2020;9(2):14.
5. Ben-Hur A, Weston J. A User's Guide to Support Vector Machines. In: Carugo O, Eisenhaber F, editors. Data mining techniques for the Life sciences. Totowa, NJ: Humana Press; 2010. p. 223–39.
6. Han X, Zhu X, Pedrycz W, et al. A three-way classification with fuzzy decision trees. Appl Soft Comput 2023;132:109788.
7. Janikow CZ, editor. Exemplar learning in fuzzy decision trees. Proceedings of IEEE 5th International Fuzzy Systems; IEEE; 1996.
8. Hassanzadeh R, Farhadian M, Rafieemehr H. Hospital mortality prediction in traumatic injuries patients: comparing different SMOTE-based machine learning algorithms. BMC Med Res Methodol 2023;23(1):1–15.
9. Moassefi M, Faghani S, Khosravi B, et al. Artificial Intelligence in Radiology: Overview of Application Types, Design, and Challenges. Semin Roentgenol 2023;58(2):170–7.
10. Hill AJ, Basourakos SP, Lewicki P, et al. Incidence of Kidney Stones in the United States: The Continuous National Health and Nutrition Examination Survey. J Urol 2022;207(4):851–6.
11. Sokolovskaya E, Shinde T, Ruchman RB, et al. The Effect of Faster Reporting Speed for Imaging Studies

on the Number of Misses and Interpretation Errors: A Pilot Study. J Am Coll Radiol 2015;12(7):683–8.

12. Patel SR, Stanton P, Zelinski N, et al. Automated renal stone volume measurement by noncontrast computerized tomography is more reproducible than manual linear size measurement. J Urol 2011; 186(6):2275–9.

13. Parakh A, Lee H, Lee JH, et al. Urinary Stone Detection on CT Images Using Deep Convolutional Neural Networks: Evaluation of Model Performance and Generalization. Radiol Artif Intell 2019;1(4):e180066.

14. Yildirim K, Bozdag PG, Talo M, et al. Deep learning model for automated kidney stone detection using coronal CT images. Comput Biol Med 2021;135:104569.

15. Islam MN, Hasan M, Hossain MK, et al. Vision transformer and explainable transfer learning models for auto detection of kidney cyst, stone and tumor from CT-radiography. Scientific Rep 2022;12(1):11440.

16. De Perrot T, Hofmeister J, Burgermeister S, et al. Differentiating kidney stones from phleboliths in unenhanced low-dose computed tomography using radiomics and machine learning. Eur Radiol 2019; 29(9):4776–82.

17. Längkvist M, Jendeberg J, Thunberg P, et al. Computer aided detection of ureteral stones in thin slice computed tomography volumes using Convolutional Neural Networks. Comput Biol Med 2018;97:153–60.

18. Jendeberg J, Thunberg P, Lidén M. Differentiation of distal ureteral stones and pelvic phleboliths using a convolutional neural network. Urolithiasis 2021;49(1): 41–9.

19. Lee HJ, Kim KG, Hwang SI, et al. Differentiation of urinary stone and vascular calcifications on non-contrast CT images: an initial experience using computer aided diagnosis. J Digit Imaging 2010;23(3):268–76.

20. Assimos D, Krambeck A, Miller NL, et al. Surgical Management of Stones: American Urological Association/Endourological Society Guideline, PART I. J Urol 2016;196(4):1153–60.

21. Türk C, Petřík A, Sarica K, et al. EAU Guidelines on Interventional Treatment for Urolithiasis. Eur Urol 2016;69(3):475–82.

22. Babajide R, Lembrikova K, Ziemba J, et al. Automated Machine Learning Segmentation and Measurement of Urinary Stones on CT Scan. Urology 2022;169:41–6.

23. Elton DC, Turkbey EB, Pickhardt PJ, et al. A deep learning system for automated kidney stone detection and volumetric segmentation on noncontrast CT scans. Med Phys 2022;49(4):2545–54.

24. Panthier F, Ventimiglia E, Berthe L, et al. How much energy do we need to ablate 1 mm3 of stone during Ho:YAG laser lithotripsy? An in vitro study. World J Urol 2020;38(11):2945–53.

25. Andreeva V, Vinarov A, Yaroslavsky I, et al. Preclinical comparison of superpulse thulium fiber laser and a holmium:YAG laser for lithotripsy. World J Urol 2020;38(2):497–503.

26. Traxer O, Keller EX. Thulium fiber laser: the new player for kidney stone treatment? A comparison with Holmium:YAG laser. World J Urol 2020;38(8):1883–94.

27. Doizi S, Keller EX, De Coninck V, et al. Dusting technique for lithotripsy: what does it mean? Nat Rev Urol 2018;15(11):653–4.

28. Jeffrey Johnson MM, Han David, Pingle Srinath-Reddie, et al. Comparative Analysis and Ablation Efficacy of Thulium Fiber Laser by Stone Composition. The J Urol 2023;209. No. 4S, Supplement.

29. Kazemi Y, Mirroshandel SA. A novel method for predicting kidney stone type using ensemble learning. Artif Intell Med 2018;84:117–26.

30. Abraham A, Kavoussi NL, Sui W, et al. Machine Learning Prediction of Kidney Stone Composition Using Electronic Health Record-Derived Features. J Endourol 2022;36(2):243–50.

31. Kriegshauser JS, Silva AC, Paden RG, et al. Ex Vivo Renal Stone Characterization with Single-Source Dual-Energy Computed Tomography: A Multiparametric Approach. Acad Radiol 2016;23(8):969–76.

32. Zhang GM, Sun H, Shi B, et al. Uric acid versus non-uric acid urinary stones: differentiation with single energy CT texture analysis. Clin Radiol 2018;73(9):792–9.

33. Große Hokamp N, Lennartz S, Salem J, et al. Dose independent characterization of renal stones by means of dual energy computed tomography and machine learning: an ex-vivo study. Eur Radiol 2020;30(3):1397–404.

34. Black KM, Law H, Aldoukhi A, et al. Deep learning computer vision algorithm for detecting kidney stone composition. BJU Int 2020;125(6):920–4.

35. Estrade V, Daudon M, Richard E, et al. Towards automatic recognition of pure and mixed stones using intra-operative endoscopic digital images. BJU Int 2022;129(2):234–42.

36. Kawahara T, Miyamoto H, Ito H, et al. Predicting the mineral composition of ureteral stone using non-contrast computed tomography. Urolithiasis 2016; 44(3):231–9.

37. Estrade V, Denis de Senneville B, Meria P, et al. Toward improved endoscopic examination of urinary stones: a concordance study between endoscopic digital pictures vs microscopy. BJU Int 2021;128(3):319–30.

38. Bergot C, Robert G, Bernhard JC, et al. The basis of endoscopic stones recognition, a prospective monocentric study. Prog Urol 2019;29(6):312–7.

39. Estrade V, Daudon M, Richard E, et al. Deep morphological recognition of kidney stones using intra-operative endoscopic digital videos. Phys Med Biol 2022;67(16).

40. Rebuck DA, Macejko A, Bhalani V, et al. The Natural History of Renal Stone Fragments Following Ureteroscopy. Urology 2011;77(3):564–8.

41. Johnston SS, Chen BP, Rai P, et al. Incremental Healthcare Cost Implications of Retreatment Following Ureteroscopy or Percutaneous Nephrolithotomy for Upper Urinary Tract Stones: A Population-Based Study of Commercially-Insured US Adults. Med Devices (Auckl) 2022;15:371–84.

42. de la Rosette J, Denstedt J, Geavlete P, et al. The clinical research office of the endourological society ureteroscopy global study: indications, complications, and outcomes in 11,885 patients. J Endourol 2014;28(2):131–9.

43. de la Rosette J, Assimos D, Desai M, et al. The Clinical Research Office of the Endourological Society Percutaneous Nephrolithotomy Global Study: indications, complications, and outcomes in 5803 patients. J Endourol 2011;25(1):11–7.

44. Thomas K, Smith NC, Hegarty N, et al. The Guy's stone score—grading the complexity of percutaneous nephrolithotomy procedures. Urology 2011; 78(2):277–81.

45. Smith A, Averch TD, Shahrour K, et al. A nephrolithometric nomogram to predict treatment success of percutaneous nephrolithotomy. J Urol 2013;190(1):149–56.

46. Aminsharifi A, Irani D, Tayebi S, et al. Predicting the Postoperative Outcome of Percutaneous Nephrolithotomy with Machine Learning System: Software Validation and Comparative Analysis with Guy's Stone Score and the CROES Nomogram. J Endourology 2019;34(6):692–9.

47. Alghafees MA, Abdul Rab S, Aljurayyad AS, et al. A retrospective cohort study on the use of machine learning to predict stone-free status following percutaneous nephrolithotomy: An experience from Saudi Arabia. Ann Med Surg (Lond) 2022;84:104957.

48. Shabaniyan T, Parsaei H, Aminsharifi A, et al. An artificial intelligence-based clinical decision support system for large kidney stone treatment. Australas Phys Eng Sci Med 2019;42(3):771–9.

49. Aminsharifi A, Irani D, Pooyesh S, et al. Artificial Neural Network System to Predict the Postoperative Outcome of Percutaneous Nephrolithotomy. J Endourol 2017;31(5):461–7.

50. de la Rosette JJ, Laguna MP, Rassweiler JJ, et al. Training in percutaneous nephrolithotomy–a critical review. Eur Urol 2008;54(5):994–1001.

51. Taguchi K, Hamamoto S, Okada A, et al. A Randomized, Single-Blind Clinical Trial Comparing Robotic-Assisted Fluoroscopic-Guided with Ultrasound-Guided Renal Access for Percutaneous Nephrolithotomy. J Urol 2022;208(3):684–94.

52. Wang J, Wang D, Wang Y, et al. Predicting narrow ureters before ureteroscopic lithotripsy with a neural network: a retrospective bicenter study. Urolithiasis 2022;50(5):599–610.

53. Choo MS, Uhmn S, Kim JK, et al. A Prediction Model Using Machine Learning Algorithm for Assessing Stone-Free Status after Single Session Shock Wave Lithotripsy to Treat Ureteral Stones. J Urol 2018;200(6):1371–7.

54. Gomha MA, Sheir KZ, Showky S, et al. Can we improve the prediction of stone-free status after extracorporeal shock wave lithotripsy for ureteral stones? A neural network or a statistical model? J Urol 2004;172(1):175–9.

55. Poulakis V, Dahm P, Witzsch U, et al. Prediction of lower pole stone clearance after shock wave lithotripsy using an artificial neural network. The J Urol 2003;169(4):1250–6.

56. Seckiner I, Seckiner S, Sen H, et al. A neural network-based algorithm for predicting stone-free status after ESWL therapy. Int braz j urol 2017;43:1110–4.

57. Xu ZH, Zhou S, Jia CP, et al. Prediction of Proximal Ureteral Stones Clearance after Shock Wave Lithotripsy Using an Artificial Neural Network. Urol J 2021;18(5):491–6.

58. Rice P, Pugh M, Geraghty R, et al. Machine Learning Models for Predicting Stone-Free Status after Shockwave Lithotripsy: A Systematic Review and Meta-Analysis. Urology 2021;156:16–22.

59. Michaels EK, Niederberger CS, Golden RM, et al. Use of a neural network to predict stone growth after shock wave lithotripsy. Urology 1998;51(2):335–8.

60. Muller S, Abildsnes H, Østvik A, et al. Can a Dinosaur Think? Implementation of Artificial Intelligence in Extracorporeal Shock Wave Lithotripsy. Eur Urol Open Sci 2021;27:33–42.

61. Sun CC, Chang P. Prediction of unexpected emergency room visit after extracorporeal shock wave lithotripsy for urolithiasis - an application of artificial neural network in hospital information system. AMIA Annu Symp Proc 2006;2006:1113.

62. Skolarikos A, de la Rosette J. Prevention and treatment of complications following percutaneous nephrolithotomy. Curr Opin Urol 2008;18(2):229–34.

63. Chen M, Yang J, Lu J, et al. Ureteral calculi lithotripsy for single ureteral calculi: can DNN-assisted model help preoperatively predict risk factors for sepsis? Eur Radiol 2022;32(12):8540–9.

64. Cummings JM, Boullier JA, Izenberg SD, et al. Prediction of spontaneous ureteral calculous passage by an artificial neural network. J Urol 2000;164(2):326–8.

65. Solakhan M, Seckiner SU, Seckiner I. A neural network-based algorithm for predicting the spontaneous passage of ureteral stones. Urolithiasis 2020;48:527–32.

66. Dal Moro F, Abate A, Lanckriet G, et al. A novel approach for accurate prediction of spontaneous passage of ureteral stones: support vector machines. Kidney Int 2006;69(1):157–60.

67. Katz JE, Abdelrahman L, Nackeeran S, et al. The Development of an Artificial Intelligence Model Based Solely on Computer Tomography Successfully Predicts Which Patients Will Pass Obstructing Ureteral Calculi. Urology 2023;174:58–63.

68. Park JS, Kim DW, Lee D, et al. Development of prediction models of spontaneous ureteral stone passage through machine learning: Comparison with conventional statistical analysis. PloS one 2021; 16(12):e0260517.

69. Scales CD Jr, Smith AC, Hanley JM, et al. Prevalence of kidney stones in the United States. Eur Urol 2012;62(1):160–5.

70. Antonelli JA, Maalouf NM, Pearle MS, et al. Use of the National Health and Nutrition Examination Survey to Calculate the Impact of Obesity and Diabetes on Cost and Prevalence of Urolithiasis in 2030. Eur Urol 2014;66(4):724–9.

71. Chiang D, Chiang HC, Chen WC, et al. Prediction of stone disease by discriminant analysis and artificial neural networks in genetic polymorphisms: a new method. BJU Int 2003;91(7):661–6.

72. Dussol B, Verdier J-M, Le Goff J-M, et al. Artificial neural networks for assessing the risk of urinary calcium stone among men. Urol Res 2006;34:17–25.

73. Pearle MS, Goldfarb DS, Assimos DG, et al. Medical management of kidney stones: AUA guideline. J Urol 2014;192(2):316–24.

74. Türk C, Petřík A, Sarica K, et al. EAU Guidelines on Diagnosis and Conservative Management of Urolithiasis. Eur Urol 2016;69(3):468–74.

75. Milose JC, Kaufman SR, Hollenbeck BK, et al. Prevalence of 24-hour urine collection in high risk stone formers. J Urol 2014;191(2):376–80.

76. Kavoussi NL, Floyd C, Abraham A, et al. Machine Learning Models to Predict 24 Hour Urinary Abnormalities for Kidney Stone Disease. Urology 2022; 169:52–7.

77. Otto BJ, Bozorgmehri S, Kuo J, et al. Age, Body Mass Index, and Gender Predict 24-Hour Urine Parameters in Recurrent Idiopathic Calcium Oxalate Stone Formers. J Endourol 2017;31(12):1335–41.

78. Wu S, Chen X, Pan J, et al. An Artificial Intelligence System for the Detection of Bladder Cancer via Cystoscopy: A Multicenter Diagnostic Study. J Natl Cancer Inst 2022;114(2):220–7.

79. Mutaguchi J, Ki Morooka, Kobayashi S, et al. Artificial Intelligence for Segmentation of Bladder Tumor Cystoscopic Images Performed by U-Net with Dilated Convolution. J Endourology 2022;36(6): 827–34.

80. Yoo JW, Koo KC, Chung BH, et al. Deep learning diagnostics for bladder tumor identification and grade prediction using RGB method. Scientific Rep 2022; 12(1):17699.

81. Iwaki T, Akiyama Y, Nosato H, et al. Deep Learning Models for Cystoscopic Recognition of Hunner Lesion in Interstitial Cystitis. Eur Urol Open Sci 2023;49:44–50.

82. Barry MJ, Fowler FJ Jr, O'Leary MP, et al. The American Urological Association symptom index for benign prostatic hyperplasia. The Measurement Committee of the American Urological Association. J Urol 1992;148(5):1549–57 [discussion: 64].

83. Lerner LB, McVary KT, Barry MJ, et al. Management of Lower Urinary Tract Symptoms Attributed to Benign Prostatic Hyperplasia: AUA GUIDELINE PART I-Initial Work-up and Medical Management. J Urol 2021;206(4):806–17.

84. Habes M, Bahr J, Schiller T, et al. New technique for prostate volume assessment. World J Urol 2014; 32(6):1559–64.

85. Rouvière O, Moldovan PC, Vlachomitrou A, et al. Combined model-based and deep learning-based automated 3D zonal segmentation of the prostate on T2-weighted MR images: clinical evaluation. Eur Radiol 2022;32(5):3248–59.

86. Sonke GS, Heskes T, Verbeek AL, et al. Prediction of bladder outlet obstruction in men with lower urinary tract symptoms using artificial neural networks. J Urol 2000;163(1):300–5.

87. Torshizi AD, Zarandi MH, Torshizi GD, et al. A hybrid fuzzy-ontology based intelligent system to determine level of severity and treatment recommendation for Benign Prostatic Hyperplasia. Comput Methods Programs Biomed 2014;113(1):301–13.

88. Tzelves L, Feretzakis G, Kalles D, et al. Cluster Analysis Assessment in Proposing a Surgical Technique for Benign Prostatic Enlargement. Stud Health Technol Inform 2022;295:466–9.

89. Fusco F, D'Anzeo G, Henneges C, et al. Predictors of Individual Response to Placebo or Tadalafil 5mg among Men with Lower Urinary Tract Symptoms Secondary to Benign Prostatic Hyperplasia: An Integrated Clinical Data Mining Analysis. PLoS One 2015;10(8):e0135484.

90. Mourmouris P, Tzelves L, Feretzakis G, et al. The use and applicability of machine learning algorithms in predicting the surgical outcome for patients with benign prostatic enlargement. Which model to use? Arch Ital Urol Androl 2021;93(4):418–24.

91. Strubell E. Energy and policy consideratons for modern deep learning research. Proc AAAI Conf Artif intelligence 2020;34(9):13693–6.

92. Sivasubramani S, Mattela V, Pal C, et al. Dipole coupled magnetic quantum-dot cellular automata-based efficient approximate nanomagnetic subtractor and adder design approach. Nanotechnology 2020;31(2):025202.

93. Gartside JC, Vanstone A, Dion T, et al. Reconfigurable magnonic mode-hybridisation and spectral control in a bicomponent artificial spin ice. Nat Commun 2021;12(1):2488.

Artificial Intelligence in Pediatric Urology

Hsin-Hsiao Scott Wang, MD, MPH, MBAn[a],*, Ranveer Vasdev, MD, MS[b],
Caleb P. Nelson, MD, MPH[c]

KEYWORDS

- Artificial intelligence • Machine learning • Prediction • Model • Algorithm • Pediatric urology

KEY POINTS

- Artificial intelligence (AI) methodologies can provide new angles to enhance clinical care.
- Applications in pediatric urology are increasing.
- Learning the challenges specific to pediatric urology in AI applications.
- Knowledge to critically appraise new studies using AI in pediatric urology is the key to high-quality and high-impact research.

INTRODUCTION

Application of artificial intelligence (AI) is one of the hottest topics in medicine. There is an abundance of evidence of exponentially increasing urologic publications using AI methodology in recent years.[1] Machine Learning (ML) theory has been developed in the field of computer science for decades. In recent years, ML emerged as a powerful tool due to significant performance improvement due to substantial hardware and software innovations and wider data availability. Modern ML techniques may be useful to improve clinical care. By analyzing vast amounts of medical data, including electronic health records, images, and biomedical data, ML algorithms can uncover hidden yet highly complex patterns, helping to identify risk factors, make treatment recommendations, improve patient monitoring, and assess prognosis. Unlike traditional methods, ML rarely relies on statistical assumptions. Through continuous learning and adaptation, ML algorithms can refine their performance over time, leading to improved accuracy and reliability.

Under the modern definition of AI, ML refers to a group of modeling methodologies that can train the computer to perform specific tasks. Several AI/ML models are particularly relevant in pediatric urology. Prediction models leverage patient data and make predictions about disease outcomes, surgical/medical treatment responses, or even clinical operation efficiency. Prescription models utilize ML to assist in the optimization of medication prescriptions, considering factors such as patient characteristics, medical history, and treatment guidelines. Computer vision models excel in analyzing medical images, such as ultrasound, axial imaging (computed tomography [CT] and/or MRI), and radiographic images (eg, voiding cystourethrogram [VCUG]), to assist in accurate diagnosis and prognosis. Natural language processing (NLP) models help extract meaningful information from unstructured medical texts, such as clinical notes or radiology reports, aiding in clinical decision support, data mining, and literature reviews. Signal processing and pattern recognition models specialize in analyzing physiologic signals, such as biophysical data, electrocardiograms or electroencephalograms, or urodynamic study (UDS), to detect abnormalities, monitor treatment response, and provide real-time feedback. Each of these ML offers unique capabilities and has the potential to

a Computational Healthcare Analytics Program, Department of Urology, Boston Children's Hospital, 300 Longwood Avenue, Boston, MA, USA; b Department of Urology, Mayo Clinic Rochester, 200 1st Street Southwest, Rochester, MN 55905, USA; c Clinical and Health Services Research, Department of Urology, Boston Children's Hospital, 300 Longwood Avenue, Boston, MA, USA
* Corresponding author. Computational Healthcare Analytics Program, Department of Urology, Boston Children's Hospital, 300 Longwood Avenue, HU390 Boston, MA.
E-mail address: scottwang3@gmail.com

Urol Clin N Am 51 (2024) 91–103
https://doi.org/10.1016/j.ucl.2023.08.002
0094-0143/24/© 2023 Elsevier Inc. All rights reserved.

enhance patient care, improve accuracy, and facilitate medical research. As the field of ML in medicine continues to advance, these models hold promise for further innovation and development, supporting health care professionals in their quest for improved diagnosis, treatment, and patient outcomes.

In this review, the authors will review the most recent AI/ML innovations being applied in pediatric urology. The authors aim to introduce these articles and address the knowledge gap between the pediatric urology and data science communities, promoting further understanding of AI/ML in pediatric urology.

MATERIALS AND METHODS
Search Methods

The authors performed a comprehensive search of *Medical Literature Analysis and Retrieval System Online (*MEDLINE) and Excerpta Medica Database (Embase) databases for published manuscripts written in English and relating to AI in pediatric urology using the keywords in **Box 1**. The search was performed on March 31, 2023, and all studies published before this date were evaluated. Abstracts and articles in-press were not included.

Study Selection

Title, author, and year published information for manuscripts were exported from MEDLINE and Embase databases. R (v0.4.0) was used to remove duplicates as identified using the matching title, first author last name, and year of publication. One of the authors (RMSV) independently scanned titles and abstracts of the remaining manuscripts to determine if studies were pertinent to urology and artificial intelligence. A secondary review of

the remaining records was performed to examine the full-text articles and ensure only pediatric patients were used in each study's cohort. After excluding non-pediatric studies, the authors performed a post-hoc review of a similar pediatric urology artificial intelligence systematic review for studies referenced but not identified in their initial database search. These unique studies were then added to theirr finalized cohort of studies. Documentation of study selection and the total number identified can be found in a modified Preferred Reporting Items for Systematic Reviews and Meta-Analyses (PRISMA) flow chart (**Fig. 1**).

Data Management and Extraction

For each included study, one of the 3 authors (RMSV, HHSW, CPN) independently reviewed and extracted key information from each full-text study. Any disagreements or concerns about missing data were resolved by joint review. Study information was extracted including authors, title, country of the corresponding author, journal, and publication date. Each article was manually categorized by the corresponding pathology or clinical relevance (ex. renal segmentation). Study characteristics included the clinical question answered outcome definition, variable selection, sample o patient population, use of multi-institutional data training/test/validation cohorts & methods, category of computational analysis (prediction, prescription, computer vision, or spectral vision), specific of machine learning algorithm type used (ex. Neural Network, Random Forrest, Support Vector Machine), and model performance.

RESULTS
Search Results

A total of 497 articles were retrieved from MEDLINE and 47 were retrieved from Embase. After excluding duplicate and non-urologic articles, 424 remaining records were screened for relevance to AI/ML, revealing 81 studies. A survey of the full-text version of these 81 records revealed that 39 were relevant to pediatric urology. Five studies, not previously identified, were added from the references of a contemporary review of pediatric urology and AI/ML, resulting in a final cohort of 44 studies (**Table 1**).[2–45]

Article Characteristics

The most commonly investigated topic was vesicoureteral reflux (N = 10 [24%] VUR) followed by a 3-way tie of 5 (12%) articles investigating either lower urinary tract dysfunction, urinary tract infections (UTI), or hydronephrosis (**Fig. 2**).

Box 1
Key words used in MEDLINE and EMBASE

MEDLINE

((Urology) AND ((Pediatric) OR (Children)) AND ((Artificial Intelligence) OR (Machine Learning) OR (Deep Learning) OR (Computer Vision) OR (Boosted Trees) OR (Random Forrest) OR (Neural Network) OR (Natural Language Processing))

EMBASE

(Urology and (Pediatric or Children) and (Artificial Intelligence or Machine Learning or Deep Learning) and (Computer Vision or Natural Language Processing or Neural Network or Random Forrest or Boosted Trees)

The most common journal of publication was the Journal of Urology (n = 9), followed by the Journal of Pediatric Urology (n = 6), and Urology (n = 5). There was an increasing trend in the number of AI-related pediatric urology articles published per year with the highest count of 10 articles in 2022 (**Fig. 3**).

Prediction Models

The vast majority of articles (N = 23) included in this review were related to prediction models; these are algorithms that take various clinical or research data to predict patient outcomes in either future or concurrent test data sets. Notable articles from this category include an article by Kwon and colleagues[25] who aimed to predict long-term complications of males with posterior urethral valves (PUV) using medical and anatomic features from a multi-institutional cohort. Using a random forest model, the authors were able to predict chronic kidney disease (CKD), kidney transplant, and the need for clean intermittent catheterization(CIC) using external data with c-indexes of 0.78, 0.98, and 0.64, respectively. Tokar and colleagues[21] analyzed the data of 8071 school-age children and their clinical characteristics to develop a model to predict enuresis in children. Another group[32] developed a decision tree–based (optimal tree) model to predict UTI recurrence and VUR anatomy from the Randomized Intervention for Children with Vesico-Ureteral Reflux (RIVUR) and

Careful Urinary Tract Infection Evaluation (CUTIE) study patients, which demonstrated an area under the curve (AUC) of 0.82. Finally, Wang and colleagues aimed to predict time spent with patient and efficiency in a pediatric urology clinic. Using a random forest model and simulation, they were able to accurately predict time with the doctor within 3.6 minutes for new patients and 5.0 minutes for returning patients.[17]

Computer Vision

Computer vision is a field that investigates ways that computers can visualize and interpret images or videos. This is applicable to the daily practice of pediatric urologists, who routinely utilize multiple imaging modalities to appropriately evaluate, treat, and monitor patients. In theory, well-designed and well-trained models can offer superior accuracy and reliability with continual improvements. Using ultrasound, for example, several articles developed methods of segmenting renal parenchyma,[11,12] estimating the volume of hydronephrosis relative to the kidney,[5] classifying Society for Fetal Urology (SFU) hydronephrosis grade,[6] predicting the need of mercaptoacetyltriglycine (MAG3) renal scan,[2] and identification of congenital urologic abnormalities.[3,4] Camera images have also been investigated as a data source in the setting of classifying hypospadias phenotypes.[8] Additionally, 1 article developed a model for capturing urethral stricture on retrograde urethrograms.[13] Similarly, 2 articles

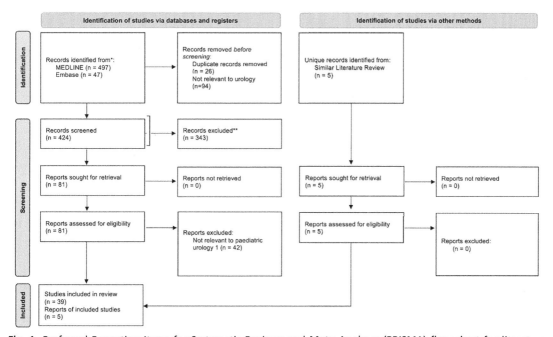

Fig. 1. Preferred Reporting Items for Systematic Reviews and Meta-Analyses (PRISMA) flow chart for literature review.

Table 1
List of final included pediatric urology AI/ML articles

Authors	Type of Model	Topic	Clinical Question	Sample Size	AI/ML Method Utilized	Test, Training, or Cross Validation Method	Performance
Cerrolaza et al,[2] 2016	Computer Vision	Hydronephrosis	Predict mercaptoacetyltriglycine (MAG3) T1/2 by ultrasound study in children with hydronephrosis	50 patients	Support vector machine, Logistic Regression	leave-one-out cross-validation	Area under the curve (AUC) ranging from 0.94 to 0.98
Yin et al,[3] (2020)	Computer Vision	Hydronephrosis	Identify children with congenital anomalies of the kidney and urinary tract (CAKUT) from based on ultrasound	182 patients	Neural Network	In sample testing	AUC >0.95, accuracy (ACC) >0.91.
Yin et al,[4] 2020	Computer Vision	Hydronephrosis	Identification of posterior urethral valves (PUV) on US	157 patients	Neural Network	5-fold leave-one-out cross-validation	AUCs ranging from 0.949 to 0.961
Song et al,[5] 2022	Computer Vision	Hydronephrosis	Segmentation of hydronephrotic and renal paranchyma on US	168 patients	Neural Network	In the cross-validation, the fold ratio of training, validation, and test sets was 2:1:1, and their composition was changed in the order of cyclic permutations.	3 models with dice similarity coefficient (DSCs) >0.9 (DeepLabV3+ with EfficientNet- B4 highest mean DSC of 0.9087)
Smail et al,[6] 2022	Computer Vision	Hydronephrosis	Predict Society for Fetal Urology (SFU) hydronephrosis grade using US	687 patients (2492 images)	Neural Network	5-fold leave-one-out cross-validation	Mean accuracy (F1) 78% (0.78) for differentiating mild vs severe HN; mean accuracy (F1) of 71% (0.71) for differentiating moderate grades (SFU II and III).
Weaver et al,[7] 2023	Computer Vision	Hydronephrosis	Predict renal complications in children with prenatal hydro using use mercaptoacetyltriglycine (MAG3) scans	152 patients	Neural Network, Decision tree (Random Forest)	80:20 training-to-test split	Neural Network Model AUC of 0.78; RF Model AUC of 0.67
Fernandez et al,[8] 2021	Computer Vision	Hypospadias	Recognize images of hypospadias	1198 patients	Neural Network	97:3 training-to-test split with 2 rounds of training	Accuracy of 90%

Study	Category	Topic	Description	Sample	Model	Validation	Results
Zhu et al,[9] 2023	Computer Vision	Oncology	Differentiate Wilms' tumor from non-Wilms' tumors using computed tomography (CT)	364 patients	Neural Network	6:2:2 training-cross validation-test split	AUC of 0.831, accuracy of 78.1%, specificity 84.2% , and sensitivity of 56.3%
Sharaby et al,[10] 2023	Computer Vision	Oncology	Predict Wilms' tumor preoperative chemotherapy response using CT features	63 patients	Support vector machine, Neural Network, Decision Tree (Randomn Forest), Logistic Regression, Multilayer Proceptron	train-to-test split not mentioned, used both 4-fold and 10-fold cross validation	Accuracy of 95.24%, sensitivity of 95.65%, and specificity of 94.12%
Yin et al,[11] 2019	Computer Vision	Renal Segmentation	Segmentation of kidneys from renal US	100 patients (185 images)	Neural Network	missing	DICE score of 0.94; Accuracy of 98.9%
Yin et al,[12] 2020	Computer Vision	Renal Segmentation	Automated segmentation of kidneys using ultrasound	152 patients (289 images)	Neural Network, Logistic Regression	105:20:164 training-cross validation-test split	Highest DICE score of 0.9451
Kim[13] 2022	Computer Vision	Urethral Strictures	Identification of urethral stricture on retrograde urethrogram	242 images	Neural Network	90:10 training-to-test split	Accuracy of 88.5%
Lee et al,[14] 2022	Computer Vision	Urinary tract infection (UTI)	Predict UTI recurrence using renal scans	180 patients	Neural Network	66:33 training-to-test split with k-fold cross validation	AUC of 0.816
Khondker et al,[15] 2020	Computer Vision	Vesicoureteral reflux (VUR)	Grading of VUR severity using features such as novel features such as uretheral tortuosity and dilation	3144 patients	Random Forrest, Decision tree (XGBoost), Support vector machine	10-fold leave-one-out cross-validation	Mean AUC of 0.84; Accuracy of 62%
Khondker[16] 2022	Computer Vision	VUR	Differentiate high grade VUR (IV/V) from low grade (I/II/III) using VCUG imaging	41 images	Random Forrest	leave-one-out cross-validation	AUC of 0.90
Wang et al,[17] 2021	Prediction model	Clinical Workflow	Predict clinic time and efficiency during pediatric urology clinic	256 patients	Random Forrest	80:20 training-to-test split with simulation	Predicted doctor time accurately to 3.6 min (new patients) and 5.0 min (returning patients). Simulation predicted reduction of wait time by 24% to 54%.
Bagli et al,[18] 1998	Prediction model	Hydronephrosis	Predict postoperative sonography findings following pyeloplasty	100 patients	Neural Network	84:16 training-to-test split	100% sensitivity, 100% specificity

(continued on next page)

Table 1
(continued)

Authors	Type of Model	Topic	Clinical Question	Sample Size	AI/ML Method Utilized	Test, Training, or Cross Validation Method	Performance
Lorenzo[19] 2019	Prediction model	Hydronephrosis	Predict need for surgical intervention in hydronephrosis patients	557 patients	Decision Jungle	70:30 training-to-test split	AUC of 0.9, accuracy of 0.87, and precision of 0.80,
Fernandez et al,[20] 2023	Prediction model	Hypospadias	Determine correlation of genotypes and hypospadias phenotypes from literature review	1731 patients (126 studies)	Neural Network	70:30 training-to-test split	Varying AUC depending on hypospadius type ranging from 0.892 to 0.9782
Tokar et al,[21] 2021	Prediction model	lower urinary tract dysfunction (LUTD)	Predict enuresis in children using demographic information and patient/family characteristics	8071 patients	Logistic Regression, Decision tree (XGBoost), Neural Netowrk, Random Forrest, SVC, Multilayer Proceptron, Naïve Bayes, Regression Trees	70:30 training-to-test split	Accuracy of 81.3%.
Babajide et al,[22] 2022	Prediction model	Nephrolithiasis	Identify stones and stone characteristics using computed tomography (CT)	94 patients	Neural Network	37:7 training-to-test split	100% sensitivity, 100% specificity
Bhambavanii et al,[23] 2020	Prediction model	Oncology	Predict 5-y survival rates in pediatric patients with genitourinary (GU) rhabdomyosarcoma	277 patients	Neural Network	80:20 training-to-test split	Disease-Specific Survival AUC of 0.91; Overall Survival AUC 0.93
Abdovic et al,[24] 2019	Prediction model	PUV	Predicting late presenting PUV in males based on uroflow	408 patients	Neural Network	80:20 training-to-test split with k-fold cross validation	AUC of 0.98; Accuracy of 92.7%
Kwong et al,[25] 2022	Prediction model	PUV	Predict long-term complications of males with PUV using early kidney and anatomic features	152 patients	Decision tree (Random Forrest)	80:20 training-to-test split with k-fold cross validation	Chronic kidney disease (CKD) progression (c-index = 0.77; external C-index = 0.78), KRT (c-index = 0.95; external C-index = 0.89); and indicated CIC (c-index = 0.70; external C-index = 0.64)

Study	Type	Condition	Purpose	Patients	Model	Validation	Results
Weaver et al,[26] 2023	Prediction model	PUV	Predict progression of chronic kidney disease (CKD) among children with PUV	225 patients	Neural Network, Decision tree (Random Forrest)	80:20 training-test split with 5-fold cross validation	c-index ranging from 0.79 to 0.82; AUC ranging from 0.65, to0.82
Santori et al,[27] 2007	Prediction model	Transplant	Predict delayed decrease of serum creatinine in pediatric patients undergoing renal transplant	148 patients	Neural Network, Logistic Regression	107:41 training-to-test split	Highest accuracy of 89.1%,
Seckiner et al,[28] 2011	Prediction model	ureteropelvic junction obstruction (UPJO)	Predict UPJO outcomes	53 patients	Neural Network	37:8:8 training-cross validation-test split	Sensitivity of 75% and specificity of 77%
Drysdale et al,[29] 2022	Prediction model	UPJO	Predict those at risk for UPJO recurrence after dismembered pyleopasty	543 patients	Penalized regreesion (Least absolute shrinkage and selection operator [LASSO])	In sample	AUC of 0.86 for prediction of reoperation; AUC of 0.78 for predicted the time to re-intervention
Arlen et al,[30] 2016	Prediction model	UTI	Prediction of breakthrough UTI in children with VUR	255 patients	Neural Network, Logistic Regression	3:1 training-to-test split	DICE score of 0.94; Accuracy of 98.9%
Ozkan et al,[31] 2018	Prediction model	UTI	Identify UTI from history, clinical examination, urinalysis, and ultrasonography	59 patients	Decision Tree, Support vector machine (SVM), Random Forrest, Neural Network	80:20 training-test split with 5-fold cross validation	Model accuracies ranging from 93.22% to 98.30%
Advanced Analytics Group of Pediatric Urology[32] 2019	Prediction model	UTI	Predict UTI recurrence and VUR in children with a history of UTI	500 patients	Decision Tree (Optimal classification tree)	85:15 training-to-test split	AUC of 0.761
Serrano-Durbá et al,[33] 2004	Prediction model	VUR	Predict deflux outcome for patients with VUR	261 patients	Neural Network	174:87 training-to-test split	AUC of 0.77
Knudson et al,[34] 2007	Prediction model	VUR	Prediction of VUR resolution within 1–2 y of diagnosis	205 patients	Neural Network, SVM, Logistic Regression	31:10 training-to-test split	AUC 0.86 (VUR resolution at 2 y)
Seckiner et al,[35] 2008	Prediction model	VUR	Predict resolution of VUR with varying treatment modalities (abx ppx, deflux, or reimplant)	96 patients	Neural Network	99:23:22 training-cross validation-test split	Sensitivity of 98.5% and specificity of 92.5%
Kirsch et al,[36] 2014	Prediction model	VUR	Predict spontaneous resolution of primary VUR	229 patients	Decision tree (Random Forrest), Cox Hazard Regression	In sample	Five RF normalized categories had improvement/ resolution rates of 89%, 69%, 53%, 16%, and 11%, respectively.

(continued on next page)

Table 1
(continued)

Authors	Type of Model	Topic	Clinical Question	Sample Size	AI/ML Method Utilized	Test, Training, or Cross Validation Method	Performance
Logvinenko et al,[37] 2015	Prediction model	VUR	Predict VUR by Renal US	2259 patients	Neural Network, Logistic Regression	In sample	AUC of 0.69 for any VUR; AUC of 0.67 for VUR grade > II; and AUC of 0.79 for VUR grade > III.
Keskinoglu et al,[38] 2020	Prediction model	VUR	Predict VUR vs UTI using clinical data	611 patients	Neural Network	10-fold leave-one-out cross-validation	Highest AUC of 0.806
Eroglu et al,[39] 2021	Prediction model	VUR	Grade VUR using VCUG imaging	1228 patients	Neural Network	80:20 training-to-test split	Accuracy of 96.9
Bertsimas et al,[40] 2021	Prescription model	VUR	Predict UTI recurrence rate among children with VUR	600 patients	Decision Tree	80:20 training-to-test split	AUC of 0.82
Wang et al,[41] 2021	Signal Analysis	LUTD	Detection of detrusor overactivity (DO) on urodynamic study (UDS)	799 patients	Manifold learning, dynamic time warping	5-fold leave-one-out cross-validation	AUC of 0.84
Ge et al,[42] 2022	Signal Analysis	LUTD	Estimate bladder compliance using intravesical pressure	52 patients	Support vector machine, Random Forest, Logistic Regression, Perceptron, Decision tree (XGBoost), and Naïve Bayes	leave-one-out cross-validation	AUC 0.688–0.873 (SVM was the highest)
Hobbs et al,[43] 2022	Signal Analysis	LUTD	Identification of DO on UDS	546 patients (805 UDS)	Support vector machine	85:15 training-to-test split with 3-fold cross validation	Maximum AUC of 90.5
Weaver et al,[44] 2023	Signal Analysis	LUTD	Categorize bladder dysfunction severity using videourodynamics	256 patients (306 studies)	Neural Network, Decision tree (Random Forrest)	80:20 training-to-test split with stratified 5-fold cross validation	Clinical Model AUC 0.51–0.68; UDS Tracing Model AUC 0.56–0.87; Imaging Model AUC 0.64–0.86; Ensemble Model 0.64–0.89
Blum et al,[45] 2018	Signal Analysis	UPJO	Identify clinical relevant UPJO from diuresis renogram compared to T1/2 and C30 values	55 patients	Support vector machine	In sample	AUC of 0.96; Accuracy of 93%

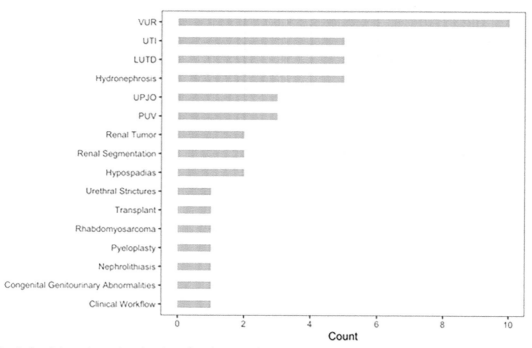

Fig. 2. Breakdown by topics of reviewed pediatric urology artificial intelligence (AI) literature.

used voiding cystourethrogram (VCUG) images to investigate VUR. Khondker and colleagues[16] developed a model to differentiate high-grade and low-grade VUR with an AUC of 0.90; this same group[15] used features such as ureteral tortuosity and dilation as input to predict the grading of VUR with a mean AUC of 0.84. Though the utility of CT scans in children is limited, it is indicated in the evaluation of oncologic conditions. While Zhu and colleagues[9] utilized neural network model to differentiate between Wilms' and non-Wilms' tumor on CT, Sharaby and colleagues[10] used a cohort of patients with known Wilms' tumor and used multiple models to predict chemotherapy response using CT features. Finally, there is a range of ML articles utilizing nuclear imaging, especially renal scans. Weaver and colleagues[7] used renal scans of patients with prenatal hydronephrosis to

predict further complications with neural network model AUC of 0.78 and a random forest model AUC of 0.67. Alternatively, Lee and colleagues[14] used renal scans to predict UTI recurrence with an AUC of 0.82.

Signal Analysis

Signal analysis is a related field of electrical engineering that investigates time series data forms such as music, speech, or seismic activity. One of the most commonly encountered time series data relevant to urology are cystometrogram recordings as part of urodynamic studies, which report pressure and volume over time. Hobbs and colleagues[43] and Wang and colleagues[41] have used signal analysis and machine learning methodology to identify detrusor overactivity (DO) in cystometrogram. Hobbs used support vector machine model and the fast Fourier transform, a signal processing technique to describe signals by their frequency components, to predict DO with an AUC of 0.905. Alternatively, Wang and colleagues utilized manifold learning, and dynamic time warping methodology to identify DO events with an AUC of 0.84. Ge and colleagues predicted bladder compliance categories using features generated from intravesical pressure signal analysis with the highest AUC of 0.87.[42] Weaver and colleagues[44] took clinical and videourodynamic data (tracings and cystograms) to categorize expert-defined lower

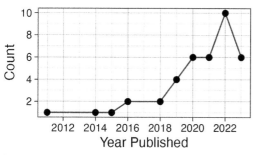

Fig. 3. Pediatric urology AI published manuscript counts by year.

urinary tract dysfunction (LUTD) severity from the ensemble model ranging from AUC of 0.64 to 0.89.

Signal analysis methods can also be used on drainage curves of nuclear diuresis renogram. Blum and colleagues[45] extracted drainage curves features from diuresis renograms and input them into predictive ML models to identify ureteropelvic junction obstruction (UPJO) surgical cases.

Prescription Studies

Prescription models refer to algorithms that provide not only predictions but also treatment recommendation (prescriptions). The decision for the treatment is usually based on patients' predicted outcome with or without treatment. Since in most cases, the observed data can only happen in one way (the patient underwent surgery or did not) for each patient (factuals), prescription models need to be able to estimate the outcomes for the scenario that did not actually happen (counter-factuals) to evaluate the treatment benefit. For example, Bertsimas and colleagues utilized the Randomized Intervention for Children with Vesicoureteral Reflux (RIVUR) trial data to predict the risk of recurrent febrile urinary tract infection risk with or without antibiotic prophylaxis to inform individualized recommendation for children with VUR.[40]

DISCUSSION

Our review shows a vast variety of promising and growing AI pediatric studies across disciplines in pediatric urology such as hydronephrosis, UPJO, VUR, UTI, neurogenic bladder/lower tract dysfunction, transplant, and oncology. Among numerous potential benefits, the capabilities of these models can potentially enable other clinicians to identify high-risk conditions or anatomy, personalize treatment plans, and allocate resource effectively in a scalable and reliable fashion.

On the other hand, there are several notable challenges for AI, especially in pediatric urology. For example, for pediatric urologic conditions, obtaining large and diverse datasets can be difficult due to factors such as privacy concerns, limited populations, or rarity of the diseases. When training ML models with small sample sizes, there is an increased risk of overfitting, where the model becomes too specific to the limited data it was trained on, leading to poor generalization on unseen data and unstable model performance (the good or bad results are due to chance instead of actual, newly discovered patterns). Many have proposed best practices to mitigate this issue such as providing confidence interval estimates[46,47] in model evaluation metrics, more robust model training methodologies such as bootstrapping samples, enhanced data splitting, cross-validations, or collaborations between multiple institutions to generate larger cohorts. Additionally, small sample sizes can result in imbalanced classes, making it difficult for the model to learn meaningful patterns and correlations. Furthermore, most pediatric urologists lack training and education in principles of data science and AI/ML. This knowledge gap can hinder the effective utilization of ML, including the ability to interpret and critically appraise the results produced by these algorithms. Without clear quality control guidelines with data science experts and pediatric urologists, the responsibility to present the best quality of study with the most generalizable model can be heavy in the authors' and editors' hands.

The "black-box" reputation of most of the AI/ML model also poses a significant challenge for pediatric urology applications. The interpretability and explainability of prediction models are critical to health care professionals to understand the factors influencing the predictions, enabling trust and facilitating adoption in clinical practice. This aspect is most unique to medicine due to the implicit trust between the clinicians and families, as well as the underlying medicolegal risk. With ongoing advancements in ML algorithms, new methodologies to provide more interpretability provide more promise in AI/ML for medicine.

Selecting appropriate study design for AI/ML study can also be difficult. As most current AI/ML studies utilized "supervised" learning, defined as training the algorithm to learn the "ground-truth" provided by the researchers and clinicians (as opposed to unsupervised learning that does not require "true" labels), it can be difficult to structure the study to provide generalizable result. If the desired outcome of modeling is still unclear or highly debated, using the new AI/ML methodology might not be helpful. For example, if one wishes to model a chance that a patient receives a specific surgery, or classify bladder hostility categories, even if a stable and highly accurate model can be trained, the result can be a moot point since it is learning from a debatable label (examples might include variable surgical indications across different surgeons or institutions, or variable interpretation/criterion of "hostile bladder" on urodynamic studies by different urologists).

Despite the potential of AI/ML in pediatric urology, certain areas, such as NLP and reinforcement learning, are not fully utilized in the field.

NLP techniques have shown promise in extracting valuable information from unstructured medical texts. However, the adoption of NLP in health care settings faces challenges related to data availability from electronic health records, and interoperability between institutions. Integrating NLP into clinical workflows and electronic health record systems remains a complex task. Similarly, reinforcement learning, which involves training models to make sequential decisions through trial and error, holds great potential in optimizing personalized treatment. However, the application of reinforcement learning in medicine is still limited, partly due to the complexity and risks associated with clinical decision-making. Addressing these challenges and expanding the utilization of new AI/ML techniques require interdisciplinary collaboration, robust data infrastructure, and the development of governance and ethical guidelines to ensure patient safety, privacy, and fairness.

The future of ML in pediatric urology is filled with excitement and promise. ML techniques have the potential to revolutionize various aspects of this specialized field, spanning multiple disciplines. From diagnostic imaging and surgical planning to treatment optimization and patient outcomes, ML can enhance the precision and effectiveness of pediatric urologic interventions. Advanced imaging analysis algorithms can aid in the accurate detection and classification of congenital anomalies, tumors, and urinary tract abnormalities, enabling early interventions and personalized treatment plans. ML models can assist surgeons in preoperative planning, optimizing surgical approaches, and predicting surgical outcomes. As the accessibility and availability of pediatric urologic data and multi-institutional collaborations continue to grow, AI/ML algorithms can learn from diverse datasets, leading to improved predictive accuracy and personalized interventions. Ultimately, the integration of ML into pediatric urology has the potential to improve patient outcomes, reduce health care costs, and drive advancements in this our field.

SUMMARY

The authors' review showed a clear growing interest in AI/ML for pediatric urology. The published studies cover various clinical areas in our field. While these studies show great promise for better understanding of disease and patient care, we should be realistic about the challenges arising from the nature of pediatric urologic conditions and practice, in order to continue to produce high-impact research.

CLINICS CARE POINTS

- AI pediatric urologic applications can potentially provide direct and actionable insight to clinicians.
- Important to understand the stregth and weakness when planning for AI implementation in clinical use.
- New AI applications are powerful but requires careful and critical considerations.

FUNDING SOURCE

None. No financial relationships to disclose for all authors.

REFERENCES

1. Chen J, Remulla D, Nguyen JH, et al. Current status of artificial intelligence applications in urology and their potential to influence clinical practice. BJU Int 2019;124(4):567–77.
2. Cerrolaza JJ, Peters CA, Martin AD, et al. Quantitative Ultrasound for Measuring Obstructive Severity in Children with Hydronephrosis. J Urol 2016;195(4 Pt 1):1093–9.
3. Yin S, Peng Q, Li H, et al. Computer-Aided Diagnosis of Congenital Abnormalities of the Kidney and Urinary Tract in Children Using a Multi-Instance Deep Learning Method Based on Ultrasound Imaging Data. Proc IEEE Int Symp Biomed Imaging 2020;2020:1347–50.
4. Yin S, Peng Q, Li H, et al. Multi-instance Deep Learning of Ultrasound Imaging Data for Pattern Classification of Congenital Abnormalities of the Kidney and Urinary Tract in Children. Urology 2020;142: 183–9.
5. Song SH, Han JH, Kim KS, et al. Deep-learning segmentation of ultrasound images for automated calculation of the hydronephrosis area to renal parenchyma ratio. Investig Clin Urol 2022;63(4):455–63.
6. Smail LC, Dhindsa K, Braga LH, et al. Using Deep Learning Algorithms to Grade Hydronephrosis Severity: Toward a Clinical Adjunct. Front Pediatr 2020;8:1.
7. Weaver JK, Logan J, Broms R, et al. Deep learning of renal scans in children with antenatal hydronephrosis. J Pediatr Urol 2023;S1477-5131(22): 00632–5.
8. Fernandez N, Lorenzo AJ, Rickard M, et al. Digital Pattern Recognition for the Identification and Classification of Hypospadias Using Artificial Intelligence vs Experienced Pediatric Urologist. Urology 2021; 147:264–9.

9. Zhu Y, Li H, Huang Y, et al. CT-based identification of pediatric non-Wilms tumors using convolutional neural networks at a single center. Pediatr Res 2023; 94(3):1104–10.

10. Sharaby I, Alksas A, Nashat A, et al. Prediction of Wilms' Tumor Susceptibility to Preoperative Chemotherapy Using a Novel Computer-Aided Prediction System. Diagnostics 2023;13(3):486.

11. Yin S, Zhang Z, Li H, et al. Fully-Automatic Segmentation of Kidneys in Clinical Ultrasound Images Using a Boundary Distance Regression Network. Proc IEEE Int Symp Biomed Imaging 2019;2019:1741–4.

12. Yin S, Peng Q, Li H, et al. Automatic kidney segmentation in ultrasound images using subsequent boundary distance regression and pixelwise classification networks. Med Image Anal 2020;60:101602.

13. Kim JK, McCammon K, Robey C, et al. Identifying urethral strictures using machine learning: a proof-of-concept evaluation of convolutional neural network model. World J Urol 2022;40(12):3107–11.

14. Lee H, Yoo B, Baek M, et al. Prediction of Recurrent Urinary Tract Infection in Paediatric Patients by Deep Learning Analysis of (99m)Tc-DMSA Renal Scan. Diagnostics 2022;12(2):424.

15. Khondker A, Kwong JCC, Yadav P, et al. Multi-institutional Validation of Improved Vesicoureteral Reflux Assessment With Simple and Machine Learning Approaches. J Urol 2022;208(6):1314–22.

16. Khondker A, Kwong JCC, Rickard M, et al. A machine learning-based approach for quantitative grading of vesicoureteral reflux from voiding cystourethrograms: Methods and proof of concept. J Pediatr Urol 2022;18(1):78 e71.

17. Wang HS, Cahill D, Panagides J, et al. A Machine Learning Model to Maximize Efficiency and Face Time in Ambulatory Clinics. Urol Pract 2021;8(2): 176–82.

18. Bagli DJ, Agarwal SK, Venkateswaran S, et al. Artificial neural networks in pediatric urology: prediction of sonographic outcome following pyeloplasty. J Urol 1998;160(3 Pt 2):980–3. discussion 994.

19. Lorenzo AJ, Rickard M, Braga LH, et al. Predictive Analytics and Modeling Employing Machine Learning Technology: The Next Step in Data Sharing, Analysis, and Individualized Counseling Explored With a Large, Prospective Prenatal Hydronephrosis Database. Urology 2019;123:204–9.

20. Fernandez N, Chua M, Villanueva J, et al. Neural network non-linear modeling to predict hypospadias genotype-phenotype correlation. J Pediatr Urol 2023;19(3):288 e281.

21. Tokar B, Baskaya M, Celik O, et al. Application of Machine Learning Techniques for Enuresis Prediction in Children. Eur J Pediatr Surg 2021;31(5): 414–9.

22. Babajide R, Lembrikova K, Ziemba J, et al. Automated Machine Learning Segmentation and Measurement of Urinary Stones on CT Scan. Urology 2022;169:41–6.

23. Bhambhvani HP, Zamora A, Velaer K, et al. Deep learning enabled prediction of 5-year survival in pediatric genitourinary rhabdomyosarcoma. Surg Oncol 2021;36:23–7.

24. Abdovic S, Cuk M, Cekada N, et al. Predicting posterior urethral obstruction in boys with lower urinary tract symptoms using deep artificial neural network. World J Urol 2019;37(9):1973–9.

25. Kwong JC, Khondker A, Kim JK, et al. Posterior Urethral Valves Outcomes Prediction (PUVOP): a machine learning tool to predict clinically relevant outcomes in boys with posterior urethral valves. Pediatr Nephrol 2022;37(5):1067–74.

26. Weaver JK, Milford K, Rickard M, et al. Deep learning imaging features derived from kidney ultrasounds predict chronic kidney disease progression in children with posterior urethral valves. Pediatr Nephrol 2023;38(3):839–46.

27. Santori G, Fontana I, Valente U. Application of an artificial neural network model to predict delayed decrease of serum creatinine in pediatric patients after kidney transplantation. Transplant Proc 2007; 39(6):1813–9.

28. Seckiner I, Seckiner SU, Bayrak O, et al. Use of artificial neural networks in the management of antenatally diagnosed ureteropelvic junction obstruction. Can Urol Assoc J 2011;5(6):E152–5.

29. Drysdale E, Khondker A, Kim JK, et al. Personalized application of machine learning algorithms to identify pediatric patients at risk for recurrent ureteropelvic junction obstruction after dismembered pyeloplasty. World J Urol 2022;40(2):593–9.

30. Arlen AM, Alexander SE, Wald M, et al. Computer model predicting breakthrough febrile urinary tract infection in children with primary vesicoureteral reflux. J Pediatr Urol 2016;12(5):288 e281.

31. Ozkan IA, Koklu M, Sert IU. Diagnosis of urinary tract infection based on artificial intelligence methods. Comput Methods Programs Biomed 2018;166:51–9.

32. Advanced Analytics Group of Pediatric U, Group ORCPM. Targeted Workup after Initial Febrile Urinary Tract Infection: Using a Novel Machine Learning Model to Identify Children Most Likely to Benefit from Voiding Cystourethrogram. J Urol 2019;202(1):144–52.

33. Serrano-Durba A, Serrano AJ, Magdalena JR, et al. The use of neural networks for predicting the result of endoscopic treatment for vesico-ureteric reflux. BJU Int 2004;94(1):120–2.

34. Knudson MJ, Austin JC, Wald M, et al. Computational model for predicting the chance of early resolution in children with vesicoureteral reflux. J Urol 2007;178(4 Pt 2):1824–7.

35. Seckiner I, Seckiner SU, Erturhan S, et al. The use of artificial neural networks in decision support in

vesicoureteral reflux treatment. Urol Int 2008;80(3): 283–6.

36. Kirsch AJ, Arlen AM, Leong T, et al. Vesicoureteral reflux index (VURx): a novel tool to predict primary reflux improvement and resolution in children less than 2 years of age. J Pediatr Urol 2014;10(6): 1249–54.

37. Logvinenko T, Chow JS, Nelson CP. Predictive value of specific ultrasound findings when used as a screening test for abnormalities on VCUG. J Pediatr Urol 2015;11(4):176 e171–e177.

38. Keskinoğlu A, Özgür S. The Use of Artificial Neural Networks for Differential Diagnosis between Vesicoureteral Reflux and Urinary Tract Infection in Children. J Pediatr Res 2020;7(3):230–5.

39. Eroglu Y, Yildirim K, Cinar A, et al. Diagnosis and grading of vesicoureteral reflux on voiding cystourethrography images in children using a deep hybrid model. Comput Methods Programs Biomed 2021; 210:106369.

40. Bertsimas D, Li M, Estrada C, et al. Selecting Children with Vesicoureteral Reflux Who are Most Likely to Benefit from Antibiotic Prophylaxis: Application of Machine Learning to RIVUR. J Urol 2021;205(4): 1170–9.

41. Wang HS, Cahill D, Panagides J, et al. Pattern recognition algorithm to identify detrusor overactivity on urodynamics. Neurourol Urodyn 2021;40(1): 428–34.

42. Ge Z, Tang L, Peng Y, et al. Design of a rapid diagnostic model for bladder compliance based on real-time intravesical pressure monitoring system. Comput Biol Med 2022;141:105173.

43. Hobbs KT, Choe N, Aksenov LI, et al. Machine Learning for Urodynamic Detection of Detrusor Overactivity. Urology 2022;159:247–54.

44. Weaver JK, Martin-Olenski M, Logan J, et al. Deep Learning of Videourodynamics to Classify Bladder Dysfunction Severity in Patients With Spina Bifida. J Urol 2023;209(5):994–1003.

45. Blum ES, Porras AR, Biggs E, et al. Early Detection of Ureteropelvic Junction Obstruction Using Signal Analysis and Machine Learning: A Dynamic Solution to a Dynamic Problem. J Urol 2018;199(3):847–52.

46. Gengsheng Q, Hotilovac L. Comparison of nonparametric confidence intervals for the area under the ROC curve of a continuous-scale diagnostic test. Stat Methods Med Res 2008;17(2):207–21.

47. LeDell E, Petersen M, van der Laan M. Computationally efficient confidence intervals for cross-validated area under the ROC curve estimates. Electronic Journal of Statistics 2015;9(1):1583–607.

Surgical Artificial Intelligence in Urology
Educational Applications

Mitchell G. Goldenberg, MBBS, PhD, FRCSC

KEYWORDS

- Surgical education • Machine learning • Artificial intelligence • Surgical simulation • Surgical skill

KEY POINTS

- Medical education is undergoing a paradigm shift toward more objective and iterative evaluation of trainee competency, with increasing demand for frequent and evidence-based assessments.
- Evaluation of surgical trainee skill in the operating room has become a focus of artificial intelligence research in academic surgery.
- Acceptance and implementation of machine learning in surgical education faces specific challenges that may be addressed through improved transparency related to algorithm outcomes and improved understanding of the strengths and limitations of the technology in academic settings.

BACKGROUND

Surgical education is undergoing a paradigm shift.[1] Throughout the educational continuum from medical school to surgical practice, policy makers have mandated that curricula are outcome-focused.[2] This new archetype, commonly referred to as competency-based medical education (CBME), is rooted in the idea that medical providers must demonstrate an ability to perform cognitive, communicative, and procedural tasks to a satisfactory standard.[1] This approach to medical education requires routine evaluation of trainee's performance across several competencies, to ensure that some level of proficiency has been reached before accreditation and independent practice.[3] The nature of these assessments varies between jurisdictions,[4,5] but all use some form of benchmark that must be achieved before a trainee can progress through their curriculum.

It is worth firstly reflecting on the concept of competency regarding surgical training, specifically relating to surgical procedural skills. This idea arose as a result of internal and external pressure on the profession to produce physicians who have met an acceptable level of ability that will ensure they provide their patients with adequate medical care.[6] Included in this broad mandate is the notion that doctors will also be effective communicators, leaders, and remain up-to-date with innovations and updates in their specialty or area of care. In the United States, this is all encapsulated by the Accreditation Council for Graduate Medical Education (ACGME) "Core Competency" framework.[7] This framework outlines the qualities all physicians should demonstrate at the conclusion of their training, across all disciplines. To aid in curricular design, the ACGME introduced the Milestone Project,[5] an initiative that had each specialty meticulously design a list of the skills or abilities that make up each of these competencies in their respective fields. What evolved from these efforts were specialty-specific and subcategorized units of professional practice that trainees must be tested on and demonstrate their ability to carry out this standard of competency. Each of these entrustable professional activities (EPA) then required their own definitions that were specific

Catherine & Joseph Aresty Department of Urology, USC Institute of Urology, University of Southern California, 1441 Eastlake Avenue, Suite 7416, Los Angeles, CA 90033, USA
E-mail address: Mitchell.goldenberg@med.usc.edu

Urol Clin N Am 51 (2024) 105–115
https://doi.org/10.1016/j.ucl.2023.06.003
0094-0143/24/© 2023 Elsevier Inc. All rights reserved.

and reproducible to ensure that trainees being evaluated by different clinicians and in different residency programs could be reliably compared[8]; this has created an educational landscape that is rich in data but prone to the limitations and inherent biases of peer evaluation.

The demand for frequent and standardized assessments in surgical training has posed specific challenges to stakeholders in this field. First and foremost, completing meaningful evaluations of surgical residents is a time and energy-consuming undertaking.[7,9] Compared with other professions, physicians invest a great deal of their cognitive bandwidth toward the education of future colleagues, and the self-regulative nature of medicine demands this. In an already time-constrained work environment, this unsurprisingly leads to mental fatigue among educators, sometimes referred to as "rater burnout," which leads to inconsistency among evaluators and heterogeneity in the standards to which residents of similar training levels are held.[10,11] Secondly, there is significant variability between educators in their definitions of "competency" or "entrustability," informed by their own subconscious biases, clinical experience, or personal training backgrounds; this leads to the well-known divide between "hawks" and "doves," that is those who provide more or less favorable ratings of performance, respectively, compared with their colleagues.[12] Although variability among evaluators is not always a detriment to trainees, such as during low-stakes or formative assessments aimed at providing feedback, this lack of objectivity may be detrimental when related to high-stakes decisions around progression through training or credentialing practices.

Another limitation of the existing framework for evaluating trainee performance is a lack of understanding of the relationship between assessment and real-world outcomes. According to Messick's contemporary framework of validity, *consequences evidence* is a central tenet of educational assessment validation.[13] In the context of surgical skill evaluations, this refers to the potential impact that a trainee's score or pass/fail status on a high-stakes, summative assessment has on their own career, their patient's well-being, and society at large.[14] Specific sources of evidence have been studied in the literature, most notably the relationship between ratings of performance and patient outcomes following a procedure.[15,16] Across multiple procedures and surgical specialties, this relationship has been demonstrated and externally validated. In urology, this is most evident in the robotic-assisted radical prostatectomy (RARP) literature, where multiple groups have previously shown correlations between human expert ratings of skill and postoperative outcomes such as continence, potency, and surgical margin status.[16,17] These studies have generally used video-based assessment strategies to quantify surgical skill, relying on expert surgeons or trained raters to evaluate the quality of the observed surgeon or trainee's movements, interaction with tissue, and ability to safely progress through steps of the surgery.

The ACGME has worked for years on instituting the current competency-based framework into surgical and medical training, requiring an overhaul in the curriculum and administration of residency programs across all disciplines nationally. However, recent literature exploring the fallout from this implementation has revealed that these changes are not accepted by all educators and trainees, who point to the persistent lack of data supporting tangible benefits of a much more assessment-heavy educational structure.[18] The term "assessment fatigue" has become more pervasive in the medical education literature, and without a clear understanding of the benefits that much more frequent trainee evaluation has on educational outcomes, it is becoming harder to justify their use.[19] Some have gone as far to say that CBME's reliance on assessment data has led to a shift away from learner-centeredness and toward the "one-size-fits-all" approach, which is antithetical to the purpose of a competency-based curriculum.[20]

This combination of factors has become a barrier to wider acceptance and implementation of outcome-based education in surgical training, and these challenges require innovative solutions to be overcome.[21] Artificial intelligence (AI) has been injected into many aspects of health care delivery, and surgical education is no exception.[22-24] Adoption of machine learning (ML) and computer vision (CV) analyses across all facets of the health care sciences has been spurred by encouraging results, notably the objective, autonomous analysis of large quantities of data, and the ability to make accurate predictions through data manipulation not possible with traditional statistical modeling. Stakeholders in medical education see AI as a potential solution to many of the highlighted limitations here, with relevance to the scalability of skill and performance assessments in surgical training.[25]

The data on assessments of technical performance form most of the published literature in this space. As with other high-reliability industries, the quantification of performance is essential for standardization of training, providing readily analyzed metrics that allow comparison between individuals. Quantification of performance also enables standards to be set, providing benchmarks that can be used to ensure trainees reach a minimum predetermined benchmark before progressing through a curriculum.[26] Current methods of quantifying surgical skill involve the use expert surgeons and educators to make decisions based on a scoring rubric, often using some type of ordinal or Likert-type scale. These "global rating scales (GRS)" are validated primarily through interrater reliability or correlation with variables such as operative time or patient outcomes.[27] Although usually methodologically robust, there is an innate level of bias that is introduced when a human expert is providing a rating of technical skill, despite conventional mitigating steps such as blinding.[28] Surgeons can be influenced by their own education, preferences regarding intraoperative decision-making, and incorrect assumptions regarding best practices.[29] Furthermore, when observing the video of a procedure alone, the lack of context regarding nontechnical factors that may influence technical execution of a procedural task is missed.[30]

In this article, the various applications of AI in the education of urologists and urologic trainees are discussed, both in the existing literature as well as ongoing and future innovative uses of AI to improve the quality of surgical training.

APPLICATIONS OF ARTIFICIAL INTELLIGENCE IN UROLOGIC EDUCATION

Urologic education is a broad term that includes preresidency training, specialty and subspecialty education, as well as accreditation and recertification. Participation spans medical school to independent practice, and this often makes studying this population challenging. Furthermore, the type of data that are accumulated over the course of this educational timeline is diverse and includes written, audiovisual, and even biophysiological and kinematic information. It is important to remember that AI's current role in this space has not been to necessarily change the way in which we are training surgeons, but rather to automate and objectify the current processes that exist in the training curriculum. These processes include quantification and evaluation of surgical technical and nontechnical skills, identifying and ranking optimal candidates for residency selection, and optimizing simulation for ex vivo training of surgeons without compromising patient safety. AI has also been used to improve our ability to predict surgical outcomes, and this has important implications for educational efforts as we better understand what

clinically important aspects of intraoperative performance can be targeted for educational interventions.

TECHNICAL SKILLS ASSESSMENT
Simulation Setting

Simulation provides surgical educators with the ability to replicate clinical environments, where real-life surgical procedures and complications can be fabricated within a safe and controlled setting. The ability to provide a low-stakes and safe training environment to both trainees learning surgical principles and practicing surgeons practicing novel surgical techniques is invaluable.[31] The ability to standardize and manipulate all external nontest factors during the simulation such as human anatomy, surgical team composition, and distractions allows for direct comparisons in performance made between trainees.[32]

The current utilization of AI in surgical simulation predominantly revolves around virtual reality (VR) training platforms, where performance evaluation typically relies on computer-generated kinematic data.[33] AI seamlessly aligns with simulation-based education, as it allows for the collection of large volumes of data that do not require preannotation or labeling. These raw datasets serve as valuable learning resources for ML algorithms, demonstrating the capability to discern varying skill levels and exhibiting strong correlation with expert-based ratings.[34–36] Simulator-generated data were in fact one of the earliest forays into the world of AI for surgical educators. For instance, an Italian group in 2006 used a hidden Markov model (HMM) to create an "expert" algorithm, enabling the establishment of a "similarity" metric to distinguish high-performing individuals in laparoscopic VR tasks.[37] Similarly, Rosen and colleagues conducted an HMM in an animal model simulation setting to develop learning curves for intracorporeal knot tying, derived from trainees and surgeons with differing levels of expertise.[38] Using kinematic data obtained from instruments tracking, their models exhibited favorable comparison to subjective performance ratings.

The University of Southern California group explored the use of ML in assessing technical performance during laparoscopic knot tying and needle-driving in a simulated setting. They developed a multivariate autoregressive model, surpassing the performance of a traditional HMM in classifying skill levels with better sensitivity and specificity.[39] In addition, Ershad and colleagues used crowdsourced assessment of video recordings from VR tasks to create an algorithm that classified participants based on a lexicon of adjectives related to the Global Evaluation Assessment of Robotic Skills (GEARS) score.[40] By correlating kinematic data from the VR platform and physical sensors with crowd ratings, meaningful metrics were identified to construct an ML algorithm capable of accurately categorizing participants based on their skill levels. Although these studies pursue the same objective of using AI to enhance the evaluation of technical performance in a simulation setting, they each approach it from a different angle, laying the foundation for future work and the integration of this technology into simulation platforms and surgical curricula.

CV models, which derive their information from visual rather than graphical data, can be used for evaluating traditional "open" surgery when endoscopic camera images are not available. The challenge here lies in capturing high-quality video from these procedures in a scalable manner.[41] Because of these challenges, current efforts in this area outside of urology have mainly focused on ex vivo assessments in the simulation environment. An Atlanta-based collaboration examined the use of a CV technique called spatio-temporal interest points, correlating AI-generated skill ratings from a suturing and knot-tying simulation with expert rater–derived Objective Structured Assessment of Technical Skills (OSATS) scores.[42] The algorithm achieved high accuracy in classifying videos across the 6 OSATS domains. Similarly, an Australian study trained a convolutional neural network (CNN) on knot-tying data collected through sensor-equipped hands and applied the algorithm to the JIGSAW dataset, an open-source collection of preannotated videos from robotic simulations.[43] The CNN accurately classified performance in these datasets containing a diversity of data and outperformed traditional ML algorithms trained on each individual set. Finally, a Canadian group used kinematic and image-based ResNet models to evaluate trainee and surgeon knot tying and found it was able to accurately classify participants both in level of training and according to their expert-provided skill rating with the OSATS score.[44] Although exciting and innovative, researchers remain faced with the challenge of developing low-profile, operating room (OR) compatible means of gathering video to train CV algorithms with.

However, the development of ML algorithms to analyze the vast amount of data generated by surgical simulators presents a challenge for educators. In the absence of AI, statistical techniques are used to identify key variables for inclusion in predictive models, often in an a priori manner. ML presents a unique opportunity by allowing algorithms to select the combination of variables that maximize the overall accuracy of the model. Winkler-Schwartz and colleagues demonstrated that an ML can not only be trained to classify surgeons by skill but also sift through a sea of simulator-derived kinematic data to identify the optimal combination of metrics needed to maximize model performance.[45] This autonomous "self-optimization" has important implications for future efforts to fine-tune algorithms for classification of trainee technical skill and predicting surgical outcomes when faced with an exponentially expanding amount of available performance data.

Operating Room

Utilization of AI in the OR allows for the study of in vivo performance in the truest sense. Compared with simulation, our understanding of best practices for implementing these disruptive technologies in the clinical environment is limited. Medicolegal and patient safety concerns exist around the recording of data from the OR, and this has appropriately tempered the expansion of these technologies due to the sensitive and high-stakes nature of patient care.[46,47] However, there have been some strides made toward introducing AI into routine clinical practice, through a variety of data sources as outline later.

Anonymized data containing no patient or surgeon identifiers is a logical place to begin studying AI in the OR. Kinematic data collected from surgical equipment have been used in the creation of AI algorithms and emerged as an early disruptive application of this technology.[36] Kinematics refers to the movement of surgeons and surgical instruments in given space, with movements generally made in 3 dimensions.[48,49] Studies using kinematic data for surgical performance assessment generally capture these metrics using sensors or trackers, positioned on the individual of interest and captured with either video or equipment. These data are highly objective but can also be quite artifactual. Harnessing the power of AI algorithms to analyze this intricate kinematic data captured during surgical procedures, researchers and educators have unlocked new opportunities for objective performance assessment, personalized feedback, and enhanced training methods. AI algorithms can analyze and interpret the intricate nuances of surgical movements, providing objective metrics to assess precision, dexterity, efficiency, and other critical performance parameters. These metrics can then be contrasted against a trainee's peers and expert surgeons completing the same task. This data-driven evaluation provides educators a deeper understanding of a trainee's abilities.

Hung and colleagues pioneered work involving the extraction of raw kinematic data obtained through the surgeon console during RARP, transforming it mathematically into actionable metrics known as Automated Performance Metrics (APMs).[50] These APMs could then be readily used to train AI algorithms, including Random Forest-50 (RF-50), Support Vector Machine-Radial Basis Function (SVMRBF), and L2 Regularization (LR-L2) models. Their RF-50 model was able to predict key surgical outcomes such as postoperative length of stay. They found that camera movements during the procedure were particularly relied on by the ML model. Although these findings are not themselves evidence for APMs as educational tools, this important validation step supports the notion that a teachable subject such as surgeon movement is important to focus on during training.

Transferability of assessments of technical skill from the simulation laboratory to the OR is a key step in validation that remains underexplored. Simulation is advertised to improve patient safety by allowing the trainee to both practice and improve key surgical skills before performing these procedures on patient and shorten the learning curve by providing a low-stakes environment for repetitive and deliberate practice. The correlation between APMs derived from simulation-based training and intraoperative skill assessments has been demonstrated in the literature,[51] and this highlights their efficacy in ensuring trainees attain the required proficiency levels before engaging in real-world procedures.

Kinematic data can also be extracted from video data as well, through image-based analysis with CV models. Many examples exist in the literature of surgical video–based models that extract kinematic data based on instrument motion. These predictive models can classify surgical actions based on a reference standard provided by human expert raters, often trained, and validated on publicly available datasets.[52] These models do perform quite well, with high accuracy and area-under-the-curve (AUC) statistics but remain limited in their ability to provide surgeons with meaningful, actionable information about their performance.[53] Often these models are trained to provide a dichotomous outcome, such as "high" and "low" performances, without much additional granularity.[54] However, there are examples of algorithms that are designed to provide more nuance regarding assessments of technical skill, such as "task highlights" that identify key parts of the procedural video that contributed to their performance rating.[55]

Performance Feedback

One of the ultimate goals of AI integration into urologic education is the automation and real-time administration of surgical technical skill feedback to trainees and surgeons alike.[56] As with other uses of AI described here, early efforts to accomplish this has focused on the use of readily accessible data such as surgeon kinematics. Therefore, unsurprisingly a significant proportion of our current knowledge on this subject comes from the use of APMs as a feedback tool for surgical trainees.[57] AI algorithms can process and analyze individual performance data, identifying specific strengths and areas for improvement for each trainee. The use of a given metric both as a measure of technical ability and as an actionable tool for quality improvement makes APMs and possibly other kinematic computations ideal as educational interventions.[58,59] Offering tailored feedback and targeted interventions, educators can guide trainees toward refining their skills and addressing specific challenges. This personalized approach to feedback accelerates the learning process, fostering skill development and ultimately enhancing surgical performance.

AI can also be leveraged to provide real-time feedback during simulations, aiding in the improvement of trainee performance on procedural tasks. Mirchi and colleagues introduced an ML-generated display that presented participants with feedback on their performance relative to a predefined proficiency benchmark across various skill domains.[60] Their algorithm effectively classified participants based on skill and training levels, with the hypothesis that providing simplified, real-time feedback on technical performance would enhance technical ability without overwhelming the subjects with overly detailed feedback. Hung and colleagues used APMs to explore the effects of feedback on skill acquisition through a simulation-based clinical trial.[57] Their findings revealed that providing postprocedure feedback, based solely on data, to trainees resulted in significant improvements in technical skills over a 4-week period compared with controls; this has important implications, as it not only demonstrates the applicability of these AI models for predicting outcomes during live surgery but in addition can be used to directly affect surgical skills of training urologists.

Surgical Visualization

Although not directly related to providing a technical skills score, some researchers in this space have instead focused on algorithms that can identify key aspects of the case that are important to patient safety. Recognition of a standardized field of view during a case has educational utility for trainees, especially if obtaining these views of specific anatomic structures has been shown to directly influence patient outcomes. Examples of this include algorithms that can identify the "critical view of safety" during laparoscopic cholecystectomy to prevent cystic duct and artery injury[61] and the prostate during colorectal transanal total mesorectal excision to mitigate urethral injury.[62] Although excellent additions to the literature, using a field recognition approach for education is limited by the accepted procedural variability common to most of the surgeries, wherein differences in the visual appearance of the surgical field at a given moment may vary extensively within the accepted heterogeneity of procedural approaches.[63]

Residency Selection

The use of AI stretches beyond technical surgical performance. The selection of candidates for surgical residency holds immense significance, and urology residency sports are particularly sought-after positions for newly graduated physicians.[64] Existing methods of identifying outstanding candidates rely in large part on standardized testing such as the United States Medical Licensing Examination (USMLE), particularly the knowledge-based Step 1 Exam.[65] Evidence suggests that these test scores are in no way predictive of a student's ability to acquire clinical skills necessary to excel in a specialty.[66] Extensive literature supports the notion that many of the existing selection criteria for residency positions are inherently biased, with socioeconomic status and the type of medical school (ie, osteopathic vs allopathic) demonstrating an impact on USMLE scores.[67] Moreover, gender, race, and even physical characteristics such as weight and attractiveness can influence the medical school and residency program admission processes.[68] These glaring issues at this key juncture in the training pathway has spurred efforts to improve our ability to select the right individuals for these coveted training positions.

Recognizing the need for more objectivity in the residency selection process, ML has emerged as a potential solution. Leveraging data from the Electronic Residency Application Service (ERAS), ML algorithms have the potential to enhance the identification of optimal candidates. Burk-Rafel and colleagues, for example, developed an ML algorithm that screened applicants for an internal medicine program over a 3-year period, using an invitation to interview as the desired outcome.[69]

Remarkably, even when USMLE scores were omitted, their algorithm demonstrated a high AUC in predicting successful applicants. By designing the algorithm in this manner, they were able to discern the application elements that held the greatest importance for selection committee members. Such studies are instrumental in mitigating bias in the selection process. Another study conducted at the University of Utah used natural language processing techniques to identify candidates whose applications best aligned with the ACGME core competencies.[70] By analyzing components such as letters of reference and personal statements, the investigators emphasized the need to shift away from relying solely on USMLE scores, particularly as the exam has transitioned to a pass/fail model, limiting its utility in comparing applicants.

Nontechnical Skills

In surgical education, the evaluation of nontechnical components of operative performance is a vital aspect often overlooked in favor of assessing technical skills. Traditionally, nontechnical skills (NTS) have been assessed using instruments that rely on human ratings, including self-assessment or peer assessment.[71] The Non-Technical Skills for Surgeons (NOTSS) is a widely accepted gold-standard evaluation tool, using a 4-domain Likert GRS to assess NTS.[72] In a similar vein, evaluation of mental workload is especially important for surgical trainees. The NASA-Task Load Index (NASA-TLX), adapted from aeronautics and extensively studied in high-stakes industries beyond the OR, has been used to quantify workload among trainees in simulated high-stress OR situations.[73] Although these instruments have been incorporated into surgical literature and have broad applicability across different surgical approaches, there may be advantages to using tailored assessments specific to certain surgical techniques. Raison and colleagues developed the Interpersonal and Cognitive Assessment for Robotic Surgery (ICARS) through a Delphi Consensus process, creating a platform-specific tool that incorporates the unique aspects of the robotic surgery OR.[74]

As with the assessment of technical skills, technology enables the creation of automated methods for collecting, analyzing, and providing feedback on NTS data to surgeons and surgical teams. Leveraging existing measures that allow for the quantification of NTS performance, the responsibility lies with the education research community to adapt ML techniques to facilitate measurement and subsequent improvement of these crucial aspects of procedural competency.

Innovative platforms have been developed to collect audiovisual and sensor data from the OR environment. The OR Black Box®, for instance, generates a procedural timeline that includes video footage of the procedure, room camera recordings, interpersonal communication audio among the operative team, and input from surgical instruments and other sensors (eg, temperature, door opening).[75] These invaluable data enable stakeholders to evaluate the overall functioning of the surgical team, from the induction phase to extubation, and facilitates the study of trainee autonomy, decision-making, and communication skills.

Annotation

One challenge posed by CV AI is the annotation of video frames for developing the model. To appropriately train the model and provide "ground truth" during validation, regions of interest must be annotated or "labeled," traditionally done using human input. The Michigan Urological Surgery Improvement Collaborative (MUSIC) has explored the use of crowdsourcing as a tool for scaling their annotation efforts and evaluating surgical video.[76] Crowdsourcing involves engaging a large number of individuals, including laypeople, to provide input or information on a project, often via the Internet. In surgical education, this approach has traditionally been used to gather evaluations of surgical performance using conventional assessment tools. In one study, MUSIC leveraged crowdsourcing for rapid video annotation, where "crowdworkers" delineated surgical instruments in frames from surgical videos.[77] Twelve surgeons contributed data, and 25 peer surgeons evaluated the videos using the GEARS tool. Through the application of a linear support vector machine, a CV technique, the study demonstrated excellent accuracy in distinguishing high-performing from low-performing surgeons, as determined by peer review.

However, the process of automating data labeling is not error-proof, as evidenced by research demonstrating the misclassification of surgical gestures by human annotators. Ongoing research and refinement of labeling methods is needed to improve model performance and accuracy.[78] To enable the widespread integration of CV technology into surgical training, it is crucial to develop algorithms that preprocess the vast amounts of data required for training and validating ML algorithms; this allows new and evolving surgical procedures to be rapidly analyzed while making the entire process autonomous without human input. However, the variability in procedural steps and skills within specific surgical disciplines, such as robotics or laparoscopy, presents a challenge in building programs that are widely applicable. "Semantic segmentation" has emerged as a potential solution to this issue, allowing for rapid and autonomous annotation of surgical video.[79] Khalid and colleagues explored the use of semantic segmentation in robotic surgery using a publicly accessible dataset of simulation videos.[80] Their algorithm not only autonomously labeled surgical instruments but also categorized surgical videos by performance level with near-perfect accuracy. Adopting this approach to CV skills assessment enables algorithms to be applied not only to other robotic procedures but potentially to laparoscopic, open, or microsurgical interventions.

Predictive Analytics

The "moonshot" of AI in surgical education, among other disciplines, is intraoperative real-time procedural predictive analysis. The ability to incorporate algorithms into our daily practice as surgeons represents the ultimate goal of much of this research, and the ability for AI to combine semantic segmentation with instrument tracking and anatomy identification indicates that predicting postoperative outcomes during a surgical case may not be science fiction for long.[81]

CONCERNS AND CONSTRAINTS

One significant concern surrounding the use of AI in surgical education is the role of bias in algorithm creation. Flawed data sets and inequitable access to care can perpetuate biases in predictive ML algorithms, leading to skewed predictions based on race or gender.[82] Stakeholders must be aware of this bias and take steps to minimize its impact on decisions related to trainee performance and competency. Efforts to increase transparency in the algorithmic creation process are crucial for establishing trust in AI-based educational interventions and mitigating algorithmic bias. Addressing these concerns and ensuring transparency, fairness, and reliability in AI-based surgical education is crucial for the advancement and ethical implementation of these technologies.

Medicolegal concerns exist regarding the use of AI in surgical training, with potential implications in high-stakes decision-making regarding resident competency, as well as the potential for patient harm arising from erroneous intraoperative decision support.[83] Although this issue is not exclusive to educational applications by any means, the impact that flawed algorithms could have on the careers of individuals from medical school to independent practice must be carefully examined before implementing these technologies in the real world. Should a medical student be denied the residency or specialty of their choice, or a resident be denied progression through their curriculum, in whole or part because of the decision made by an AI algorithm, stakeholders must be able to unpack the contributing factors the model used to make a given determination. In a world where trainees already must be more diligent than ever regarding their personal liability when learning new skills in the clinical environment, introducing new and constantly evolving technology into one's daily practice should be done with extreme caution. It is up to policy makers and educators to ensure that checks and balances are in place to ensure that these technologies be used to enhance those aspects of surgical training that lead to the creation of competent urologists.

SUMMARY

Our ability to create and evaluate surgical performance measures becomes more sophisticated as we struggle to keep up with the explosion of AI-based technology around us, and it seems that many of these avenues toward the advancement of surgical education are obstructed only by our ability to collaborate across institutional and disciplinary boundaries. We in the academic community must continue to combine our data, our technology, and collective wills to maximally leverage the power of AI for the betterment of our patients.

CLINICS CARE POINTS

- AI should not be viewed as a new means of training urologists, but rather a tool to help automate and objectify existing educational initiatives across a wide range of processes including skills assessment and residency selection.

- Simulation remains a key training environment for urology residents, and the ability to standardize assessment parameters and collect large amounts of pre-annotated data while replicating real-world clinical scenarios makes it an important entry point for AI in educational innovation.

- The use of AI in the operating room to readily evaluate the efficiency, precision, and judgement of surgical trainees through computer vision machine learning techniques provides an opportunity for real-time evaluation of surgeon competency and its impact on patient safety.

- Feedback and targeted interventions for surgeon skill acquisition and optimization can be created using AI and have been shown to accelerate or shorten the learning curve for fundamental surgical skills.

- Urology resident selection may be improved with the assistance of AI, reducing bias and modeling an individual's capacity for immediate and future skill acquisition.

- Ongoing concerns about the medicolegal aspects of routine capture of surgical video and performance data may be an obstacle to the integration of AI-based technology in the operating room.

DISCLOSURE

The author has no personal or financial relationships relevant to this work to disclose.

REFERENCES

1. Frank JR, Snell LS, Cate O Ten, et al. Competency-based medical education: theory to practice. Med Teach 2010;32(8):638–45.
2. Harden RM, Crosby JR, Davis MH, et al. AMEE Guide No. 14: Outcome-based education: Part 5-From competency to meta-competency: a model for the specification of learning outcomes. Med Teach 1999;21(6):546–52.
3. Holmboe ES, Sherbino J, Long DM, et al. Collaborators for the IC. The role of assessment in competency-based medical education. Med Teach 2010;32(8):676–82.
4. The Royal College of Physicians and Surgeons of Canada. Competence by Design: Reshaping Canadian Medical Education. 2014: 1-141. Available at: https://www.royalcollege.ca/ca/en/educational-initiatives/educational-cbd-medical-education-ebook.html.
5. Swing SR. The ACGME outcome project: retrospective and prospective. Med Teach 2009;29(7):648–54.
6. Taber S, Frank JR, Harris KA, et al. Identifying the policy implications of competency-based education. Med Teach 2010;32(8):687–91.
7. Lockyer J, Carraccio C, Chan MK, et al. Core principles of assessment in competency-based medical education. Med Teach 2017;39(6):609–16.
8. Cate O Ten, Chen HC, Hoff RG, et al. Curriculum development for the workplace using Entrustable Professional Activities (EPAs): AMEE Guide No. 99. Med Teach 2015;37(11):983–1002.
9. Crooks TJ, Kane MT, Cohen AS. Threats to the Valid Use of Assessments. Assess Educ 2010;3(3):265–86.

10. Beard JD. Setting Standards for the Assessment of Operative Competence. Eur J Vasc Endovasc Surg 2005;30(2):215–8.

11. Szasz P, Bonrath EM, Louridas M, et al. Setting Performance Standards for Technical and Nontechnical Competence in General Surgery. J Am Coll Surg 2016;223(4):S132–133.

12. McManus IC, Thompson M, Mollon J. Assessment of examiner leniency and stringency ('hawk-dove effect') in the MRCP(UK) clinical examination (PACES) using multi-facet Rasch modelling. BMC Med Educ 2006;6:42.

13. Messick S. Validity of Psychological Assessment.; 1994. http://books.google.ca/books?id=LE-nXwAACAAJ&dq=intitle:Validity+of+Psychological+Assessment&hl=&cd=2&source=gbs_api.

14. Goldenberg MG, Garbens A, Szasz P, et al. Systematic review to establish absolute standards for technical performance in surgery. Br J Surg 2017;104(1).

15. Birkmeyer JD, Finks JF, O'Reilly A, et al. Surgical Skill and Complication Rates after Bariatric Surgery. N Engl J Med 2013;369(15):1434–42.

16. Goldenberg MG, Goldenberg L, Grantcharov TP. Surgeon Performance Predicts Early Continence after Robot-Assisted Radical Prostatectomy. J Endourol 2017;31(9). https://doi.org/10.1089/end.2017.0284.

17. Hung A, Chen J, Che Z, et al. Utilizing machine learning and automated performance metrics to evaluate robot-assisted radical prostatectomy performance and predict outcomes. J Endourol/Endourological Society 2018. https://doi.org/10.1089/end.2018.0035. 0035.

18. Shalhoub J, Vesey AT, Fitzgerald JEF. What Evidence is There for the Use of Workplace-Based Assessment in Surgical Training? J Surg Educ 2014;71(6):906–15.

19. Ott MC, Pack R, Cristancho S, et al. "The Most Crushing Thing": Understanding Resident Assessment Burden in a Competency-Based Curriculum. J Grad Med Educ 2022;14(5):583–92.

20. Dagnone JD, Bandiera G, Harris K. Re-examining the value proposition for Competency-Based Medical Education. Can Med Educ J 2021;12(3):155–8.

21. He J, Baxter SL, Xu J, et al. The practical implementation of artificial intelligence technologies in medicine. Nat Med 2019;25(1):30–6.

22. Norori N, Hu Q, Aellen FM, et al. Addressing bias in big data and AI for health care: A call for open science. Patterns 2021;2(10):100347.

23. Vedula SS, Ghazi A, Collins JW, et al. Artificial Intelligence Methods and Artificial Intelligence-Enabled Metrics for Surgical Education: A Multidisciplinary Consensus. J Am Coll Surg 2022; 234(6):1181–92.

24. Paranjape K, Schinkel M, Panday RN, et al. Introducing Artificial Intelligence Training in Medical Education. JMIR Med Educ 2019;5(2). https://doi.org/10.2196/16048.

25. Cacciamani GE, Anvar A, Chen A, et al. How the use of the artificial intelligence could improve surgical skills in urology: state of the art and future perspectives. Curr Opin Urol 2021;31(4):378–84.

26. Yudkowsky R, Park YS, Lineberry M, et al. Setting Mastery Learning Standards. Acad Med 2015; 90(11):1495–500.

27. Schatz A, Kogan B, Feustel P. Assessing Resident Surgical Competency in Urology Using a Global Rating Scale. J Surg Educ 2014;71(6):790–7.

28. Williams RG, Verhulst S, Colliver JA, et al. A template for reliable assessment of resident operative performance: assessment intervals, numbers of cases and raters. Surgery 2012;152(4):517–24 [discussion: 524-7].

29. Williams RG, Klamen DA, McGaghie WC. Cognitive, social and environmental sources of bias in clinical performance ratings. Teach Learn Med 2003;15(4): 270–92.

30. Ahmed K, Brunckhorst O. Standardising and structuring of robotic surgery curricula: validation and integration of non-technical skills is required. BJU Int 2014;113(5):687–9.

31. Borgersen NJ, Naur TMH, Sørensen SMD, et al. Gathering Validity Evidence for Surgical Simulation: A Systematic Review. Ann Surg 2018;267(6):1063–8.

32. Cook DA, Zendejas B, Hamstra SJ, et al. What counts as validity evidence? Examples and prevalence in a systematic review of simulation-based assessment. Adv Health Sci Educ Theory Pract 2014;19(2):233–50.

33. Palter VN, Grantcharov TP. Virtual reality in surgical skills training. Surg Clin North Am 2010;90(3): 605–17.

34. Turner AE, Abu-Ghname A, Davis MJ, et al. Role of Simulation and Artificial Intelligence in Plastic Surgery Training. Plast Reconstr Surg 2020;146(3): 390E–1E.

35. Winkler-Schwartz A, Bissonnette V, Mirchi N, et al. Artificial Intelligence in Medical Education: Best Practices Using Machine Learning to Assess Surgical Expertise in Virtual Reality Simulation. J Surg Educ 2019;76(6):1681–90.

36. Ismail Fawaz H, Forestier G, Weber J, et al. Evaluating Surgical Skills from Kinematic Data Using Convolutional Neural Networks. Lect Notes Comput Sci 2018;214–21, 11073 LNCS.

37. Megali G, Sinigaglia S, Tonet O, et al. Modelling and evaluation of surgical performance using hidden Markov models. IEEE Trans Biomed Eng 2006; 53(10):1911–9.

38. Rosen J, Brown JD, Chang L, et al. Generalized approach for modeling minimally invasive surgery as a stochastic process using a discrete Markov model. IEEE Trans Biomed Eng 2006;53(3):399–413.

39. Loukas C, Georgiou E. Multivariate autoregressive modeling of hand kinematics for laparoscopic skills assessment of surgical trainees. IEEE Trans Biomed Eng 2011;58(11):3289–97.

40. Ershad M, Rege R, Fey AM. Meaningful Assessment of Robotic Surgical Style using the Wisdom of Crowds. Int J Comput Assist Radiol Surg 2018; 13(7):1037–48.

41. Saun TJ, Zuo KJ, Grantcharov TP. Video Technologies for Recording Open Surgery: A Systematic Review. Surg Innov 2019;26(5):599–612.

42. Zia A, Sharma Y, Bettadapura V, et al. Video and accelerometer-based motion analysis for automated surgical skills assessment. Int J Comput Assist Radiol Surg 2018;13(3):443–55.

43. Anh NX, Nataraja RM, Chauhan S. Towards near real-time assessment of surgical skills: A comparison of feature extraction techniques. Comput Methods Progr Biomed 2020;187. https://doi.org/10.1016/J.CMPB.2019.105234.

44. Kasa K, Burns D, Goldenberg MG, et al. Multi-Modal Deep Learning for Assessing Surgeon Technical Skill. Sensors 2022;22(19):7328.

45. Winkler-Schwartz A, Yilmaz R, Mirchi N, et al. Machine Learning Identification of Surgical and Operative Factors Associated With Surgical Expertise in Virtual Reality Simulation. JAMA Netw Open 2019. https://doi.org/10.1001/jamanetworkopen.2019.8363.

46. Silas MR, Grassia P, Langerman A. Video recording of the operating room–is anonymity possible? J Surg Res 2015;197(2):272–6.

47. Langerman A, Grantcharov TP. Are We Ready for Our Close-up?: Why and How We Must Embrace Video in the OR. Ann Surg 2017. https://doi.org/10.1097/sla.0000000000002232.

48. Mayer H, Nagy I, Knoll A, et al. Adaptive control for human-robot skilltransfer: trajectory planning based on fluid dynamics. In: Proceedings 2007 IEEE International Conference on robotics and automation. Rome, Italy: IEEE; 2007. p. 1800–7. https://doi.org/10.1109/ROBOT.2007.363583.

49. Brydges R, Sidhu R, Park J, et al. Construct validity of computer-assisted assessment: quantification of movement processes during a vascular anastomosis on a live porcine model. Am J Surg 2007;193(4):523–9.

50. Hung AJ, Chen J, Che Z, et al. Utilizing Machine Learning and Automated Performance Metrics to Evaluate Robot-Assisted Radical Prostatectomy Performance and Predict Outcomes. J Endourol 2018; 32(5):438–44.

51. Sanford DI, Ma R, Ghoreifi A, et al. Association of Suturing Technical Skill Assessment Scores Between Virtual Reality Simulation and Live Surgery. J Endourol 2022;36(10):1388–94.

52. Ismail Fawaz H, Forestier G, Weber J, et al. Accurate and interpretable evaluation of surgical skills from kinematic data using fully convolutional neural networks. Int J Comput Assist Radiol Surg 2019; 14(9):1611–7.

53. Azari DP, Frasier LL, Quamme SRP, et al. Modeling Surgical Technical Skill Using Expert Assessment for Automated Computer Rating. Ann Surg 2019; 269(3):574–81.

54. Lam K, Chen J, Wang Z, et al. Machine learning for technical skill assessment in surgery: a systematic review. NPJ Digit Med 2022;5(1):24.

55. Baloul MS, Yeh VJH, Mukhtar F, et al. Video Commentary & Machine Learning: Tell Me What You See, I Tell You Who You Are. J Surg Educ 2022; 79(6):e263–72.

56. Watling CJ, Ginsburg S. Assessment, feedback and the alchemy of learning. Med Educ 2019;53(1): 76–85.

57. Ma R, Lee RS, Nguyen JH, et al. Tailored Feedback Based on Clinically Relevant Performance Metrics Expedites the Acquisition of Robotic Suturing Skills-An Unblinded Pilot Randomized Controlled Trial. J Urol 2022. https://doi.org/10.1097/JU.0000000000002691.

58. Bing-You R, Hayes V, Varaklis K, et al. Feedback for Learners in Medical Education: What Is Known? A Scoping Review. Acad Med 2017;92(9):1346–54.

59. Trehan A, Barnett-Vanes A, Carty MJ, et al. The impact of feedback of intraoperative technical performance in surgery: a systematic review. BMJ Open 2015;5(6). https://doi.org/10.1136/BMJOPEN-2014-006759.

60. Mirchi N, Bissonnette V, Yilmaz R, et al. The virtual operative assistant: An explainable artificial intelligence tool for simulation-based training in surgery and medicine. PLoS One 2020;15(2). https://doi.org/10.1371/JOURNAL.PONE.0229596.

61. Mascagni P, Vardazaryan A, Alapatt D, et al. Artificial intelligence for surgical safety: Automatic assessment of the critical view of safety in laparoscopic cholecystectomy using deep learning. Ann Surg 2021. https://doi.org/10.1097/SLA.0000000000004351.

62. Kitaguchi D, Takeshita N, Matsuzaki H, et al. Computer-assisted real-time automatic prostate segmentation during TaTME: a single-center feasibility study. Surg Endosc 2021;35(6):2493–9.

63. Apramian T, Cristancho S, Watling C, et al. "Staying in the Game": How Procedural Variation Shapes Competence Judgments in Surgical Education. Acad Med 2016;91(11):S37–43. Association of American Medical Colleges Learn Serve Lead: Proceedings of the 55th Annual Research in Medical Education Sessions).

64. Huang MM, Clifton MM. Evaluating Urology Residency Applications: What Matters Most and What Comes Next? Curr Urol Rep 2020;21(10):37.

65. Weissbart SJ, Stock JA, Wein AJ. Program directors' criteria for selection into urology residency. Urology 2015;85(4):731–6.

66. McGaghie WC, Cohen ER, Wayne DB. Are United States Medical Licensing Exam Step 1 and 2 scores valid measures for postgraduate medical residency selection decisions? Acad Med 2011;86(1):48–52.

67. Burk-Rafel J, Pulido RW, Elfanagely Y, et al. Institutional differences in USMLE Step 1 and 2 CK performance: Cross-sectional study of 89 US allopathic medical schools. PLoS One 2019;14(11). https://doi.org/10.1371/JOURNAL.PONE.0224675.

68. Ghaffari-Rafi A, Lee RE, Fang R, et al. Multivariable analysis of factors associated with USMLE scores across U.S. medical schools. BMC Med Educ 2019;19(1). https://doi.org/10.1186/s12909-019-1605-z.

69. Burk-Rafel J, Reinstein I, Feng J, et al. Development and Validation of a Machine Learning-Based Decision Support Tool for Residency Applicant Screening and Review. Acad Med 2021;96(11S):S54–61.

70. CREATING A VALUES-BASED APPROACH TO RESIDENCY SELECTION USING MACHINE LEARNING - SHM Abstracts | Society of Hospital Medicine. Accessed June 18, 2022. https://shmabstracts.org/abstract/creating-a-values-based-approach-to-residency-selection-using-machine-learning/.

71. Sharma B, Mishra A, Aggarwal R, et al. Non-technical skills assessment in surgery. Surg Oncol 2011;20(3):169–77.

72. Yule S, Flin R, Maran N, et al. Surgeons' Non-technical Skills in the Operating Room: Reliability Testing of the NOTSS Behavior Rating System. World J Surg 2008;32(4):548–56.

73. Lowndes BR, Forsyth KL, Blocker RC, et al. NASA-TLX Assessment of Surgeon Workload Variation across Specialties. Ann Surg 2020;271(4):686–92.

74. Raison N, Wood T, Brunckhorst O, et al. Development and validation of a tool for non-technical skills evaluation in robotic surgery-the ICARS system. Surgical Endoscopy And Other Interventional Techniques 2017;7(7):403–8.

75. Goldenberg MG, Jung J, Grantcharov TP. Using data to enhance performance and improve quality and safety in surgery. JAMA Surg 2017;152(10).

76. Prebay ZJ, Peabody JO, Miller DC, et al. Video review for measuring and improving skill in urological surgery. Nature Publishing Group 2019;38:1362.

77. Ghani K, Liu Y, Law H, et al. Video analysis of skill and technique (VAST): Machine learning to assess the technical skill of surgeons performing robotic prostatectomy. Eur Urol Suppl 2017;16(3):e1927–8.

78. Hung AJ, Rambhatla S, Sanford DI, et al. Road to automating robotic suturing skills assessment: Battling mislabeling of the ground truth. Surgery 2022; 171(4):915–9.

79. Tanzi L, Piazzolla P, Porpiglia F, et al. Real-time deep learning semantic segmentation during intra-operative surgery for 3D augmented reality assistance. Int J Comput Assist Radiol Surg 2021;16(9):1435–45.

80. Khalid S, Goldenberg M, Grantcharov T, et al. Evaluation of Deep Learning Models for Identifying Surgical Actions and Measuring Performance. JAMA Netw Open 2020;3(3).

81. Colborn K, Brat G, Callcut R. Predictive Analytics and Artificial Intelligence in Surgery—Opportunities and Risks. JAMA Surg 2023;158(4):337.

82. Ledford H. Millions of black people affected by racial bias in health-care algorithms. Nature 2019; 574(7780):608–9.

83. Jovanovic I. AI in endoscopy and medicolegal issues: the computer is guilty in case of missed cancer? Endosc Int Open 2020;8(10):E1385–6.

Artificial Intelligence in Urology
Current Status and Future Perspectives

Rayyan Abid[a], Ahmed A. Hussein, MD[b], Khurshid A. Guru, MD[b],*

KEYWORDS

- Artificial intelligence • Machine learning • Natural language processing • Computer vision

KEY POINTS

- Artificial intelligence (AI) has made significant progress in multiple facets of surgery over the past decade including diagnostics, outcome prediction, and robotics.
- Autonomous surgery must be interpretable to its users and patients, and its ethical concerns regarding racial bias, consideration of treatment implications, and consent must be addressed.
- For robotic surgery to progress from assisting surgeons to eventually reaching autonomous procedures, there must be advancements in machine learning, natural language processing, and computer vision.

INTRODUCTION

Urology is increasingly trending toward the incorporation of artificial intelligence (AI) into surgical practice, including some or even complete autonomy of imaging and pathology interpretation and surgical robots. Nevertheless, practical, ethical, monetary, and safety concerns exist raising a broader question regarding the future of AI in urology, and what are the potential advantages, implications, limitations, and how, specifically, should it be applied within the field.

Surgical robots were introduced into surgical practice with the aim of improving precision, magnification, and improved surgical dexterity allowing surgeons to perform delicate and complex procedures with more precision, flexibility, and control. For patients, robot-assisted surgery is less invasive procedures with shorter recovery times, less pain, and blood loss without compromising surgical or functional outcomes compared with conventional open surgery.[1] Robotic autonomy in surgical procedures would potentially allow distant and remote interventions even from separate locations. Currently, complete autonomy has not yet been achieved, but its application in surgical procedures promises certain advantages over humans (insusceptibility to fatigue, resistance to tremors, scalable motion, greater range of axial motion, and others).[2,3] Thus, combining the advantages of surgical robotics with AI could significantly reduce technical errors and operative times and allow for unprecedented noninvasive surgeries.[4]

It is important, however, to create a distinction between robot-assisted surgery and AI. Automation and autonomy exist on a spectrum, whereas total autonomy is the most refined form. Automatic machines are, to some extent, under the control of its operator. Their behaviors are totally predictable and follow established theories. Any variation in the behaviors of automatic systems is due solely to small adaptations that still follow predetermined parameters based on external conditions. If variations in its expected environment are too large, an automatic system would be incapable of adapting and fail. Autonomy implies the ability to fulfill these large adaptations and changes to its environment without the input of an external user. This is done by "planning" its tasks, requiring wider sets of

[a] Case Western Reserve University, 10900 Euclid Avenue, Cleveland, OH 44106, USA; [b] Department of Urology, Roswell Park Comprehensive Cancer Center

* Corresponding author. A.T.L.A.S (Applied Technology Laboratory for Advanced Surgery) Program, Roswell Park Comprehensive Cancer Center, Elm & Carlton St, Buffalo, NY 14263.
E-mail address: Khurshid.guru@roswellpark.org

Urol Clin N Am 51 (2024) 117–130
https://doi.org/10.1016/j.ucl.2023.06.005

data and the use of cognitive tools not found in automatic systems.[5] Degrees of surgical autonomy can be organized into six levels. Levels 4 and 5 are mostly theoretic and do not yet have examples of standardized application (**Table 1**).[6,7]

Definitions and Terminology

To better understand AI, its current applications, and future perspectives, it is critical to understand some definitions, including artificial neural network (ANN), computer vision (CV), convolutional neural network (CNN), deep learning, machine learning, natural language processing (NLP), and others (**Table 2**).

MACHINE LEARNING

Before discussing the existing applications of AI, it is important to discuss one of its most fundamental components. Machine learning is an application of AI that uses computational algorithms to simulate intellectual processes. This allows machines to perform reasoning, learning, and problem-solving tasks without the aid of outside influence. More specifically, these algorithms are not preprogrammed with any specific objective or rules. Rather, sample data allow algorithms to address risk stratification, diagnoses, treatment decisions, and survival predictions in real time. High-quality large data sets are critical to training these algorithms. This allows models to continuously improve with new data and limit the number of cofounders, missing data points and biases that could affect the algorithm. These improvements, or "incremental learning," allow trainable neural networks to adjust outdated software or techniques. Humans also offer potential opportunities for algorithms to learn. Adaptations during real-life surgeries that go beyond textbook data would only improve machine learning tools (**Fig. 1**).

Current research into machine learning tools has focused on machine vision, clinical matching for diagnoses, treatments, risk assessment, intraoperative assistance, and performance evaluation.[11] For example, a machine learning project trained on Pythia was designed in a study by Corey and colleagues to predict the risk of postoperative complications using patient electronic health record (EHR) data. This information included demographics, smoking status, current medications, comorbidities, and other surgical details, assisting surgeons in determining whether a patient is a suitable candidate for surgery.[8] Bihorac and colleagues developed a tool to predict eight different postoperative complications and death within 1 year. MySurgeryRisk accurately predicts acute kidney injury, sepsis, venous thromboembolism, and intensive care unit admission within 48 hours and mechanical ventilation within 48 hours with area under the curve (AUC) values between 0.82 and 0.94. When predicting the likelihood of death, it produced AUC values ranging between 0.77 and 0.83, both exceeding typical predictions by surgeons and traditional risk calculations.[9]

Machine learning has also been used in predicting the efficacy of treatments such as nephrolithiasis. Aminsharifi and colleagues designed and evaluated an ANN to predict postoperative stone-free rates (SFR) following percutaneous nephrolithotomies. With a set of 200 patients, the system predicted the success of outcomes with an AUC of 0.92 compared with an AUC of 0.62 for a traditional Guy's stone score.[10] Tanaka and colleagues used a machine learning algorithm to determine the malignancy of small cell renal masses using a data set of 1807 image sets from 159 lesions. The algorithm predicted malignancy with an accuracy of approximately 80%.[12]

Other researchers have applied machine learning to measure surgeon performance and

Table 1
Levels of autonomy

Level	Description	Example
0	No autonomy	Robots directly translate human movements[7]
1	Robot assistance	da Vinci surgical system[8]
2	Task autonomy	Autonomous prostate brachytherapy seed placement[9]
3	Conditional autonomy	Aqua ablation of the prostate using the AquaBeam system[10]
4	High autonomy	Human supervision: robot plans and performs operation[7]
5	Full autonomy	No human involvement: robot plans and performs operation independently[7,11]

Table 2
Definitions of commonly used terms relating to artificial intelligence

Term	Definition
Algorithm	A set of instructions to be followed in calculations or other operations
Artificial neural network (ANN)	Computing systems inspired by the biological neural networks that constitute animal brains; an ANN is based on a collection of connected units or nodes called artificial neurons, which loosely model the neurons in a biological brain
Computer vision (CV)	A field of artificial intelligence (AI) that enables computers and systems to derive meaningful information from digital images, videos and other visual inputs and take actions or make recommendations based on that information
Convolutional neural network (CNN)	A class of artificial neural network most commonly applied to analyze visual imagery. CNNs use a mathematical operation called convolution in place of general matrix multiplication in at least one of their layers
Dataset	A collection of data that is used to train the model; a data set acts as an example to teach the machine learning algorithm how to make predictions
Deep learning	A type of machine learning based on artificial neural networks in which multiple layers of processing are used to extract progressively higher level features from data
Machine learning	The semiautomated extraction of knowledge and insight from data. Developed within the fields of statistics, computer science, and artificial intelligence, it allows the training of algorithms that can discover and identify complex patterns and relationships faster than conventional statistical models that focus on only a handful of patient variables
Natural language processing (NLP)	The branch of AI concerned with giving computers the ability to understand text and spoken words in much the same way human beings can

better predict patient outcomes. Hung and colleagues combined procedure-specific performance metrics with algorithms that could objectively assess a surgeon's performance during a robotic surgery. To compensate for any biases, misinformation, or misdiagnoses of performance, the algorithm drew from large amounts of data sets from multiple institutions to create a sufficiently accurate and consistent model. Naturally, this has also allowed surgeons to learn from the algorithm's critiques and refine any mistakes, either through video clips or virtual reality.[13] Baghdadi and colleagues also developed an automated assessment of surgical performance of pelvic lymph node dissection that was comparable to manual expert-based assessments.[14]

No technologies that support accurate, consisted, autonomous intraoperative interventions exist today. A successful application would involve developing a multifaceted AI platform that could identify patient anatomy and equipment while tracking the movement of both in an operative environment. However, many studies have laid the groundwork for the development of this technology. For example, Nosrati and colleagues developed a multimodal approach to see through

instruments, blood, and adipose tissues during dissection. More specifically, they were able to align preoperative data with intraoperative endoscopic imaging during partial nephrectomy. This was accomplished using subliminal cues such as vessel pulsation patterns, color, and texture information to orient the workspace.[15] PROCEPT BioRobitics has introduced the first example of fully automated system for prostate adenoma ablation. Trials have shown that this technology might be safe for treating benign prostatic hypertrophy.[16] Although neither of these applications currently includes adaptability, they and other existing research are promising for the future of machine learning in surgery.

Thus, AI offers a unique advantage in terms of specificity. As opposed to one-size-fits-all statistical models, tools such as machine learning algorithms learnt the data sets they are given, pick up on specific patterns, and provide better interpretations of data sets they are given.

ARTIFICIAL NEURAL NETWORK

ANNs are computing systems inspired by the biological neural networks that constitute animal

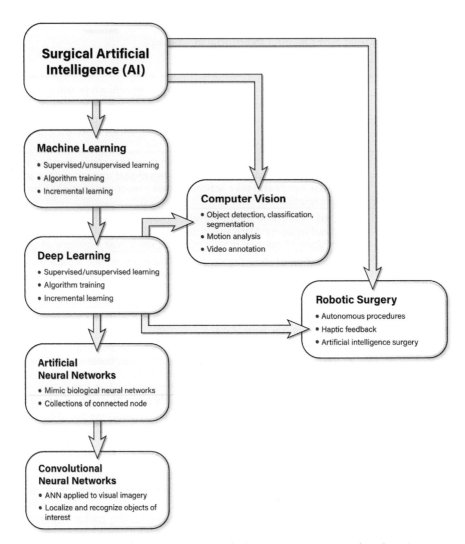

Fig. 1. AI in surgery is made up of machine learning which in turn encompasses deep learning. Computer vision and robotics both rely on deep learning and rely on one another to generate components of autonomous surgery like motion analysis and nonvisual data points.

brains; an ANN is based on a collection of connected units or nodes called artificial neurons, which loosely model the neurons in a biological brain. Although ANNs are a relatively recent addition to medicine, they offer many potential applications. So far, they have been used in imaging, surgical procedures, and prognoses and been used to diagnose appendicitis, dementia, myocardial infarction, and other disorders.[17]

ANNs have been particularly useful in the prediction of postoperative outcomes. For example, Lam and Choi used clinicopathological data from the urology unit of a hospital in Hong Kong to predict the morbidities and mortalities of radical cystectomy. Their ANN used the same risk factors used with traditional statistical models but slightly exceeded these methods. More sophisticated

advancements to ANNs thus offer the potential for even greater accuracy.[18] Aminsharifi and colleagues also developed an ANN that could "learn" the relationship between variables such as kidney stone burden and stone morphometry that predict SFR, the need for blood transfusions, and postpercutaneous nephrolithotomy (PCNL) ancillary procedures with accuracies ranging from 81.0% to 98.2%.

COMPUTER VISION AND DEEP LEARNING

Advancements in CV have developed methods of processing, recognizing, and analyzing images and video with human-like recognition.[19] Although this tool has become a fundamental aspect of semiautonomous machines such as self-driving cars, CV is also critical to medical image analysis and potential autonomous surgeries.[20]

Traditionally, CV algorithms have been based on general features of images or videos, including color, edges, and points of interest.[21] Until the development of deep learning and CNN, there were few innovations in CV. Today's routine tasks were considered tenuous, time-consuming, and challenging.[22] Methods relying on general features relied on the quality of the analyzed images and it was often difficult to filter out unimportant or superfluous features. Moreover, these methods were dependent on domain, noise, light, and orientation in the surrounding environment.

Deep learning has far surpassed past methods, learning the representations behind images in a more holistic fashion, unlike traditional piecemeal interpretation of features. As shown below in **Fig. 2**, deep learning changes CV from a multistep process of extraction, sifting, and algorithmic interpretation to a longitudinal map of raw pixels that can lead to a particular outcome.[23]

CONVOLUTIONAL NEURAL NETWORK

A class of ANN most commonly applied to analyze visual imagery. CNNs use a mathematical operation called convolution in place of general matrix multiplication in at least one of their layers.

CNN-based methods have revolutionized the capability of AI to localize and recognize objects of interest. For example, Esteva and colleagues were able to train a CNN model with a data set of over 125,000 images of skin diseases. This model could identify diseases with similar proficiency to experts.[23] Typically, these kinds of models rely heavily on transfer learning or taking advantage of existing deep models. This is due to the impracticality of repeatedly collecting and annotating massive amounts of images and video. Transfer learning has been especially helpful to diagnosing cancers. Levine and colleagues showed that a CNN-based method relying on transfer learning could complete radiology and pathology-like tasks with proficiency similar to medical experts.[24]

CNNs have also allowed for significant advancement in object localization. In addition to traditional methods' ability to classify an image as normal or abnormal, CNN-based methods can locate and highlight the abnormal area. Schwab and colleagues applied these methods to recognizing findings in chest x-rays using a multi-instance learning (MIL) method that used both classification and detections. MIL is a method that divides images into a patchwork and uses prior data to determine which sections of the positive images are negative.[25]

Three factors are ultimately responsible for this revolution in the ability of CV. The development of neural networks and deep CNNs have allowed for an entirely new methodology of interpreting images and videos. Raw computing power has also increased significantly in the last decade, allowing deep models to consume massive amounts of data, images, and narrative text. Finally, increased access to these images has also allowed for the significant data sets necessary for deep learning.[22]

However, it is important to emphasize the temporal nature of surgery. It is a process in which past events influence future ones and is, thus, best represented by video rather than images. Thus, many researchers run into limitations when applying image recognition techniques to surgical videos. Computers do not have the capability to contextualize the point in time that they were watching. Although their CNNs were able to conceive of what was occurring, they had no "memory" of what step came before another. Thus, this shortcoming was remedied by adding long short-term memory (LSTM) to neural networks.[26] Combining CNNs and LSTM provides computers with the visual and temporal context necessary to understand surgery. The next steps

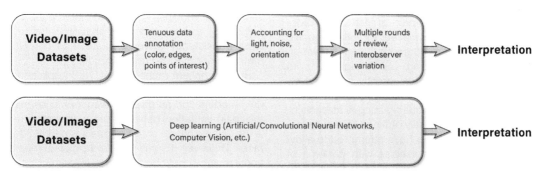

Fig. 2. A comparison of traditional computer vision methods (top) versus deep learning methods (bottom).

toward autonomy include the identification of the surgical phase and instruments. Although this skill is not inherently valuable, these algorithms require this next set of contexts to reach a higher surgical understanding.[27]

Teaching CNNs to understand and recognize the sequence of operative events is at the forefront of surgical AI research. Like medical student training, researchers began by training algorithms to identify surgical phases at a given point in time. Traditional methods struggled to complete this task without computer-friendly data streams such as annotated binary.[28] The application of machine learning techniques to laparoscopic surgery, cholecystectomy, and hysterectomies yielded some early success. They also included some basic video to categorize visually distinct events.[28]

Although traditional machine learning methods were incapable of processing the large quantities of data contained in video, CNNs have allowed researchers to create algorithms that accurately recognize surgical phases. Twinanda and colleagues, for example, developed EndoNet, capable of consistently accurate phase recognition in laparoscopic cholecystectomy.[29] These researchers were the first to recognize the importance of temporal context to help with identification through LSTMs. After this large milestone, most research has focused on gradual improvements to existing CNN and LSTM algorithms.[29] Others have begun to address a lack of available data. Too few videos currently exist to continue feeding CNNs and each new piece of data must be annotated by surgeons so that algorithms may learn from them. Some researchers have begun feeding some algorithms unannotated video so that it may independently recognize general patterns.[30] Others allow machines to teach themselves, feeding machine-generated annotations to themselves, surprisingly leading to improved performance.[31]

Like the identification of surgical phases, AI detection of instruments was revolutionized by deep learning and CNNs. After applying these methods to tracking surgical tooltips during retinal surgery, consistent detection of instrument presence in videos was achieved for other laparoscopic and cataract surgeries.[32] As shown in surgical phase, including LSTM algorithms to form a memory component greatly improved visual only models.[32] However, this process is just as time intensive as annotating images as each instrument must be manually outlined by a surgeon. Again, some researchers have attempted to allow machines to teach themselves with patterns of relevant features, reducing the need for annotations by 75%.[33]

NATURAL LANGUAGE PROCESSING

NLP is a branch of AI that synthesizes AI with linguistics. Today, NLP has evolved from basic, word-to-word, approaches to a more complex method of coding words and sentences within specific meanings and context. Thus, algorithms are capable of interpreting large amounts of human communication rather than simply reporting and directly comparing it. Within health care, EHRs offer the most potential for surgical treatment. NLP allows for collection and organization of massive amounts of narrative data without time-consuming, biased, and misleading manual reviewing of these documents. Thus, the application of NLP to EHRs promises massive untapped value for big data analytical system. Currently, data regarding symptoms, risk factors, and outcomes are trapped in these records, coming in the form of unstructured narrative. Translation of these data could allow for more precise screening, surgical plans, and postoperative care. Koleck and colleagues used NLP to interpret EHRs to potentially normalize symptoms to controlled vocabularies that could avoid overlap of synonyms and redundancy. However, despite oncology remaining a key area of study for AI, only 11% of the studies in this review analyzed patients with cancer. Moreover, signs and symptoms were often construed as the same variable, muddying interpretation.[34]

Applied to surgery, NPL has been pushed heavily toward improving preoperative planning and comparing postoperative complications such as surgical site infection (SSI). Bucher and colleagues developed an NPL model that could predict SSI by analyzing over 21,000 patient EHRs with only text-based documents describing history, physical conditions, operative and progress notes, and discharge summaries.[35] Although the model had a sensitivity of 79%, its most significant finding was the absolute reliable negative predicted value. In fact, NLP models have proven to be far more accurate in ruling out specific surgical outcomes than non-NLP models. For example, studies of deep venous thrombosis, myocardial infarction, and pulmonary embolism showed that NLP methods were consistently more accurate than non-NLP methods of detecting complications.[36]

Beyond patient management, NLP applications could also be used to validate existing predictive risk models for surgical procedures. However, the main limitation behind more widespread use is the diverse nature of NLP models and EHR interfaces. However, if some standardization of the national registry could be designed, algorithms could be verified on a variety of populations. NLP could also benefit surgeons as well, especially within surgical education. Decoding, compiling, and standardizing intraoperative conversations between residents, nurses, attendings, and other faculty would create standard data sets that could be studied like a hands-on textbook. Moreover, NLP could be used to analyze Entrustable Professional Activities (EPAs). EPAs catalog the behaviors of residents, and compiling this information could offer a guide to understanding their training and provide an even greater set of data for surgical autonomy.[37]

Current Applications

Before discussing the potential for high or complete autonomy, it is important to discuss the current state of AI in urology. There is a wide range of possible applications including diagnostics, patient education and decision-making tools, surgical training and evaluation, robot-assisted surgery, and others.

Diagnosis

Prostate cancer is unique in that it already contains rich data sets of diagnostic approaches. Thus, it is an ideal candidate for the application of AI; multiparametric MRI (mpMRI), extensive mapping prostate biopsies, analytics from robotic surgical systems, and genomic sequencing all offer an abundance of data.[38]

Acquisition of mpMRI data generates large amounts of 2D images that contain trends and indications imperceptible to the human eye. Thus, "radiomics" has emerged as the study of the data extracted from these images.[39] Multiple studies have shown considerable interobserver variation among radiologists in the interpretation of mpMRI, where AI can play a significant role. The ability to render the mpMRI images and to fuse them in real time with the live transrectal ultrasound images allowed for a targeted biopsy approach. This approach has been associated with improved detection of clinically significant cancers compared with the traditional random biopsy approach.[40]

In addition, multiple examples exist of AI outperforming humans in both detecting prostate cancer and estimating correct Gleason scores.[41] The current diagnosis of prostate cancers relies on the subjective diagnosis of multiple pathologists reviewing specimen slides that may differ in their interpretations or suffer from intra-observer bias.[42,43] Radiomics and AI-assisted image analysis uses image recognition, examination, and evaluation of tissue specimen, yielding standardized diagnoses.[42] For example, Nguyen and

colleagues developed a machine learning algorithm capable of calculating Gleason scores with different AUC scores for tissue samples exhibiting and not exhibiting cancer. The algorithm had a score of 0.97 for cancerous specimen and a score of 0.87 for noncancerous specimen. It was also capable of performing more refined diagnoses, yielding an AUC score of 0.82 when distinguishing between Gleason 3 and Gleason 4 cancer.[41] Kwak and colleagues performed two studies that applied AI in diagnosing prostate cancer.[43,44] First, the researchers developed an algorithm capable of detecting cancers in optical pathology images. When given segmented prostate specimen images, the algorithm achieved an accuracy of over 97%.[43] In a second study, the researchers developed an ANN with data of the nuclear morphology of prostatic epithelial cells. They surpassed the diagnostic accuracy of handcrafted nuclear engineering technologies with an AUC score of 0.97 for the diagnosis of prostate cancer.[44]

For urothelial cancers, both radiomic imaging and urinary metabolite markers have been combined to diagnose bladder cancers. Xu and colleagues used mpMRI characteristics to develop machine learning algorithms capable of differentiating bladder tumors and normal bladder wall tissue.[45] Shao and colleagues instead used biomarkers to develop prediction trees that achieved an accuracy of 76.6%, a sensitivity of 71.8%, and a specificity of 86.6% when diagnosing urothelial cancer.[46] Garapati and colleagues used computed tomography (CT) urography morphologic and textural features to determine the stage of bladder cancer development. Their algorithm achieved an AUC of 0.7 to 0.9 in prediction.[47] Ikeda and colleagues used "transfer learning" to enable detection of anomalies in tissue by using gastroscopic images to extract information that applies to cystoscopic images. With a data set of 22 cystoscopic images, the model was capable of outperforming urologists and medical students with a median time of diagnosis of 5 seconds to the observer's time of 634 seconds. The algorithm also achieved a 0.930 score for Youden's index.[48] AI may also play a role in assisting Vesical Image Reporting and Data System (VI-RADS) scores. A study done by Taguchi and colleagues assessed the utility of denoising deep learning reconstruction. When used alongside VI-RADS scores, deep learning reconstruction provided higher accuracy for diagnosing muscle invasion in patients with bladder cancer before transurethral resection of bladder tumor than VI-RADS score alone.[49]

The early detection of renal cell cancer (RCC) is critical to effective treatment but can be challenging. AI allowed clinicians to use metabolomic data and Raman spectra to build models that can diagnose RCC before or during surgery.[50] Zheng and colleagues applied this methodology, using a nuclear magnetic resonance-based serum metabolite biomarker cluster to diagnose RCC. More specifically, the investigators used ANNs to group patients' serum metabolites as either healthy or exhibiting RCC and then used these data to individually diagnose them. ANNs were also applied to patients following a nephrectomy, expecting that those who were initially classified as exhibiting RCC would now present as health.[50] Similarly, Haifer and colleagues used Raman spectra from RCC tissue and healthy tissue to train an AI model to differentiate between benign and malignant tissue during surgery. This model represents an improvement over current identification methods which rely on frozen section pathology.[51] Baghdadi and colleagues developed a CNN trained on 192 patients to differentiate CD117(+) oncocytoma from the chromophobe subtype of renal cell carcinoma. This automated tumor-to-cortex peak early-phase enhancement ratio (PEER) achieved 95% accuracy in tumor type classification compared with manual PEER score by radiologists.[52]

AI can also be applied to a variety of other urologic diseases besides oncology. Blum and colleagues used renogram features to train a machine learning model to detect hydronephrosis. The model displayed improved diagnostic accuracy with only half-time and 30 minutes of clearance.[53] Cerrolaza and colleagues also developed machine learning models to predict renal obstructions but used ultrasound features instead.[54] Logvinenko and colleagues used to ultrasonography data to develop an AI capable of predicting vesicoureteral reflux on voiding cystourethrogram with slightly increased accuracy over multivariate logistic regression.[55] Urolithiasis will also likely be drastically affected by AI. Kazemi and colleagues used multiple algorithms such as the Bayesian model, decision trees, and ANNs to predict the development of kidney stones with an accuracy of 97.1%, which could drastically improve the detection and prevention of kidney stones.[56] Längkvist and colleagues built a CNN based on CT scans that could detect ureteral stones with a specificity of 100% and an AUC score of 0.9971.[57]

Male infertility is a multifaceted disorder with factors such as genetic mutations, lifestyle choices, and other comorbidities all contributing to infertility. Thus, AI techniques have been used to predict fertility and reduce the costs of genetic and fertility tests. Gil and colleagues developed an algorithmic model capable of using factors such as lifestyle and environment to determine semen quality with an accuracy of about 86% for sperm concentration and 73% to 76% for motility.[58] Akinsal and colleagues used ANNs to predict candidates for additional genetic evaluation from a group of azoospermic patients. The networks identified patients with and without chromosomal abnormalities with an accuracy of 95%.[59] In addition to genetic analysis, Thirumalarjaju and colleagues also used ANNs to avoid time-consuming and expensive semen analysis and analyze the sperm morphology itself. Their network used a data set with thousands of sperm images annotated by 10 laboratory technicians to diagnose individual abnormal sperm samples with 100% accuracy. The network was also tested on nine slides from the American Association of Bioanalytics Proficiency Testing Service database and again exhibited complete accuracy.[60]

Outcome Prediction

Existing outcome predictions are heavily reliant on developing statistical models that can interpret massive amounts of data. However, like diagnoses, the creation and analysis of these models are typically dependent on human interpretation. Thus, AI could allow for increased accuracy and complexity in these large swaths of data found in clinical and biological data.[61]

Urologic oncology once again has seen the most significant changes from the advent of AI. Patient clinicopathological characteristics are most commonly used to help AI models create patterns for outcomes. Wong and colleagues, for example, used clinicopathological data to predict early biochemical recurrence following prostatectomies. They used three machine learning algorithms, including K-nearest neighbor (KNN), random forest classifier, and logistic regression, which exhibited an accuracy of 95% to 98% and an AUC of 0.9 to 0.94, surpassing the prediction performance of the traditional Cox regression analysis.[62] Although Cox regressions assume proportional hazards and linearity, ML models such as KNN derive their parameters from data itself to find relationships. This better represents the complex relationships between predictors and biochemical recurrence than linear models. Other existing parameters for predicting outcomes include tissue morphometric data and imaging radiomic features.[42,63]

Surgical performance itself can impact outcomes. Hung and colleagues generated AI algorithms to predict the duration of patient recovery and hospital stays following robot-assisted radical prostatectomy with an accuracy of 87.2%.[64] Thus, AI can be used to analyze every facet of outcomes from recurrences to prognoses to hospital stays. Baghdadi and colleagues developed an automated assessment of surgical performance of pelvic lymph node dissection as part of robot-assisted radial cystectomy using console-feed videos of live surgery. After being given fourteen procedures, the algorithm assigned pelvic lymphadenectomy appropriateness and completion evaluation sores to six procedures, predicting expert-based scores with an accuracy of 83.3%. This is another example of surgical performance evaluation during endoscopic robotic surgeries.[14]

Because urothelial cancers have a high chance of recurrence, AI systems are uniquely applicable to predicting recurrence and survival. Wang and colleagues created an AI algorithm to estimate survival 5 years post-radical cystectomy consistent with existing statistical methods.[65] Sapre and colleagues used a machine learning classifier with urinary microRNA to diagnose bladder cancers in patients before they arose.[66]

Although treatments such as PCNL and shockwave lithotripsy (SWL) are commonly used treatments for urolithiasis, success rates vary significantly and often entail repeat procedures. Aminsharifi and colleagues used ANNs to predict the presence of stones following PCNLs with an accuracy of 82.8% and the need for repeat PCNLs with an accuracy of 97.7%.[10] Mannil and colleagues developed a study focusing on individual patients, using their body mass index (BMI), the texture and scale of the stones, and distance of the scale to skin to estimate the efficacy of SWL. Their algorithms registered AUC values between 0.79 and 0.85.[22]

Robot-Assisted Surgery

AI offers significant promise in improving and developing new surgical techniques. These typically entail minimally invasive procedures involving surgical robots. Although the goal of AI is to eventually achieve high or complete autonomy, current applications of AI are more limited. These typically include informing best practices by analyzing patterns and aiding in reducing technical and human error.

Robot-assisted surgery has been widely adopted in urology, including most oncologic and reconstructive procedures. Robot-assisted surgery has been associated with significant benefits for the surgeon (improved dexterity, ergonomics, magnification, three-dimensional visualization, allows access to deep areas such as the pelvis and others), and also to patients (improved recovery, shorter hospital stay, less perioperative complications, and others).

Some challenges exist with the current surgical robotic systems. First is the cost. With the increased popularity of surgical robots, several robots are currently available in the market that hopefully will decrease the associated cost and make the technology available all over the world. Second, the lack of haptics, which can be crucial especially in oncologic surgery in the setting of locally advanced malignancies. Third is the human–robotic interaction, which can have some learning curve and comes with its own challenges.

Paths Toward Autonomy and Barriers

Although the above applications of AI are promising for the future of urology, they are undoubtedly distinct from surgery itself. These applications are relatively static and do not exhibit the dynamic nature of surgical procedures. To achieve autonomous surgical action and eventual total autonomy, machine learning, deep learning, CV, and natural language processing offer the most plausible path (**Fig. 2**).

Although machine learning, natural language processing, and CV all play a crucial role in implementing AI in surgery, total autonomous surgery is far more complex. Each of these processes presents their own challenges and, thus, ensures that autonomy is a somewhat distant reality. Although there are several factors involved, two key barriers prevent widespread development of total AI in surgery along with its associated ethical concerns.

Data

Although a significant amount of EHR, image, and video data sets has been made available in the last decade, few are designed with autonomous or semiautonomous surgery in mind. These data sets are critical to providing algorithms with sufficient information to learn and make independent decisions.[67] Hashimoto and colleagues provide an example of a data set prepared for artificially intelligent surgery by collecting video of entire laparoscopic surgeries. With neural networks, they were able to determine operative steps of the surgery with 85.6% accuracy.[68]

As mentioned earlier, these data must also be annotated so that it may be interpreted by algorithms. Marking these areas of interest is incredibly time and labor intensive, requiring experts to individually label large quantities of images or video. For full surgical procedures, this task becomes even more complex. There are also no standard protocols in place for annotations, leading to a wide variety in detail, poor inter-annotator reproducibility, and discord in what constitutes significant recordable events within a surgery.[69]

Although AI has occasionally proven that it can teach itself to recognize necessary markers for the surgical phase, these methods are not always reliable. For example, a National Institutes of Health (NIH) data set of chest x-rays was shown to generate algorithms capable of making diagnoses. Specifically, an NLP used radiology reports to label chest x-rays and these labels were used to teach a deep learning network to recognize pathology and were especially proficient at identifying pneumothorax.[70] However, another analysis of data sets from Oakden-Rayner showed that these algorithms often labeled pneumothorax with chest tube presence, raising concerns that these instances were misdiagnosed.[71] Moreover, validating algorithms within their own data sets eliminates any external validity.

Interpretability

Another important issue regarding the future of AI applications is their interpretability. Naturally, surgeons and patients often want to know why an algorithm or neural network may have reached a certain decision. Although neural networks allow algorithms to detect patterns missed by humans, they rarely provide explanations or justification for how these solutions are achieved. Thus, many surgeons are skeptical of the lack of accountability of algorithms, the reproducibility of automated analyses, and the implications of analysis of human–machine interactions on clinical practice.[72] Thus, surgeons often refer to these algorithms as indecipherable "black boxes."

Although these issues have been recognized, attempts to remedy them are still in their infancy. One proposed technique includes attention mechanisms that highlight periods in processing in which model inputs contribute disproportionately to output. This was done by correlating pairwise similarities between data points between phenotypic clusters. Moreover, training models were used on labeled patient data to create a linear gradient boosting so that the model assigned relative importance to patient data input features.[73]

Connectivity

Autonomous and distance surgeries may also be hindered by high-latency and low-bandwidth communication networks. Mere milliseconds of delay between surgical input and machine response can have critical consequences to surgical outcomes. Moreover, higher network latency is associated with higher error rates and task completion times.[74] For example, in a study analyzing laparoscopic knot tying using an analog delay device that varied data transmission delay from no delay to 0.40 seconds. In increments of 0.05 seconds, increasing the time delay created a near linear increase in rates of error and median time to complete the task.[75] Even the fastest available networks have proven that delays are unavoidable when performing long-distance communications between surgeons and robots.[74]

However, even these issues may be resolved further by machine learning. Delay-tolerant Semi-autonomous Robot Teleoperation for Surgery is a developmental military technology that uses a learning-enabled closed-loop system to address the effects of connectivity delayed surgeries. The surgeon's movements are encoded into unit instructions (surgemes) and interpreted by a robot mediator. Moreover, the surgeon uses a simulator rather than a live video stream while a robot acts as a mediator between the surgeon and surgery in real time, eliminating the need to encode video frames. A feedback module transmits all relevant information in the environment back to the surgeon. This system outperformed the same laparoscopic procedure analyzed in the previous study that used traditionally time-delayed robotic procedures.[76]

Ethical Implications

The application of AI in surgery poses several ethical questions. First, autonomous surgery would be totally under the influence of the data sets it is provided. Thus, biased data sets would yield biased algorithms. For example, an algorithm trained with a data set consisting primarily of a single demographic may be inaccurate when applied to another. The Framingham heart study, including mostly white participants, showed this phenomenon by neglecting risk factors in patients that varied based on race or ethnicity.[77] As discussed above, it may also be difficult to assign accountability or localize this bias to correct or blame specific algorithms.

Another issue is the algorithm's insensitivity to the impact of a false negative or positive test. Typically, when provided with malignant and benign lesions, human and machine learning systems often find it difficult to discriminate between the two. However, human experts tend to err on the side of caution and are more likely to administer false positives. Thus, algorithms must be adjusted to consider the implications of their diagnoses rather than their accuracy alone.[78]

Ethical issues also arise when attempting to apply large amounts of data to natural language processing or CV. Without attaining permissions from each owner of these data, large-scale application may not be possible. Consent must also be attained to record procedures done on patients and for them to be included in larger data sets. Skepticism regarding AI or its uses for patients or physicians alike poses an ethical issue that could slow its application.

SUMMARY

AI has made a significant progress in multiple facets of surgery over the past decade including diagnostics, outcome prediction, and robotics. However, many obstacles still exist before urology can achieve fully autonomous surgery. Autonomous actions will require a complex network of machine learning, natural language processing, and CV. Each of these facets requires large amounts of data in the form of EHRs, images, and videos that all must be annotated. Thus, the future of urologic surgery must focus on data collection, preparation, and annotation. Other questions must also be answered before AI becomes widespread in surgery. Autonomous surgery must be interpretable to its users and patients, and its ethical concerns regarding racial bias, consideration of treatment implications, and consent must be addressed.

CLINICS CARE POINTS

- Despite significant advancements in previous decades, machines capable of performing totally autonomous surgeries without human assistance are still many years away. Moreover, it remains to be seen whether replacing traditional or partially autonomous surgery with totally autonomous surgery will ever be economically viable.

- Totally and partially autonomous surgery is largely reliant on the development of secure and viable networks and connectivity. Lifelike haptic feedback, protection of patient confidentiality, and acceptable limitations of error are not possible with existing network latency. However, current bandwidth capabilities still allow for regular use of Level 1 autonomous surgery, treating millions annually.

- Patient acceptance of autonomous surgery remains in question. With increasingly complicated procedures, it may become difficult to adequately provide informed consent, fairly distribute healthcare resources, or develop protocols for errors during surgery. Thus, ethical and social concerns must be considered alongside technological advancement.

ACKNOWLEDGMENTS

Roswell Park Alliance Foundation.

REFERENCES

1. Patel SR, Moran ME, Nakada SY. The history of technologic advancements in urology. Springer, New York, NY; 2018.
2. Zaman M, Buchholaz N, Bach C. Robotic Surgery and Its Application in Urology: A Journey Through Time. European Medical Journal Urology 2021; 9(1):72–82.
3. Lanfranco AR, Castellanos AE, Desai JP, et al. Robotic surgery: a current perspective. Ann Surg 2004;239(1):14–21.
4. Panesar S, Cagle Y, Chander D, et al. Artificial Intelligence and the Future of Surgical Robotics. Ann Surg 2019;270(2):223–6.
5. Attanasio A, Scaglioni B, De Momi E, et al. Autonomy in surgical robotics. Annual Review of Control, Robotics, and Autonomous Systems 2021;4:651–79.
6. Yang GZ, Cambias J, Cleary K, et al. Medical robotics-Regulatory, ethical, and legal considerations for increasing levels of autonomy. Sci Robot 2017; 2(4):eaam8638.
7. Connor MJ, Dasgupta P, Ahmed HU, et al. Autonomous surgery in the era of robotic urology: friend or foe of the future surgeon? Nat Rev Urol 2020; 17(11):643–9.
8. Corey KM, Kashyap S, Lorenzi E, et al. Development and validation of machine learning models to identify high-risk surgical patients using automatically curated electronic health record data (Pythia): A retrospective, single-site study. PLoS Med 2018; 15(11):e1002701.
9. Bihorac A, Ozrazgat-Baslanti T, Ebadi A, et al. MySurgeryRisk: Development and Validation of a Machine-learning Risk Algorithm for Major Complications and Death After Surgery. Ann Surg 2019; 269(4):652–62.
10. Aminsharifi A, Irani D, Pooyesh S, et al. Artificial neural network system to predict the postoperative outcome of percutaneous nephrolithotomy. J Endourol 2017;31(5):461–7.
11. Ngiam KY, Khor IW. Big data and machine learning algorithms for health-care delivery. Lancet Oncol 2019;20(5):e262–73.
12. Tanaka T, Huang Y, Marukawa Y, et al. Differentiation of Small (</= 4 cm) Renal Masses on Multiphase Contrast-Enhanced CT by Deep Learning. AJR Am J Roentgenol 2020;214(3):605–12.
13. Hung AJ, Chen J, Gill IS. Automated Performance Metrics and Machine Learning Algorithms to Measure Surgeon Performance and Anticipate Clinical Outcomes in Robotic Surgery. JAMA Surg 2018; 153(8):770–1.

14. Baghdadi A, Hussein AA, Ahmed Y, et al. A computer vision technique for automated assessment of surgical performance using surgeons' console-feed videos. Int J Comput Assist Radiol Surg 2019;14(4):697–707.

15. Nosrati MS, Amir-Khalili A, Peyrat JM, et al. Endoscopic scene labelling and augmentation using intraoperative pulsatile motion and colour appearance cues with preoperative anatomical priors. Int J Comput Assist Radiol Surg 2016;11(8):1409–18.

16. Roehrborn CG, Teplitsky S, Das AK. Aquablation of the prostate: a review and update. Can J Urol 2019;26(4 Suppl 1):20–4.

17. Wei JT, Zhang Z, Barnhill SD, et al. Understanding artificial neural networks and exploring their potential applications for the practicing urologist. Urology 1998;52(2):161–72.

18. Lam KM, He XJ, Choi KS. Using artificial neural network to predict mortality of radical cystectomy for bladder cancer. Paper presented at: 2014 International Conference on Smart Computing; 3-5, Novermber 3, 2014 in Hong Kong, Hong Kong.

19. Krizhevsky A, Sutskever I, Hinton GE. ImageNet classification with deep convolutional neural networks. Commun ACM 2017;60(6):84–90.

20. Vyborny CJ, Giger ML. Computer vision and artificial intelligence in mammography. AJR Am J Roentgenol 1994;162(3):699–708.

21. Noble WS. What is a support vector machine? Nat Biotechnol 2006;24(12):1565–7.

22. Mannil M, von Spiczak J, Hermanns T, et al. Three-dimensional texture analysis with machine learning provides incremental predictive information for successful shock wave lithotripsy in patients with kidney stones. J Urol 2018;200(4):829–36.

23. Esteva A, Kuprel B, Novoa RA, et al. Dermatologist-level classification of skin cancer with deep neural networks. Nature 2017;542(7639):115–8.

24. Levine AB, Schlosser C, Grewal J, et al. Rise of the Machines: Advances in Deep Learning for Cancer Diagnosis. Trends Cancer 2019;5(3):157–69.

25. Schwab E, Gooßen A, Deshpande H, et al. Localization of Critical Findings in Chest X-Ray Without Local Annotations Using Multi-Instance Learning. IEEE 17th International Symposium on Biomedical Imaging (ISBI) 2020;1879–82.

26. Donahue J, Hendricks LA, Rohrbach M, et al. Long-Term Recurrent Convolutional Networks for Visual Recognition and Description. IEEE Trans Pattern Anal Mach Intell 2017;39(4):677–91.

27. Vercauteren T, Unberath M, Padoy N, et al. CAI4CAI: The Rise of Contextual Artificial Intelligence in Computer Assisted Interventions. Proc IEEE Inst Electr Electron Eng 2020;108(1):198–214.

28. Padoy N, Blum T, Feussner H, et al. On-line recognition of surgical activity for monitoring in the operating room. Chicago, Illinois: Proceedings of the 20th national conference on Innovative applications of artificial intelligence; 2008.

29. Twinanda AP, Shehata S, Mutter D, et al. EndoNet: A Deep Architecture for Recognition Tasks on Laparoscopic Videos. IEEE Trans Med Imaging 2017;36(1):86–97.

30. Bodenstedt S, Rivoir D, Jenke A, et al. Active learning using deep Bayesian networks for surgical workflow analysis. Int J Comput Assist Radiol Surg 2019;14(6):1079–87.

31. Yu T, Mutter D, Marescaux J, et al. Learning from a tiny dataset of manual annotations: a teacher/student approach for surgical phase recognition. ArXiv 2018;abs/1812:00033.

32. Hu X, Yu L, Chen H, Qin J, Heng P-A. AGNet: Attention-Guided Network for Surgical Tool Presence Detection. 2017; Cham.

33. Ross T, Zimmerer D, Vemuri A, et al. Exploiting the potential of unlabeled endoscopic video data with self-supervised learning. Int J Comput Assist Radiol Surg 2018;13(6):925–33.

34. Koleck TA, Dreisbach C, Bourne PE, et al. Natural language processing of symptoms documented in free-text narratives of electronic health records: a systematic review. J Am Med Inform Assoc 2019;26(4):364–79.

35. Bucher BT, Shi J, Ferraro JP, et al. Portable Automated Surveillance of Surgical Site Infections Using Natural Language Processing: Development and Validation. Ann Surg 2020;272(4):629–36.

36. Mellia JA, Basta MN, Toyoda Y, et al. Natural Language Processing in Surgery: A Systematic Review and Meta-analysis. Ann Surg 2021;273(5):900–8.

37. Stahl CC, Jung SA, Rosser AA, et al. Natural language processing and entrustable professional activity text feedback in surgery: A machine learning model of resident autonomy. Am J Surg 2021;221(2):369–75.

38. Brodie A, Dai N, Teoh J, et al. 1109 Artificial Intelligence in Urological Oncology. Br J Surg 2021;108(Supplement_6). znab259. 947.

39. Gillies RJ, Kinahan PE, Hricak H. Radiomics: images are more than pictures, they are data. Radiology 2016;278(2):563–77.

40. Fehr D, Veeraraghavan H, Wibmer A, et al. Automatic classification of prostate cancer Gleason scores from multiparametric magnetic resonance images. Proc Natl Acad Sci USA 2015;112(46):E6265–73.

41. Nguyen TH, Sridharan S, Macias V, et al. Automatic Gleason grading of prostate cancer using quantitative phase imaging and machine learning. J Biomed Opt 2017;22(3):036015.

42. Hameed BZ, Dhavileswarapu AV, Raza SZ, et al. Artificial intelligence and its impact on urological

diseases and management: A comprehensive review of the literature. J Clin Med 2021;10(9):1864.

43. Kwak JT, Hewitt SM. Multiview boosting digital pathology analysis of prostate cancer. Comput Methods Progr Biomed 2017;142:91–9.

44. Kwak JT, Hewitt SM. Nuclear architecture analysis of prostate cancer via convolutional neural networks. IEEE Access 2017;5:18526–33.

45. Xu X, Zhang X, Tian Q, et al. Three-dimensional texture features from intensity and high-order derivative maps for the discrimination between bladder tumors and wall tissues via MRI. Int J Comput Assist Radiol Surg 2017;12:645–56.

46. Shao C-H, Chen C-L, Lin J-Y, et al. Metabolite marker discovery for the detection of bladder cancer by comparative metabolomics. Oncotarget 2017;8(24):38802.

47. Garapati SS, Hadjiiski L, Cha KH, et al. Urinary bladder cancer staging in CT urography using machine learning. Medical physics 2017;44(11):5814–23.

48. Ikeda A, Nosato H, Kochi Y, et al. Support system of cystoscopic diagnosis for bladder cancer based on artificial intelligence. J Endourol 2020;34(3):352–8.

49. Taguchi S, Watanabe M, Tambo M, et al. Proposal for a New Vesical Imaging-Reporting and Data System (VI-RADS)-Based Algorithm for the Management of Bladder Cancer: A Paradigm Shift From the Current Transurethral Resection of Bladder Tumor (TURBT)-Dependent Practice. Clin Genitourin Cancer 2022;20(4):e291–5.

50. Zheng H, Ji J, Zhao L, et al. Prediction and diagnosis of renal cell carcinoma using nuclear magnetic resonance-based serum metabolomics and self-organizing maps. Oncotarget 2016;7(37):59189.

51. Haifler M, Pence I, Sun Y, et al. Discrimination of malignant and normal kidney tissue with short wave infrared dispersive Raman spectroscopy. J Biophot 2018;11(6):e201700188.

52. Baghdadi A, Aldhaam NA, Elsayed AS, et al. Automated differentiation of benign renal oncocytoma and chromophobe renal cell carcinoma on computed tomography using deep learning. BJU Int 2020;125(4):553–60.

53. Blum ES, Porras AR, Biggs E, et al. Early detection of ureteropelvic junction obstruction using signal analysis and machine learning: a dynamic solution to a dynamic problem. J Urol 2018;199(3):847–52.

54. Cerrolaza JJ, Peters CA, Martin AD, et al. Quantitative ultrasound for measuring obstructive severity in children with hydronephrosis. J Urol 2016;195(4 Part 1):1093–9.

55. Logvinenko T, Chow JS, Nelson CP. Predictive value of specific ultrasound findings when used as a screening test for abnormalities on VCUG. J Pediatr Urol 2015;11(4):176 e171–e176 e177.

56. Kazemi Y, Mirroshandel SA. A novel method for predicting kidney stone type using ensemble learning. Artif Intell Med 2018;84:117–26.

57. Längkvist M, Jendeberg J, Thunberg P, et al. Computer aided detection of ureteral stones in thin slice computed tomography volumes using Convolutional Neural Networks. Comput Biol Med 2018;97:153–60.

58. Gil D, Girela JL, De Juan J, et al. Predicting seminal quality with artificial intelligence methods. Expert Syst Appl 2012;39(16):12564–73.

59. Akinsal EC, Haznedar B, Baydilli N, et al. Artificial neural network for the prediction of chromosomal abnormalities in azoospermic males. Urol J 2018;15(3):122–5.

60. Thirumalaraju P, Bormann C, Kanakasabapathy M, et al. Automated sperm morpshology testing using artificial intelligence. Fertil Steril 2018;110(4):e432.

61. Cosma G, Brown D, Archer M, et al. A survey on computational intelligence approaches for predictive modeling in prostate cancer. Expert Syst Appl 2017;70:1–19.

62. Wong NC, Lam C, Patterson L, et al. Use of machine learning to predict early biochemical recurrence after robot-assisted prostatectomy. BJU Int 2019;123(1):51–7.

63. Chen J, Remulla D, Nguyen JH, et al. Current status of artificial intelligence applications in urology and their potential to influence clinical practice. BJU Int 2019;124(4):567–77.

64. Hung AJ, Chen J, Ghodoussipour S, et al. A deep-learning model using automated performance metrics and clinical features to predict urinary continence recovery after robot-assisted radical prostatectomy. BJU Int 2019;124(3):487–95.

65. Wang G, Lam K-M, Deng Z, et al. Prediction of mortality after radical cystectomy for bladder cancer by machine learning techniques. Comput Biol Med 2015;63:124–32.

66. Sapre N, Macintyre G, Clarkson M, et al. A urinary microRNA signature can predict the presence of bladder urothelial carcinoma in patients undergoing surveillance. British journal of cancer 2016;114(4):454–62.

67. Madapana N, Rahman MM, Sanchez-Tamayo N, et al. DESK: a robotic activity dataset for dexterous surgical skills transfer to medical robots. IEEE/RSJ International Conference on Intelligent Robots and Systems (IROS), Macau, China 2019;6928–34.

68. Hashimoto DA, Rosman G, Witkowski ER, et al. Computer Vision Analysis of Intraoperative Video: Automated Recognition of Operative Steps in Laparoscopic Sleeve Gastrectomy. Ann Surg 2019;270(3):414–21.

69. Ward TM, Fer DM, Ban Y, et al. Challenges in surgical video annotation. Comput Assist Surg (Abingdon) 2021;26(1):58–68.

70. Wang X, Peng Y, Lu L, et al. "ChestX-Ray8: Hospital-Scale Chest X-Ray Database and Benchmarks on Weakly-Supervised Classification and Localization of Common Thorax Diseases". 2017 IEEE Conference on Computer Vision and Pattern Recognition (CVPR), Honolulu, HI, USA 2017;3462–71. https://doi.org/10.1109/CVPR.2017.369.

71. Oakden-Rayner L. Exploring Large-scale Public Medical Image Datasets. Acad Radiol 2020;27(1):106–12.

72. Cabitza F, Rasoini R, Gensini GF. Unintended Consequences of Machine Learning in Medicine. JAMA 2017;318(6):517–8.

73. Che Z, Purushotham S, Khemani R, et al. Interpretable Deep Models for ICU Outcome Prediction. AMIA Annu Symp Proc 2016;2016:371–80.

74. Anvari M, Broderick T, Stein H, et al. The impact of latency on surgical precision and task completion during robotic-assisted remote telepresence surgery. Comput Aided Surg 2005;10(2):93–9.

75. Kim T, Zimmerman PM, Wade MJ, et al. The effect of delayed visual feedback on telerobotic surgery. Surgical Endoscopy And Other Interventional Techniques 2005;19(5):683–6.

76. Gonzalez G, Agarwal M, Balakuntala MV, et al. DESERTS: DElay-tolerant SEmi-autonomous Robot Teleoperation for Surgery. Paper presented at: 2021 IEEE International Conference on Robotics and Automation (ICRA); 30 May-5. 2021, 2021.

77. Gijsberts CM, Groenewegen KA, Hoefer IE, et al. Race/Ethnic Differences in the Associations of the Framingham Risk Factors with Carotid IMT and Cardiovascular Events. PLoS One 2015;10(7):e0132321.

78. Heba T, Vincent G, Sherifa T, Andrew G. The challenges of deep learning in artificial intelligence and autonomous actions in surgery: a literature review. The challenges of deep learning in artificial intelligence and autonomous actions in surgery: a literature review. 2022;2(3):144-158.

Comprehensive Assessment of MRI-based Artificial Intelligence Frameworks Performance in the Detection, Segmentation, and Classification of Prostate Lesions Using Open-Source Databases

Lorenzo Storino Ramacciotti, MD[a,b,c,1], Jacob S. Hershenhouse, BS[a,b,c,1],
Daniel Mokhtar, BS[a,b,c], Divyangi Paralkar, MD[a,b,c],
Masatomo Kaneko, MD, PhD[a,b,c,d], Michael Eppler, BA[a,b,c],
Karanvir Gill, BA[a,b,c], Vasileios Mogoulianitis, MS[e], Vinay Duddalwar, MD[f],
Andre L. Abreu, MD[a,b,c,f], Inderbir Gill, MD[a,b,c],
Giovanni E. Cacciamani, MSc, MD, FEBU[a,b,c,f,*]

KEYWORDS

- Artificial intelligence - MRI - Prostate cancer - Open-source data sets - Grand challenge
- Machine learning - Deep learning - Prostate biopsy

KEY POINTS

- Open-source data sets are extensively used for both training and validation of MRI Artificial Intelligence–based frameworks in tasks like prostate lesion detection, segmentation, and classification.
- Automated and semiautomated tasks using these Artificial Intelligence frameworks have demonstrated promising performance.
- The heterogeneity in data reporting and lack of usage of the same sample could limit the reproducibility and comparability of findings.

[a] USC Institute of Urology and Catherine and Joseph Aresty Department of Urology, Keck School of Medicine, University of Southern California, Los Angeles, CA, USA; [b] Artificial Intelligence Center at USC Urology, USC Institute of Urology, University of Southern California, Los Angeles, CA, USA; [c] Center for Image-Guided and Focal Therapy for Prostate Cancer, Institute of Urology and Catherine and Joseph Aresty Department of Urology, Keck School of Medicine, University of Southern California, Los Angeles, CA, USA; [d] Department of Urology, Graduate School of Medical Science, Kyoto Prefectural University of Medicine, Kyoto, Japan; [e] Ming Hsieh Department of Electrical and Computer Engineering, University of Southern California, Los Angeles, CA, USA; [f] Department of Radiology, University of Southern California, Los Angeles, CA, USA
[1] Contributed equally to the study.
* Corresponding author. 1441 Eastlake Avenue, NOR 7416, Los Angeles, CA 90033-9178.
E-mail address: Giovanni.cacciamani@med.usc.edu

Urol Clin N Am 51 (2024) 131–161
https://doi.org/10.1016/j.ucl.2023.08.003

INTRODUCTION

Prostate cancer (PCa) detection via MRI exhibits both intrareader and interreader[1,2] variability. The adoption of Artificial Intelligence (AI)–powered automated or semiautomated MRI interpretation has emerged as a promising strategy to streamline this process, enhancing performance[3–5] through a collaborative approach between AI and radiology.[6]

Numerous AI frameworks have been designed for prostate lesion detection, segmentation, and classification (radiological or pathologic).[7]

AI frameworks generally require large, well-curated data sets for effective training and reliable validation.[8] Optimal performance and the ability to generalize depend on data diversity, ideally from multiple sources.[9] However, much of the AI literature reveals a common practice of using small, single-source data sets for training, potentially limiting the models' real-world effectiveness owing to reduced robustness and generalization. Therefore, to comparatively evaluate these frameworks, it is imperative that they be tested within the same sample to ensure an equal footing for performance assessment.

Over the past decade, several open-source data sets have been released with the intention of providing freely available MRIs for the testing of diverse AI frameworks in automated or semiautomated tasks.[10] However, a thorough, comprehensive analysis of performance metrics and subsequent reporting is currently deficient.

The purpose of this study is to investigate the performance of MRI-based AI frameworks in the detection, segmentation, and classification of prostate lesions using open-source databases.

METHODS
Evidence Selection

Using the comprehensive overview of available open-source MRI prostate data sets,[10] a systematic selection process was implemented to choose appropriate data sets for the study. First, the authors selected only data sets whose primary objectives encompassed disease classification or cancer detection, as defined in later discussion. Afterward, a comprehensive citation analysis was then performed for each data set through Google Scholar study, as previously done.[11] When the data set's reference was absent on Google Scholar, citations were searched through the corresponding data set's Web site.

Based on the title and abstract, this pool of citations underwent an initial screening phase to filter manuscripts reporting the development of AI algorithms specifically designed for PCa detection. Meeting or conference abstracts, systematic reviews, and nonsystematic reviews were excluded during this process. After this preliminary screening, a full-text screening of the remaining manuscripts was done. Only those reporting the performance of MRI-based AI frameworks in tasks using the selected open-source data set for training, internal/external validation, or testing were included. Studies assessing the use of radiomic features[3] without using any AI framework were excluded. Details of the screening and selection process are reported in **Fig. 1**.

Tasks Identification and Performance Assessment

Studies testing AI frameworks using the selected open-source data sets were screened to identify

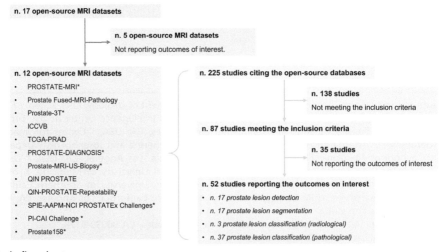

Fig. 1. Study flowchart.

the automated or semiautomated tasks (**Fig. 2**A), as defined as follows:

1. *Lesion Detection:* Automated or semiautomated algorithms for accurately identifying lesions within the prostate (**Fig. 2**B)
2. *Lesion Segmentation:* Automated or semiautomated algorithms for accurately outlining or segmenting the lesions within the prostate (**Fig. 2**C)
3. *Lesion Classification:* Automated or semiautomated algorithms for classifying lesions using 2 established criteria: (a) Prostate Imaging Reporting and Data System (PI-RADS) classification,[12–14] and (b) pathologic findings (**Fig. 2**D)

Performance was evaluated on either a per-patient or a per-lesion basis. Any performance metrics reported in the reviewed manuscripts were included. When multiple performance metrics were reported for the same task, the best-performing metric was selected for consistency.

Data Extraction and Collection

Following training supervised by a senior author (G.C.), 4 members of the study team (L.S.R., J.H., D.M., D.P.) gathered essential data. These data encompassed details regarding the specific AI frameworks used, the open-source databases incorporated, the nature of tasks performed, and the appropriate performance metrics used for evaluation.

RESULTS
Evidence Synthesis

Among the 17 open-source MRI data sets pertaining to the prostate, a total of 12 data sets were composed of case studies gathered specifically for the detection or classification of PCa.[15–26] Details are reported in **Table 1**. As shown in **Fig. 1**, an initial identification process evidenced 225 studies referencing these data sets. After the removal of duplicate records and studies with an exclusion criterion based on title/abstract review, 87 remained and were fully reviewed for inclusion.

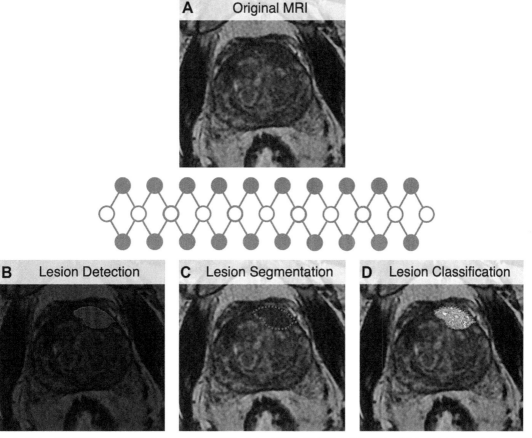

Fig. 2. Potential MRI-based AI Task Description: (*A*) original MRI, (*B*) lesion detection, (*C*) lesion segmentation, (*D*) lesion classification.

Table 1
Open-source databases included

Data Set	MRI Cases	Field Strength	Modalities	Coil Type	Scanner	Clinical Variables	Outcomes of Interest
TCGA-PRAD[26]	10	1.5 T	Axial T2W, DWI, precontrast T1W, DCE, ADC	Endorectal	Single	PSA, Gleason grade, lesion location, TNM classification	1. Disease classification 2. Cancer detection
ICCVB[21]	12	1.5 T (n = 7) 3 T (n = 5)	Axial T2W, DWI, DCE, ADC	Endorectal; phased-array surface	Multiple	NA	2. Cancer detection
QIN-PROSTATE-Repeatability[19]	15	3 T	Axial T2W, DWI, DCE, ADC	Endorectal	Single	NA	1. Disease classification
QIN PROSTATE[20]	22	3 T	Axial T2W, DWI, precontrast T1W, DCE, ADC	Endorectal	Single	NA	1. Disease classification 2. Cancer detection
PROSTATE-MRI[18]	26	3 T	Triplanar T2W, DWI, precontrast T1W, DCE	Endorectal	Single	Gleason grade	1. Disease classification
Prostate Fused-MRI-Pathology[23]	28	3 T	Triplanar T2W, DWI, precontrast T1W, DCE	Endorectal	Single	NA	1. Disease classification
Prostate-3T[22]	64	3 T	Axial T2W	Pelvic phased-array surface	Single	NA	2. Cancer detection
PROSTATE-DIAGNOSIS[17]	92	1.5 T	Axial and coronal T2W, DWI, precontrast T1W, DCE	Endorectal	Single	MRI, biopsy, specimen, treatment	1. Disease classification 2. Cancer detection
Prostate158[15]	158	3 T	Axial T2W, DWI, ADC	Phased-array surface coil	NA	NA	2. Cancer detection
SPIE-AAPM-NCI PROSTATEx Challenges[16]	346	3 T	Triplanar T2W, DWI, DCE, ADC, PDW	Pelvic phased-array surface	Multiple	Lesion location, significant/insignificant cancer, Gleason grade group	1. Disease classification 2. Cancer detection

Prostate-MRI-US-Biopsy[24]	842	MRI: 3 T (n = 807), 1.5 T (n = 35). Ultrasound: 2–10 MHz	Axial T2W	MRI: Transabdominal phased-array surface. Ultrasound: End-fire probe	Multiple	PI-RADS, PSA, Gleason grade, prostate volume, lesion location	1. Disease classification 2. Cancer detection
PI-CAI Challenge[25]	1500	1.5 T (n = 82), 3 T (n = 1418)	Triplanar T2W, DWI, ADC	Phased-array surface coil	Multiple	Age, PSA, PSA density, Gleason grade, prostate volume, histopathology type	1. Disease classification 2. Cancer detection

Abbreviations: ADC, apparent diffusion coefficient; DCE, dynamic contrast-enhanced; DWI, diffusion-weighted imaging; PDW, proton density weighted; PSA, prostate-specific antigen; T1W, T1-weighted.

Data reported as shown in Sunoqrot and colleagues[10] for ensuring consistency.

Ultimately, a total of 52 studies reporting the outcomes of interest were included in this study.[27–40,41–55,56–78] The ICCVB,[21] QIN-PROSTATE-Repeatability,[19] QIN PROSTATE,[20] and Prostate Fused-MRI-Pathology[23] data sets did not present any citing articles that met the inclusion criteria and therefore have been ultimately excluded from further assessment. Details about tasks and performance reported are reported in **Tables 2–4** and stratified by database used.

Assessment of Studies Task Reporting

In the reviewed set of 52 studies, significant variability was noted in the disclosure of performance metrics for MRI-AI–based frameworks. Each task demonstrated this inconsistency to varying degrees. Among the 17 studies that used the open-source databases for lesion detection, 5 (29.4%) omitted complete performance measures. Similarly, 6 (35.3%) of the 17 studies that used the data sets for lesion segmentation did not report any performance data. The trend persisted for the pathologic lesion classification task, where 3 (8.1%) neglected to report any performance data. In contrast, in the task of radiological lesion classification, all 3 studies provided their performance data.

SPIE-AAPM-NCI PROSTATEx Challenges

The SPIE-AAPM-NCI PROSTATEx Challenges data set[16] includes 346 MRI cases acquired on multiple 3-T scanners. A total of 44 studies reported using the open-source data set.[27–33,35–38,40–45,47–53,57,58,60–71,73–78] Of these, 32 studies used the PROSTATEx database for training, 30 for validation, and 24 for the testing of their AI frameworks. Notably, most implemented deep-learning AI models. The tasks accomplished using the data set varied. Two studies used it solely for lesion detection; 3 confined their use to lesion segmentation, whereas 24 focused exclusively on lesion classification. In addition, 2 studies used the data set for both detection and segmentation tasks, 4 for detection and classification, and 5 for segmentation and classification. Three incorporated all 3 tasks.

The SPIE-AAPM-NCI PROSTATEx data set was the only one of the 8 databases used to train, validate, or test radiological lesion classification. Out of all studies that used the data set for lesion classification, 3 reported radiological lesion classification.[45,49,65]

Task performance metrics varied across studies. For lesion detection, accuracy ranged from 80.1% to 96.2%. Regarding lesion segmentation, Dice scores spanned from 0.255 to 0.875, with Area Under the Curve (AUC) from 0.71 to 0.93. For pathologic lesion classification, the AUC values fluctuated between 0.68 and 0.96. Because of heterogeneity in the reporting for radiological lesion classification, it was not feasible to estimate a range for optimal metrics.

Prostate 3-T

The Prostate 3-T data set[22] includes 64 MRI cases acquired on a 3-T single scanner. Only one study used the data set to train and validate the transfer learning-based multiscale denoising convolutional neural network (TL-MSDCNN) algorithm, achieving accuracy rates of 99.2% and 99.3% with and without Gaussian noise insertion, respectively.[34]

TCG-PRAD

The TCG-PRAD data set[26] includes 10 MRI cases acquired on a 1.5-T single scanner. Two studies used the data set.[34,48] Both used the data set for training and validation of the AI framework, and one used it for testing. The first study used a TL-MSDCNN for lesion detection, achieving accuracy rates of 95.8% and 96.2% with and without Gaussian noise insertion, respectively.[34] The second study used a convolutional neural network (CNN) -based algorithm for lesion classification on a merged data set that included TCG-PRAD and 3 others.[48]

PROSTATE-DIAGNOSIS

The PROSTATE-DIAGNOSIS data set[17] includes 92 MRI cases acquired on a 1.5-T single scanner. A total of 2 studies using the database were included.[34,48] Both used the data set for training and internal validation. One of these also used it for testing.[48] The first study used a TL-MSDCNN for lesion detection, achieving accuracy rates of 96.6% and 96.9% with and without Gaussian noise insertion, respectively.[34] The second study used a CNN-based algorithm for lesion classification on a merged data set that included PROSTATE-DIAGNOSIS and 3 others.[48]

PI-CAI Challenge

The PI-CAI Challenge data set[25] includes 1500 MRI cases acquired on 1.5- and 3-T multiple scanners. A total of 8 studies reported using the open-source data set.[39,46,47,54,56,60,72,75] Six studies used it for training and internal validation, 3 for external validation, and 4 for testing. Four studies used the PI-CAI Challenge data set for lesion

Table 2
Prostate lesion detection performance

Study, year	Open-Source Database	Artificial Intelligence Framework	Task: Prostate Lesion Detection			
			Training Set	Validation Set (Internal)	Validation Set (External)	Testing Set
Li et al,[54] 2022	PI-CAI Challenge	CNN–SPCNet multi-task model, and 3D U-Net model	Task performed, no metrics reported	AUC 83.4%, Average Precision 66.1%	—	AUC-ROC of 86.5% and Average Precision of 68.1%.
Kan et al,[46] 2022	PI-CAI Challenge	Deep Learning	Task performed, no metrics reported	AUROC 0.918; Average Precision 0.649; Ranking Score 0.784	AUROC 0.886; Average Precision 0.593; Ranking Score 0.740	—
Karagoz et al,[47] 2023	PI-CAI Challenge	CNN	Task performed, no metrics reported	Patient-level in detecting csPCa:AUROC 0.888 Lesion-level detection: Average Precision 0.732	—	Patient-level in detecting csPCa: AUROC 0.889 Lesion-level detection: Average Precision 0.614
Li et al,[56] 2023	PI-CAI Challenge	CNN	Task performed, no metrics reported	*Lesion-based location:* before self-supervised pretraining AP 0.543 (±0.042), FROC pAUC 0.79 (±0.033); after self-supervised pretraining 0.545 (±0.06), FROC pAUC 0.803 (±0.011)	—	—
de Wilde et al,[39] 2023	PI-CAI Challenge	Deep learning	Task performed, no metrics reported	AUC 0.8	—	—
Yang et al,[72] 2023	PI-CAI Challenge	Deep Learning	—	—	AUROC = 0.827	—
Yuan et al,[75] 2022	PI-CAI Challenge	Zonal-aware Self-supervised Mesh Network with self-supervised learning technique	—	—	Ranking score [(AP + AUROC)/2] 0.8; Patient-level diagnosis AUROC 0.89; Lesion-level detection AP 0.709	Ranking score [(AP + AUROC)/2] 0.757; Patient-level diagnosis AUROC 0.881; Lesion-level detection AP 0.633

(continued on next page)

Table 2
(continued)

Study, year	Open-Source Database	Artificial Intelligence Framework	Task: Prostate Lesion Detection			
			Training Set	Validation Set (Internal)	Validation Set (External)	Testing Set
Chui et al,[34] 2022	Prostate 3-T	CNN–Transfer learning based multiscale denoising convolutional neural network	Task performed, no metrics reported	Best target model with Gaussian noise insertion: sensitivity 98.9, specificity 99.6, accuracy 99.2% Best target model without Gaussian noise insertion: sensitivity 99.1, specificity 99.7, accuracy 99.3%	—	—
Chui et al,[34] 2022	PROSTATE-DIAGNOSIS	CNN–Transfer learning based multiscale denoising convolutional neural network	Task performed, no metrics reported	Best target model with Gaussian noise insertion: sensitivity 96.9, specificity 96.2, accuracy 96.6% Best target model without Gaussian noise insertion: sensitivity 97.3, specificity 96.5, accuracy 96.9%	—	—
Li et al,[56] 2023	Prostate158	Deep Learning (self-supervised training)	—	—	—	Patient-based diagnosis: before self-supervised pretraining AUC 0.772; after self-supervised pretraining AUC 0.79 Lesion-based location: before self-supervised pretraining AP 0.363, FROC pAUC 0.403; after self-supervised pretraining 0.451, FROC pAUC 0.472

Author	Dataset	Method				
Yuan et al,[75] 2022	Prostate158	Zonal-aware Self-supervised Mesh Network with self-supervised learning technique	Task performed, no metrics reported	Task performed, no metrics reported	—	—
Chen et al,[33] 2022	PROSTATEx	CNN–Graph Convolutional Network under multi-instance learning	Task performed, no metrics reported	Task performed, no metrics reported	—	—
Duran et al,[40] 2022	PROSTATEx	Deep Learning–Deep Attention Model	Task performed, no metrics reported	ProstAttention-Net for CS (GS > 6) (whole transverse slices): 69% ± 14.5% sensitivity. 2.9 FPs per patient	—	—
Karagoz et al,[47] 2023	PROSTATEx	Deep Learning	Task performed, no metrics reported	—	—	—
Kim et al,[49] 2022	PROSTATEx	CNN–Simple convolutional neural network	Task performed, no metrics reported	—	—	—
To et al,[78] 2022	PROSTATEx	Deep learning	—	—	With ResNet50 on Institutional data: IMR + Density: 86.3% accuracy, 82.8% balanced accuracy, and 77.1% F1-score; with PROSTATEx: IMR + Density: accuracy, balanced accuracy, and F1-score of 80.2%, 81.1%, and 60.9%, respectively	—
Pastanis et al,[60] 2023	PROSTATEx	Generative Adversarial Network	Task performed, no metrics reported	—	—	—

(continued on next page)

Table 2
(continued)

Study, year	Open-Source Database	Artificial Intelligence Framework	Task: Prostate Lesion Detection			
			Training Set	Validation Set (Internal)	Validation Set (External)	Testing Set
Wang et al,[70] 2022	PROSTATEx	Deep learning	Task performed, no metrics reported	—	—	Wide-ResNet fully supervised MI-SESL: AUC: 0.869; Accuracy: 0.801; sensitivity: 0.840; Specificity: 0.76; F-score: 0.813
Yuan et al,[75] 2022	PROSTATEx	Zonal-aware Self-supervised Mesh Network with self-supervised learning technique	Task performed, no metrics reported	—	—	—
Yi et al,[73] 2022	PROSTATEx	Deep learning	Task performed, no metrics reported	—	—	On the test data set, the network had a sensitivity of 0.92, specificity of 0.90, PPV of 0.91, NPV of 0.93, and DSC of 0.84
Zong et al,[76] 2022	PROSTATEx	Deep Learning	Task performed, no metrics reported	—	—	—
Chui et al,[34] 2022	TCG-PRAD	CNN–Transfer learning based multiscale denoising convolutional neural network	Task performed, no metrics reported	Best target model with Gaussian noise insertion: sensitivity 95.4, specificity 96.3, accuracy 95.8% Best target model without Gaussian noise insertion: sensitivity 95.8, specificity 96.7, accuracy 96.2%	—	—

| Khosravi et al,[48] 2021 | TCG-PRAD + PROSTATE-DIAGNOSIS + PROSTATE-MRI + PROSTATEx (in this study the 4 data sets were used combined) | Deep Learning | Task performed, no metrics reported | Task performed, no metrics reported | — |

Results as reported from each cited references for consistency with authors findings.

Abbreviations: AUROC, area under the receiver operating characteristic; DSC, dice similarity coefficient; FP, false positive; FROC, free-response receiver operating characteristic; IMR + density, biparametric MRI and magnetic resonance–driven tissue density; NPV, negative predictive value; pAUC, partial area under the curve; PPV, positive predictive value; ROC; receiver operating characteristic.

Table 3
Prostate lesion segmentation performance

Study, year	Open-Source Database	Artificial Intelligence Framework	Task: Prostate Lesion Segmentation				
			Training Set	Validation Set (Internal)	Validation Set (External)	Testing Set	
Kan et al,[46] 2022	PI-CAI Challenge	Deep Learning	Task performed, no metrics reported	Task performed, no metrics reported	—	—	
Karagoz et al,[47] 2023	PI-CAI Challenge	CNN	Task performed, no metrics reported	Patient-level in detecting csPCa: AUROC 0.888 Lesion-level detection: Average Precision 0.732	—	Patient-level in detecting csPCa: AUROC 0.889 Lesion-level detection: Average Precision 0.614	
Li et al,[56] 2023	PI-CAI Challenge	CNN	Task performed, no metrics reported	Task performed, no metrics reported	—	—	
Yuan et al,[75] 2022	Prostate158	Zonal-aware Self-supervised Mesh Network with self-supervised learning technique	Task performed, no metrics reported	Task performed, no metrics reported	—	—	
Castillo et al,[30] 2021	PROSTATEx	Deep Learning and Radiomics	Deep Learning Model: AUC = 0.73, Accuracy = 0.71, Sensitivity = 0.70, Specificity = 0.71, F1-score = 0.65. Radiomics Model: AUC = 0.91, Accuracy = 0.85, Sensitivity = 0.72, Specificity = 0.94, F1-score = 0.85	Deep Learning AUC = 0.73; Radiomics AUC = 0.91	—	—	

Duran et al,[40] 2022	PROSTATEx	Deep Learning–Deep Attention Model	Task performed, no metrics reported	Dice 0.875	—	—	—
Hoar et al,[43] 2021	PROSTATEx	CNN–Test-time augmentation with transfer learning	—	—	—	—	Dice score of 0.59 and AUROC of 0.93
Karagoz et al,[47] 2023	PROSTATEx	Deep Learning	Task performed, no metrics reported	—	—	—	—
Lee et al,[51] 2020	PROSTATEx	CNN–cross-organ, cross-modality transfer learned network (XTL)	Task performed, no metrics reported	—	—	—	Dice coefficient of 0.72
Netzer et al,[58] 2021	PROSTATEx	Deep Learning	TD-AxP AUC = 0.82. TD-AP AUC = 0.83	PI-RADS $\geq$ 3: (Patient Based): Sensitivity = 0.97 (0.94–0.98), Specificity = 0.19 (0.16–0.23), PPV = 0.41, NPV = 0.91. PI-RADS $\geq$ 3: (Sextant Based): Sensitivity = 0.81 (75–85), Specificity = 0.71 (0.69–0.73), PPV = 0.34, NPV = 0.95	—	—	—
Pastanis et al,[60] 2023	PROSTATEx	Generative Adversarial Network	FP-GAN: AUC = 0.76 ± 0.01	FP-GAN: AUC = 0.71 ± 0.01	FP-GAN: AUC = 0.71 ± 0.04	Task performed, no metrics reported	—
Shao et al,[66] 2022	PROSTATEx	CNN–Topical Graph-Guided Multi-Instance Network	Task performed, no metrics reported	T2 + ADC: AUC = 0.801 ± 0.018	—	—	—

(continued on next page)

Table 3
(continued)

Study, year	Open-Source Database	Artificial Intelligence Framework	Training Set	Task: Prostate Lesion Segmentation			
				Validation Set (Internal)	Validation Set (External)	Testing Set
Simeth et al,[67] 2023	PROSTATEx	Deep Learning	—	—	—	Median 0.54 (IQR 0.23–0.68)
Yoshimura et al,[74] 2023	PROSTATEx	CNN	Task performed, no metrics reported	ADCmap (Normal Volume): Overall Accuracy = 69.60 ± 2.89; AUROC = 0.69 ± 0.08	—	—
Yuan et al,[75] 2022	PROSTATEx	Zonal-aware Self-supervised Mesh Network with self-supervised learning technique	Task performed, no metrics reported	—	—	—
Zong et al,[76] 2022	PROSTATEx	Deep Learning	Task performed, no metrics reported	—	—	—
Jiang et al,[45] 2023	PROSTATEx	CNN–MiniSegCaps with a gated recurrent unit (GRU)	—	—	—	The model achieved a 0.712 dice coefficient on lesion segmentation
Pellicer-Valero et al,[61] 2022	PROSTATEx	Deep Learning	Task performed, no metrics reported	—	—	0.255 PROSTATEx data set when evaluated at the 0.25 segmentation threshold, and 0.244 when evaluated at 0.5 irrespective of their GGG

| Khosravi et al,[48] 2021 | TCG-PRAD + PROSTATE-DIAGNOSIS + PROSTATE-MRI + PROSTATEx (in this study the 4 data sets were used combined) | Deep Learning | Task performed, no metrics reported | Task performed, no metrics reported | — | — |

Results as reported from each cited reference for consistency with authors findings.

Abbreviations: FP-GAN, fixed-point generative adversarial network; GAN, generative adversarial network; GGG, Gleason group grade; TD, training data.

Table 4
Prostate lesion radiological classification performance

Study, year	Open-Source Database	Artificial Intelligence Framework	Task: Prostate Lesion Radiological Classification			
			Training Set	Validation Set (Internal)	Validation Set (External)	Testing Set
Kim et al,[49] 2022	PROSTATEx	CNN–Simple convolutional neural network	Task performed, no metrics reported	—	—	AUC 0.90
Sanford et al,[65] 2020	PROSTATEx	CNN	—	The accuracy of the AI-generated PI-RADS score compared with the radiologist PI-RADS score in the validation set was 58%	—	The kappa score for the AI system vs the expert radiologist was 0.40. For the AI-derived PI-RADS scores, the rates of biopsy-positive csPCa were 0, 40, 39, and 85% for PI-RADS 2, 3, 4, and 5, respectively
Jiang et al,[45] 2023	PROSTATEx	CNN–MiniSegCaps with a gated recurrent unit (GRU)	—	—	—	89.18% accuracy, and 92.52% sensitivity on PI-RADS classification (PI-RADS ≥ 4)

Results as reported from each cited reference for consistency with authors findings.

detection only, one for lesion classification only, and 3 for both lesion detection and segmentation.

Regarding lesion detection, the internal validation lesion-based location average precision (AP) ranged from 0.543 to 0.732. The external validation AP ranged from 0.593 to 0.709, and AUC ranged from 0.827 to 0.89. The testing AP ranged from 0.614 to 0.681.

For lesion segmentation, only one study reported internal validation and testing performance metrics.[47] Patient-level identification of clinically significant PCa (csPCa) yielded an AUC that ranged from 0.888 to 0.889. Lesion-level detection AP presented a span from 0.614 to 0.732. For lesion classification, a single study reported different accuracy parameters for csPCa classification based on image cropping.[59] The highest-performing classification algorithms had an accuracy of 0.687 in the validation set and 0.756 in the testing set.

Prostate158

The Prostate158 data set[15] consists of 158 MRI cases obtained using 3-T scanners. Two studies have used this data set for developing self-supervised algorithms.[56,75] In the first study, the data set was used for training and internal validation to detect and segment lesions.[56] They achieved a lesion-based location AP of 0.363 before using self-supervised pretraining, which improved to 0.451 after self-supervised pretraining. The second study used the Prostate158 data set solely for testing the performance of lesion detection.[75] However, this study did not report specific performance metrics for lesion detection and segmentation.

Prostate-MRI-US-Biopsy

The Prostate-MRI-US-Biopsy data set[24] includes 842 cases acquired on 1.5- and 3-T different scanners. Only the T2-weighted (T2W) sequence images are available in the public access data source. One study used the data set for externally validating a 3D capsule network on lesion classification.[55] The lesion classification precision for detecting low-grade (Gleason score $\leq$6) and high-grade (Gleason score $\geq$8) was 0.9 and 0.64, respectively. The classification accuracy for all lesions was 0.85.

PROSTATE-MRI

The PROSTATE-MRI data set[18] includes 26 MRI cases acquired on a 3-T single scanner. One study reported using the data set.[48] A CNN-based model was trained and validated for lesion detection, segmentation, and classification. Results were only reported for lesion classification testing. This data set was merged with 3 other data sets (TCG-PRAD, PROSTATE-MRI, PROSTATEx, and PROSTATE-DIAGNOSIS) during the development of the model. The developed AI models presented an 81.8% accuracy in distinguishing cancerous from benign lesions and 70% in classifying high-risk versus low-risk PCa.

DISCUSSION

This comprehensive assessment of MRI-based AI frameworks using open-source PCa MRI databases demonstrates that performance in the setting of AI applications in PCa imaging is promising; however, it is affected by high heterogeneity in the reporting. The in-depth review of 52 studies revealed that MRI-based AI frameworks are being used within the medical community to automate or semiautomate tasks such as lesion detection, segmentation, and classification of prostate lesions, achieving varying degrees of success. There exists great variability in the manner and extent to which these tasks are reported, with several studies lacking standardization of reported parameters necessary to interpret their findings or not reporting the training, validation, or testing data.

Most of the cohort of studies included were designed to attempt to automatically predict the pathologic classification of a prostate lesion. This task was considerably overrepresented in the authors' comprehensive assessment because most studies used the PROSTATEx data set as participants in a scholastic challenge to create the most accurate classification model with this standard data set. This, therefore, does not signify that most open-source data sets are used for this purpose. In addition, pathologic lesion classification (**Table 5**) is the task with the greatest percentage of studies reporting performance metrics.[10]

In contrast, the least reported task was radiologic lesion classification, with 3 of the studies included in this comprehensive assessment reporting efforts to apply deep learning algorithms to radiological lesion classification. A possible reason to explain a greater focus of the scientific community on pathologic classification over radiological classification is the magnified human impact of predicting the clinical significance of a lesion, as determined by pathologic specimen evaluation.

Lesion detection and segmentation tasks were the tasks most used for training validation or testing but had the least reported performance metrics. A possible explanation for this is that the open-source databases were used primarily

Table 5
Prostate lesion pathologic classification

Study, year	Open-Source Database	Artificial Intelligence Framework	Training Set	Task: Prostate Lesion Pathologic Classification		
				Validation Set (Internal)	Validation Set (External)	Testing Set
Patsanis et al,[59] 2023	PI-CAI Challenge	ViT and CNN	Task performed, no metrics reported	Center cropping: SqueezeNet 0.666 ± 0.005 Random cropping: SqueezeNet 0.687 ± 0.004 Stride cropping: SqueezeNet 0.672 ± 0.009	—	Random cropping: the highest performance (0.756 ± 0.009) was obtained by ViT-H/14 with a cropped image size of 64×64 and a pixel spacing of 0.5 mm $\times 0.5$ mm
Yuan et al,[75] 2022	PI-CAI Challenge	Zonal-aware Self-supervised Mesh Network with self-supervised learning technique	Task performed, no metrics reported	—	—	—
Li et al,[55] 2023	PROSTATE-MRI-US-Biopsy	CNN–Capsule Network	—	—	—	3D Capsule Network: (All Lesions): Accuracy = 0.85, AUC = 0.87. (Low Grade GS $\leq$ 6): Precision = 0.90, Recall = 0.90, F1-Score = 0.90. (High Grade GS $\geq$ 8): Precision = 0.64, Recall = 0.64, F1-Score = 0.64
Cuccu et al,[36] 2020	PROSTATEx	CNN	—	—	Hydra: AUC = 0.77	Hydra: AUC = 0.80

Study	Dataset	Method				
Abraham et al,[27] 2018	PROSTATEx	Deep Learning network of stacked sparse autoencoders (SSAE), softmax classifier (SMC)	Task performed, no metrics reported	Quadratic-weighted kappa score of 0.2772. PPV of 80% in predicting clinically significant cancers (GG > 1)	—	GG > 1: quadratic-weighted kappa score of 0.2326 and PPV of 80%. GG 1: precision of 57.1% and recall of 55.6%. GG 2: precision of 49.1% and recall of 65.9%. GG 3: precision of 25% and recall of 20%. GG 4: precision of 40% and recall of 25%. Failed to classify any lesions belonging to GG 5 successfully.
Abraham et al,[28] 2019	PROSTATEx	CNN and Ordinal Class Classifier	Task performed, no metrics reported	LOPO Cross Validation: A moderate quadratic weighted kappa score of 0.4727 and 95% CI of [0.27755, 0.66785] (P value $\leq$ .001). PPV (GG > 1) = 0.9079. Standard Error = 0.09957	—	
Bleker et al,[29] 2019	PROSTATEx	Random Forest	Task performed, no metrics reported	Task performed, no metrics reported	—	Best method with T2w + DWI + DCE: AUC 0.870
Li et al,[52] 2022	PROSTATEx	CNN–novel 3D-CNN sequences	Task performed, no metrics reported	Task performed, no metrics reported	Task performed, no metrics reported	Our method + 3DResNet50: Sensitivity 0.88, Specificity 0.88, AUC 0.85, CI 0.85–0.87
Chaddad et al,[31] 2020	PROSTATEx	CNN	—	Task performed, no metrics reported	Task performed, no metrics reported	AUC for G1 vs all: 88.82; G2 vs all: 87.45; G3 vs all: 82.28; G4G5 vs all: 93.03; G1G2 vs all: 83.05

(continued on next page)

Table 5
(continued)

Study, year	Open-Source Database	Artificial Intelligence Framework	Training Set	Task: Prostate Lesion Pathologic Classification		
				Validation Set (Internal)	Validation Set (External)	Testing Set
Chen et al,[32] 2019	PROSTATEx	CNNs with transfer learning: InceptionV3 and VGG-16	Task performed, no metrics reported	InceptionV3: AUC of 0.81	—	VGG-16: AUC of 0.83 InceptionV3: AUC of 0.81
Chen et al,[33] 2022	PROSTATEx	CNN–Graph Convolutional Network under multi-instance learning	Task performed, no metrics reported	Patient-level diagnosis: Accuracy 78.34% (±1.52); F1 score 77.11% (±1.43); Sensitivity 82.5% (±2.61); Specificity 78.25% (±1.84); AUC 84.02% (±1.77)	—	—
Cuccu et al,[35] 2022	PROSTATEx	Deep Learning	Task performed, no metrics reported	AUC 0.68	—	AUC 0.87
Dai et al,[37] 2023	PROSTATEx	CNN–coarse mask-guided deep domain adaptation network (CMD2A-Net) with ensemble learning	Task performed, no metrics reported	Task performed, no metrics reported	—	AUC of 0.921, SEN 0.83, SPE 0.90 in cohort A and AUC 0.913, SEN 0.94, SPE 0.68 in cohort B
Duran et al,[40] 2022	PROSTATEx	Deep Learning–Deep Attention Model	Task performed, no metrics reported	Cohen Quadratic-Weighted Kappa Score = 0.418 ± 0.138	—	—
Fernandez-Quilez	PROSTATEx	CNN (transfer learning)	Task performed, no metrics reported	Source T2w/Target ADC Size 64 × 64– Sensitivity	—	—

Author	Dataset	Model				
et al,[41] 2021			@ 0.50.845; Specificity @ 0.50.940; AUC 0.898			
Hamm et al,[42] 2023	PROSTATEx	CNN	Task performed, no metrics reported	—		Lesion based: 1. csPCa: accuracy of 86% (95% CI: 82, 90; range, 271,297 of 330), sensitivity of 90% (95% CI: 83, 97; range, 274,320 of 330), specificity of 85% (95% CI: 80, 90; range, 265,288 of 330), and an AUROC of 0.87 (95% CI: 0.81, 0.93)
Hu et al,[44] 2022	PROSTATEx	CNN–Feature Pyramid Network	—	DAMS-Net (CBAM): K_w = 0.5413, PPV (GG > 1) = 0.9747		—
Karagoz et al,[47] 2023	PROSTATEx	Deep Learning	—			—
Lapa et al,[50] 2020	PROSTATEx	CNN	Task performed, no metrics reported	XmasNet: AUROC = 0.622 ± 0.054, AlexNet: AUROC = 1.000 ± 0.000, VGG16: AUROC = 0.729 ± 0.047, ResNet: AUROC = 0.658 ± 0.065, XmasNet-CRFpp: AUROC = 0.796 ± 0.069, CRF-XmasNet: AUROC = 0.695 ± 0.126, CRF-AlexNet: AUROC = 0.536 ± 0.191, CRF-VGG16:	—	XmasNet: AUROC = 0.517 ± 0.101, AlexNet: AUROC = 0.588 ± 0.051, VGG16: AUROC = 0.707 ± 0.050, ResNet: AUROC = 0.520 ± 0.100, XmasNet-CRFpp: AUROC = 0.388 ± 0.303, CRF-XmasNet: AUROC = 0.573 ± 0.191, CRF-AlexNet: AUROC = 0.598 ± 0.169, CRF-VGG16:

(continued on next page)

Table 5
(continued)

Study, year	Open-Source Database	Artificial Intelligence Framework	Task: Prostate Lesion Pathologic Classification			
			Training Set	Validation Set (Internal)	Validation Set (External)	Testing Set
Lee et al,[51] 2020	PROSTATEx	CNN–cross-organ, cross-modality transfer learned network (XTL)	Task performed, no metrics reported	AUROC = 0.796 ± 0.209	—	AUROC = 0.615 ± 0.147
	PROSTATEx			AUC 0.85	—	AUC (0.77–0.80)
Li et al,[53] 2022	PROSTATEx	CNN	Task performed, no metrics reported	Sensitivity: 0.84; Specificity: 0.78; AUC 0.84; CI 95% 0.78–0.84; Parameters 94.1 M	—	—
Mehrtash et al,[57] 2021	PROSTATEx	CNN–Fully convolutional network (FCN)	—	—	—	AUC 0.78 (0.72–0.84)
Pastanis et al,[60] 2023	PROSTATEx	Generative Adversarial Network	Task performed, no metrics reported	FP-GAN AUC 0.76 (0.65–0.84)	—	—
Provenzano et al,[62] 2023	PROSTATEx	Deep Learning–ResNet	Task performed, no metrics reported	0.93	—	—
Roge et al,[63] 2022	PROSTATEx	Deep Learning	R1: AUC = 0.81 ± 0.01, R2: AUC = 0.81 ± 0.01, R3: AUC = 0.83 ± 0.02, R4: AUC = 0.79 ± 0.01, R5: AUC = 0.85 ± 0.01	R1: AUC = 0.78, R2: AUC = 0.79, R3: AUC = 0.8, R4: AUC = 0.81, R5: AUC = 0.82	—	—
Saha et al,[64] 2021	PROSTATEx	Deep learning	—	—	—	MRI driven tissue density is 80.2 accurately; balance accuracy 81.1 and F1 is 60.9

Study	Dataset	Method				
Shao et al,[66] 2022	PROSTATEx	CNN–Topical Graph-Guided Multi-Instance Network	Task performed, no metrics reported	—	—	For all PCa classification: AUC 0.892, Accuracy 0.825, SEN 0.823, SPE 0.829, Precision 0.597, F-score 0.892 For Px challenge: AUC 0.95 (winner)
Vente et al,[68] 2021	PROSTATEx	Deep Learning Regression	Task performed, no metrics reported	Lesion weighted kappa = 0.13 ± 0.27	—	—
Wang et al,[71] 2020	PROSTATEx	CNN–multi-input selection network	Task performed, no metrics reported	—	—	—
Wang et al,[69] 2023	PROSTATEx	CNN	—	—	2.75D: CPM = 0.502 [0.478–0.622], AUC = 0.663 [0.0.590–0.746], 2.75Dx3: CPM = 0.545 [0.420–0.668], AUC = 0.669 [0.588–0.746], 2.75D + TL: CPM = 0.531 [0.410–0.657], AUC = 0.681 [0.608–0.754], 2.75Dx3+TL: CPM = 0.522 [0.407–0.641], AUC = 0.692 [0.621–0.759]	—
Dai et al,[38] 2022	PROSTATEx	CNN–novel mutual attention-based hybrid	Task performed, no metrics reported	—	—	MMNet18 AUC 0.92 ± 0.02, SEN 0.79 ± 0.07, SPE

(continued on next page)

Table 5
(continued)

Study, year	Open-Source Database	Artificial Intelligence Framework	Training Set	Task: Prostate Lesion Pathologic Classification		
				Validation Set (Internal)	Validation Set (External)	Testing Set
		dimensional network for MultiModal 3D medical image classification (MMNet)				0.88 ± 0.06, Accuracy 0.82 ± 0.08 MMNet34 AUC 0.94 ± 0.02, SEN 0.85 ± 0.08, SPE 0.86 ± 0.10, Accuracy 0.81 ± 0.13
Yoshimura et al,[74] 2023	PROSTATEx	CNN	Task performed, no metrics reported	Segmentation Volume (ADCmap): GS ≥ 7, Precision = 0.73 ± 0.13, GS < 7, Precision = 0.60 ± 0.11, GS ≥ 7, Recall = 0.50 ± 0.04, GS < 7, Recall = 0.82 ± 0.06. Segmentation Volume (T2WI): GS ≥ 7, Precision = 0.57 ± 0.13, GS < 7, Precision = 0.72 ± 13, GS ≥ 7, Recall = 0.53 ± 0.09, GS < 7, Recall = 0.76 ± 0.04. Normal Volume	—	—

Study	Dataset	AI approach					
Yi et al,[73] 2022	PROSTATEx	Deep learning	Task performed, no metrics reported	(ADCmap): GS ≥ 7, Precision = 0.34 ± 0.06, GS < 7, Precision = 0.88 ± 0.04, GS ≥ 7, Recall = 0.61 ± 0.07, GS < 7, Recall = 0.72 ± 0.0.02. Normal Volume (T2WI): GS ≥ 7, Precision = 0.49 ± 0.12, GS < 7, Precision = 0.73 ± 11, GS ≥ 7, Recall = 0.50 ± 0.12, GS < 7, Recall = 0.73 ± 0.05.	—	—	TPR of 0.95, TTask performed, no metrics reported of 0.82, F1-Score of 0.8920, AUC of 0.912, and accuracy of 0.885
Zong et al,[77] 2020	PROSTATEx	CNN	—	—	—	Sensitivity:1.00, Specificity: 0.83, G-mean: 0.91, AUC: 0.92, and Accuracy: 0.85	(0.87, 0.94, 0.90) for sensitivity, specificity, and G-mean, respectively
Zong et al,[76] 2022	PROSTATEx	Deep Learning	Task performed, no metrics reported	—	—	—	—
Pellicer-Valero et al,[61] 2022	PROSTATEx	Deep learning	Task performed, no metrics reported	—	—	—	At lesion-level AUC/sensitivity/ specificity for the GGG ≥ 2 significance criterion

(continued on next page)

Table 5
(continued)

		Artificial Intelligence Framework		Task: Prostate Lesion Pathologic Classification		
Study, year	Open-Source Database		Training Set	Validation Set (Internal)	Validation Set (External)	Testing Set
						of 0.96/1.00/0.79 for the ProstateX data set. At a patient level, the results are 0.87/1.00/0.375 in ProstateX
Khosravi et al,[48] 2021	TCG-PRAD + PROSTATE-DIAGNOSIS + PROSTATE-MRI + PROSTATEx (in this study the 4 data sets were used combined)	Deep Learning	Task performed, no metrics reported	Task performed, no metrics reported	—	Model 1: Distinguishing cancer patients from benign patients with an AUC of 0.89 (95% CI: [0.86–0.92]), NPV of 81.6, PPV of 81.9, specificity of 82, sensitivity of 81.5, and accuracy of 81.8 Model 2: Classifying high-risk vs low-risk (GS = 5 + 5, 5 + 4, 4 + 5, 4 + 4, 4 + 3 vs GS = 3 + 3, 3 + 4) cancer with an AUC of 0.78 (95% CI: [0.74–0.82]), NPV of 73, PPV of 67, specificity of 68.9, sensitivity of 71.3, and accuracy of 70 The performance of

Model 2 in classifying GS ≥ 8 vs GS = 3 + 3 was high (AUC = 0.86), but the ability of Model 2 to classify intermediate-risk cases (GS = 3 + 4 vs GS = 4 + 3) of PCa was lower (AUC = 0.71)

Results as reported from each cited references for consistency with authors findings.

Abbreviations: GG, group grade; Kw, weighted kappa; LOPO, Leave-One-Patient-Out; Px, PROSTAETx; SEN, sensitivity; SPE, specificity.

because of their value as an annotated and extensive sample, whereas studies may experiment the efficacy of their model applied to private or in-house data. More research is needed to investigate the scope of open-source MRI databases' applications in enhancing the performance of these algorithms.

In cases when performance is reported, the included metrics lack standardization and consistent definitions of various outcomes of interest. For instance, a common reporting item is AUC, a metric signifying a test's accuracy or, in these cases, a model's predictive diagnostic value. Nevertheless, not all studies report it, or when included, its interpretability may be suboptimal owing to insufficient context to generalize the finding. Moreover, not all studies clarify whether the results were achieved in a per-patient or per-lesion assessment.

When defining the tasks for the development of the algorithms reported in the study, authors often interchangeably use the terms PCa "detection" or "classification" to define their model's objective, even in describing the same objective, which falls squarely in one of the authors' task definitions.

The findings of this study provide evidence to support a significant deficiency in adherence to standardized guidelines, which are essential for ensuring the interpretability and reproducibility of research methodologies and findings. A call for standardization is corroborated by the variability in reporting metrics and the inconsistent frequency of disclosing training, validation, and testing performance results. Comprehensive guidelines with an associated reporting checklist for the implementation of AI in medical imaging[79] were published in 2020. The updated version of these guidelines is awaited, as the need for properly reporting performance results, along with advancing awareness and understanding of the requisite guidelines, is crucial.

Compounding these reporting challenges is the methodological issue of data overlap in open-source data sets. This problem arises when a data set, in whole or in part, incorporates cases from other publicly available data sets, such as the inclusion of PROSTATEx and Prostate-3T data sets within the PI-CAI data set. This merging of data sets, although providing a larger sample, could inadvertently generate misinterpretations and undermine the reproducibility of performance metrics, specifically for MRI-based AI frameworks leveraging more than one data set for training, validation, or testing. This highlights the necessity of careful data set selection and management of data overlap when developing an AI model.

This study is not without its limitations. The results were presented in a narrative manner without conducting a meta-analytic synthesis. Therefore, a cumulative analysis for each of the tasks considered was not provided. Furthermore, the selection of tasks was constrained to prostate lesion detection, segmentation, and classification without considering other potential tasks, resulting in a limited spectrum of evaluated tasks.

SUMMARY

Open-source data sets play a vital role in training, testing, and validating the performance of AI frameworks in detecting, segmenting, and classifying prostate lesions. However, the restricted number of these validations, coupled with the variability and heterogeneity present in the reporting of these open-source data sets, could potentially constrain the broader applicability of the developed frameworks. To address this limitation, it is imperative to invest further efforts in using larger, meticulously designed data sets that are confirmed through pathology, encompass a diverse range of cases from multiple institutions, and incorporate baseline characteristics. By embracing these comprehensive data sets, we can enhance the robustness and generalizability of AI-based systems for prostate lesion analysis.

DISCLOSURE

GPT 4.0 open AI was used for grammar correction in the introduction, methodology, and discussion. The authors take full responsibility for the information provided.

CONFLICTS OF INTEREST

Inderbir S. Gill is an unpaid advisor for Steba (Unpaid Advisor) and has equity interest in OneLine Health. Andre Luis Abreu is a consultant for Koelis and Quibim, and a speaker for EDAP. The other authors do not have any competing interests.

REFERENCES

1. Greer MD, Shih JH, Lay N, et al. Interreader Variability of Prostate Imaging Reporting and Data System Version 2 in Detecting and Assessing Prostate Cancer Lesions at Prostate MRI. AJR Am J Roentgenol 2019;212(6):1197–205.
2. Hietikko R, Kilpeläinen TP, Kenttämies A, et al. Expected impact of MRI-related interreader variability on ProScreen prostate cancer screening trial: a pre-trial validation study. Cancer Imag 2020; 20(1):72.

3. Sugano D, Sanford D, Abreu A, et al. Impact of radiomics on prostate cancer detection: a systematic review of clinical applications. Curr Opin Urol 2020;30(6):754–81.

4. Chen AB, Haque T, Roberts S, et al. Artificial Intelligence Applications in Urology: Reporting Standards to Achieve Fluency for Urologists. Urol Clin North Am 2022;49(1):65–117.

5. Checcucci E, Autorino R, Cacciamani GE, et al. Artificial intelligence and neural networks in urology: current clinical applications. Minerva Urol Nefrol 2020;72(1):49–57.

6. Cacciamani GE, Sanford DI, Chu TN, et al. Is Artificial Intelligence Replacing Our Radiology Stars? Not Yet. Eur Urol Open Sci 2023;48:14–6.

7. Goldenberg SL, Nir G, Salcudean SE. A new era: artificial intelligence and machine learning in prostate cancer. Nat Rev Urol 2019;16(7):391–403.

8. Hosseinzadeh M, Saha A, Brand P, et al. Deep learning-assisted prostate cancer detection on biparametric MRI: minimum training data size requirements and effect of prior knowledge. Eur Radiol 2022;32(4):2224–34.

9. McKinney SM, Sieniek M, Godbole V, et al. International evaluation of an AI system for breast cancer screening. Nature 2020;577(7788):89–94.

10. Sunoqrot MRS, Saha A, Hosseinzadeh M, et al. Artificial intelligence for prostate MRI: open datasets, available applications, and grand challenges. Eur Radiol Exp 2022;6(1):35.

11. Sayegh AS, Eppler M, Sholklapper T, et al. Severity Grading Systems for Intraoperative Adverse Events. A Systematic Review of the Literature and Citation Analysis. Ann Surg 2023. https://doi.org/10.1097/SLA.0000000000005883.

12. Turkbey B, Rosenkrantz AB, Haider MA, et al. Prostate Imaging Reporting and Data System Version 2.1: 2019 Update of Prostate Imaging Reporting and Data System Version 2. Eur Urol 2019;76(3):340–51.

13. Purysko AS, Rosenkrantz AB, Barentsz JO, et al. PI-RADS Version 2: A Pictorial Update. Radiographics 2016;36(5):1354–72.

14. Weinreb JC, Barentsz JO, Choyke PL, et al. PI-RADS Prostate Imaging - Reporting and Data System: 2015, Version 2. Eur Urol 2016;69(1):16–40.

15. Adams LC, Makowski MR, Engel G, et al. Prostate158-An expert-annotated 3T MRI dataset and algorithm for prostate cancer detection. Comput Biol Med 2022;148:105817.

16. Armato SG III, Huisman H, Drukker K, et al. PROSTATEx Challenges for computerized classification of prostate lesions from multiparametric magnetic resonance images. J Med Imag 2018;5(4):044501.

17. Bloch BN, Jain A, Jaffe CC. Data from prostate-diagnosis. The Cancer Imaging Archive 2015;9(10):7937.

18. Choyke P, Turkbey B, Pinto P, et al. Data from prostate-mri. The Cancer Imaging Archive 2016;9:6.

19. Fedorov A, Schwier M, Clunie D, et al. Data from QIN-PROSTATE-repeatability. Cancer Imaging Archive 2018;9.

20. Fedorov A, Tempany C, Mulkern R, et al. Data from QIN PROSTATE. The Cancer Imaging Archive; 2016.

21. Lemaitre G., Martí Marly R., Meriaudeau F., Original multi-parametric MRI images of prostate. 2016. Available at: https://dataverse.csuc.cat/dataset.xhtml?persistentId=doi:10.34810/data659.

22. Litjens G, Futterer J, Huisman H. Data from prostate-3T. Cancer Imaging Arch 2015;10:K9.

23. Madabhushi A, Feldman M. Fused Radiology-Pathology Prostate Dataset. Cancer Imaging Archive 2016;9.

24. Natarajan S, Priester A, Margolis D, et al. Prostate MRI and ultrasound with pathology and coordinates of tracked biopsy (prostate-MRI-US-biopsy). Cancer Imaging Arch 2020;10:7937.

25. Saha A, Bosma J, Twilt J, et al. Artificial Intelligence and Radiologists at Prostate Cancer Detection in MRI—The PI-CAI Challenge, Medical Imaging with Deep Learning, 2023, short paper track. Aailable at: https://openreview.net/forum?id=XfXcA9-0XxR.

26. Zuley ML, Jarosz R, Drake BF, et al. Radiology data from the cancer genome atlas prostate adenocarcinoma [tcga-prad] collection. Cancer Imaging Arch 2016;9.

27. Abraham B, Nair MS. Computer-aided classification of prostate cancer grade groups from MRI images using texture features and stacked sparse autoencoder. Comput Med Imag Graph 2018;69:60–8.

28. Abraham B, Nair MS. Automated grading of prostate cancer using convolutional neural network and ordinal class classifier. Inform Med Unlocked 2019;17:100256.

29. Bleker J, Kwee TC, Dierckx RAJO, et al. Multiparametric MRI and auto-fixed volume of interest-based radiomics signature for clinically significant peripheral zone prostate cancer. Eur Radiol 2020;30(3):1313–24.

30. Castillo TJM, Arif M, Starmans MPA, et al. Classification of Clinically Significant Prostate Cancer on Multi-Parametric MRI: A Validation Study Comparing Deep Learning and Radiomics. Cancers 2022;14(1):12.

31. Chaddad A, Kucharczyk MJ, Desrosiers C, et al. Deep Radiomic Analysis to Predict Gleason Score in Prostate Cancer. IEEE Access 2020;8:167767–78.

32. Chen Q, Hu S, Long P, et al. A Transfer Learning Approach for Malignant Prostate Lesion Detection on Multiparametric MRI. Technol Cancer Res Treat 2019;18. 1533033819858363.

33. Chen Z, Liu J, Zhu M, et al. Instance importance-Aware graph convolutional network for 3D medical diagnosis. Med Image Anal 2022;78:102421.

34. Chui KT, Gupta BB, Chi HR, et al. Transfer Learning-Based Multi-Scale Denoising Convolutional Neural Network for Prostate Cancer Detection. Cancers 2022;14(15):3687.

35. Cuccu G, Broillet C, Reischauer C, et al, editors. Typhon: parallel transfer on heterogeneous datasets for cancer detection in computer-aided diagnosis. IEEE International Conference on Big Data (Big Data); 2022.

36. Cuccu G, Jobin J, Clément J, et al, editors. Hydra: cancer detection leveraging multiple heads and heterogeneous datasets. IEEE International Conference on Big Data (Big Data); 2020.

37. Dai J, Wang X, Li Y, Liu Z, Ng Y-L, Xiao J, et al. Automatic Multiparametric Magnetic Resonance Imaging-Based Prostate Lesions Assessment with Unsupervised Domain Adaptation. Advanced Intelligent Systems:2200246.

38. Dai Y, Gao Y, Liu F, et al. Mutual attention-based hybrid dimensional network for multimodal imaging computer-aided diagnosis. arXiv; 2022. preprint arXiv:220109421.

39. de Wilde B, Saha A, ten Broek RP, et al. Medical diffusion on a budget: textual inversion for medical image generation. arXiv; 2023. preprint arXiv:230313430.

40. Duran A, Dussert G, Rouvière O, et al. ProstAttention-Net: A deep attention model for prostate cancer segmentation by aggressiveness in MRI scans. Med Image Anal 2022;77:102347.

41. Fernandez-Quilez A, Eftestøl T, Goodwin M, et al. Self-transfer learning via patches: a prostate cancer triage approach based on bi-parametric MRI. arXiv; 2021. preprint arXiv:210710806.

42. Hamm CA, Baumgärtner GL, Biessmann F, et al. Interactive Explainable Deep Learning Model Informs Prostate Cancer Diagnosis at MRI. Radiology 2023;307(4):e222276.

43. Hoar D, Lee PQ, Guida A, et al. Combined Transfer Learning and Test-Time Augmentation Improves Convolutional Neural Network-Based Semantic Segmentation of Prostate Cancer from Multi-Parametric MR Images. Comput Meth Programs Biomed 2021;210:106375.

44. Hu J, Shen A, Qiao X, et al. Dual attention guided multiscale neural network trained with curriculum learning for noninvasive prediction of Gleason Grade Group from MRI. Med Phys 2023;50(4):2279–89.

45. Jiang W, Lin Y, Vardhanabhuti V, et al. Joint Cancer Segmentation and PI-RADS Classification on Multiparametric MRI Using MiniSegCaps Network. Diagnostics 2023;13(4):615.

46. Kan H, Anhui H, Qiao L, et al. Implementation METHOD of the PI-CAI challenge (SWANGEESE team).

47. Karagoz A, Alis D, Seker ME, et al. Anatomically guided self-adapting deep neural network for clinically significant prostate cancer detection on bi-parametric MRI: a multi-center study. Insights into Imaging 2023;14(1):110.

48. Khosravi P, Lysandrou M, Eljalby M, et al. A Deep Learning Approach to Diagnostic Classification of Prostate Cancer Using Pathology–Radiology Fusion. J Magn Reson Imag 2021;54(2):462–71.

49. Kim H, Margolis DJA, Nagar H, et al. Pulse Sequence Dependence of a Simple and Interpretable Deep Learning Method for Detection of Clinically Significant Prostate Cancer Using Multiparametric MRI. Acad Radiol 2023;30(5):966–70.

50. Lapa P, Castelli M, Gonçalves I, et al. A Hybrid End-to-End Approach Integrating Conditional Random Fields into CNNs for Prostate Cancer Detection on MRI. Appl Sci 2020;10(1):338.

51. Lee J, Nishikawa RM. Cross-Organ, Cross-Modality Transfer Learning: Feasibility Study for Segmentation and Classification. IEEE Access 2020;8:210194–205.

52. Li B, Oka R, Xuan P, et al. Semi-Automatic Multiparametric MR Imaging Classification Using Novel Image Input Sequences and 3D Convolutional Neural Networks. Algorithms 2022;15(7):248.

53. Li B, Oka R, Xuan P, et al. Robust multi-modal prostate cancer classification via feature autoencoder and dual attention. Inform Med Unlocked 2022;30:100923.

54. Li X, Vesal S, Saunders S, et al. The prostate imaging: cancer AI (PI-CAI) 2022 grand challenge (PImed team).

55. Li Y, Wang J, Hu M, et al. Prostate Gleason score prediction via MRI using capsule network. SPIE; 2023.

56. Li Y, Wynne J, Wang J, et al. Cross-shaped windows transformer with self-supervised pretraining for clinically significant prostate cancer detection in Bi-parametric MRI. arXiv; 2023. preprint arXiv:230500385.

57. Prostate Cancer Diagnosis With Sparse Biopsy Data And In Presence Of Location Uncertainty. In: Mehrtash A, Kapur T, Tempany CM, et al, editors. IEEE 18th international symposium on biomedical imaging (ISBI). 2021.

58. Netzer N, Weißer C, Schelb P, et al. Fully Automatic Deep Learning in Bi-institutional Prostate Magnetic Resonance Imaging: Effects of Cohort Size and Heterogeneity. Invest Radiol 2021;56(12):799–808.

59. Patsanis A, Sunoqrot MRS, Bathen TF, et al. CROPro: a tool for automated cropping of prostate magnetic resonance images. J Med Imaging 2023;10(2):024004.

60. Patsanis A, Sunoqrot MRS, Langørgen S, et al. A comparison of Generative Adversarial Networks for automated prostate cancer detection on T2-weighted MRI. Inform Med Unlocked 2023;39:101234.

61. Pellicer-Valero OJ, Marenco Jiménez JL, Gonzalez-Perez V, et al. Deep learning for fully automatic detection, segmentation, and Gleason grade estimation of prostate cancer in multiparametric magnetic resonance images. Sci Rep 2022;12(1):2975.

62. Provenzano D, Melnyk O, Imtiaz D, et al. Machine Learning Algorithm Accuracy Using Single- versus Multi-Institutional Image Data in the Classification of Prostate MRI Lesions. Appl Sci 2023;13(2):1088.

63. Roge A, Hiremath A, Sobota M, et al. Evaluating the sensitivity of deep learning to inter-reader variations in lesion delineations on bi-parametric MRI in identifying clinically significant prostate cancer. SPIE; 2022.

64. Saha A, Bosma J, Linmans J, et al. Anatomical and Diagnostic Bayesian Segmentation in Prostate MRI $-$ Should Different Clinical Objectives Mandate Different Loss Functions? arXiv; 2021. preprint arXiv:211012889.

65. Sanford T, Harmon SA, Turkbey EB, et al. Deep-Learning-Based Artificial Intelligence for PI-RADS Classification to Assist Multiparametric Prostate MRI Interpretation: A Development Study. J Magn Reson Imag 2020;52(5):1499–507.

66. Shao L, Liu Z, Liu J, et al. Patient-level grading prediction of prostate cancer from mp-MRI via GMINet. Comput Biol Med 2022;150:106168.

67. Simeth J, Jiang J, Nosov A, et al. Deep learning-based dominant index lesion segmentation for MR-guided radiation therapy of prostate cancer. Med Phys.n/a(n/a).

68. Vente C, Vos P, Hosseinzadeh M, et al. Deep Learning Regression for Prostate Cancer Detection and Grading in Bi-Parametric MRI. IEEE Trans Biomed Eng 2021;68(2):374–83.

69. Wang X, Su R, Xie W, et al. 2.75D: Boosting learning by representing 3D Medical imaging to 2D features for small data. Biomed Signal Process Control 2023;84:104858.

70. Wang Y, Song D, Wang W, et al. Self-supervised learning and semi-supervised learning for multi-sequence medical image classification. Neurocomputing 2022;513:383–94.

71. Wang Y, Wang M. Selecting proper combination of mpMRI sequences for prostate cancer classification using multi-input convolutional neuronal network. Phys Med 2020;80:92–100.

72. Yang DD, Lee LK, Tsui JM, et al. Association Between Artificial Intelligence-Derived Tumor Volume and Oncologic Outcomes for Localized Prostate Cancer Treated with Radiation Therapy. medRxiv 2023;2023. 04.16.23288642.

73. Yi Z, Ou Z, Hu J, et al. Computer-aided diagnosis of prostate cancer based on deep neural networks from multi-parametric magnetic resonance imaging. Front Physiol 2022;13:918381.

74. Yoshimura T, Manabe K, Sugimori H. Non-Invasive Estimation of Gleason Score by Semantic Segmentation and Regression Tasks Using a Three-Dimensional Convolutional Neural Network. Appl Sci 2023;13(14):8028.

75. Yuan Y, Ahn E, Feng D, et al. A zonal-aware self-supervised mesh network for prostate cancer detection and diagnosis in bpMRI. arXiv; 2022. preprint arXiv:221205808.

76. Zong W, Carver E, Zhu S, et al. Prostate cancer malignancy detection and localization from mpMRI using auto-deep learning as one step closer to clinical utilization. Sci Rep 2022;12(1):22430.

77. Zong W, Lee JK, Liu C, et al. A deep dive into understanding tumor foci classification using multiparametric MRI based on convolutional neural network. Med Phys 2020;47(9):4077–86.

78. To MNN, Kwak JT. Biparametric MR signal characteristics can predict histopathological measures of prostate cancer. Eur Radiol 2022;32(11):8027–38.

79. Mongan J, Moy L, Charles E, et al. Checklist for Artificial Intelligence in Medical Imaging (CLAIM): A Guide for Authors and Reviewers. Radiology: Artif Intell 2020;2(2):e200029.

Printed and bound by CPI Group (UK) Ltd, Croydon, CR0 4YY

08/05/2025

01864748-0019